Dermatology: Advances on Pathophysiology and Therapies

Dermatology: Advances on Pathophysiology and Therapies

Editors

Montserrat Fernández-Guarino
Asunción Ballester-Martinez
Andrés González-García

MDPI

Basel • Beijing • Wuhan • Barcelona • Belgrade • Novi Sad • Cluj • Manchester

Editors

Montserrat Fernández-Guarino
Dermatology
Universidad Alfonso X El Sabio
Madrid
Spain

Asunción Ballester-Martinez
Dermatology
Universidad de Alcala
Madrid
Spain

Andrés González-García
Internal Medicine
Universidad de Alcala
Madrid
Spain

Editorial Office
MDPI
St. Alban-Anlage 66
4052 Basel, Switzerland

This is a reprint of articles from the Special Issue published online in the open access journal *International Journal of Molecular Sciences* (ISSN 1422-0067) (available at: www.mdpi.com/journal/ijms/special_issues/J681D4YZ2D).

For citation purposes, cite each article independently as indicated on the article page online and as indicated below:

Lastname, A.A.; Lastname, B.B. Article Title. *Journal Name* **Year**, *Volume Number*, Page Range.

ISBN 978-3-7258-0868-7 (Hbk)
ISBN 978-3-7258-0867-0 (PDF)
doi.org/10.3390/books978-3-7258-0867-0

Contents

About the Editors . . . . **vii**

Preface . . . . **ix**

Montserrat Fernández-Guarino, Stefano Bacci, Luis Alfonso Pérez González, Mariano Bermejo-Martínez, Almudena Cecilia-Matilla and Maria Luisa Hernández-Bule
The Role of Physical Therapies in Wound Healing and Assisted Scarring
Reprinted from: *Int. J. Mol. Sci.* **2023**, *24*, 7487, doi:10.3390/ijms24087487 . . . . **1**

Belen de Nicolas-Ruanes, Asuncion Ballester-Martinez, Emilio Garcia-Mouronte, Emilio Berna-Rico, Carlos Azcarraga-Llobet and Montserrat Fernandez-Guarino
From Molecular Insights to Clinical Perspectives in Drug-Associated Bullous Pemphigoid
Reprinted from: *Int. J. Mol. Sci.* **2023**, *24*, 16786, doi:10.3390/ijms242316786 . . . . **18**

María Luisa Hernández-Bule, Elena Toledano-Macías, Luis Alfonso Pérez-González, María Antonia Martínez-Pascual and Montserrat Fernández-Guarino
Anti-Fibrotic Effects of RF Electric Currents
Reprinted from: *Int. J. Mol. Sci.* **2023**, *24*, 10986, doi:10.3390/ijms241310986 . . . . **53**

Javier Perez-Bootello, Ruth Cova-Martin, Jorge Naharro-Rodriguez and Gonzalo Segurado-Miravalles
Vitiligo: Pathogenesis and New and Emerging Treatments
Reprinted from: *Int. J. Mol. Sci.* **2023**, *24*, 17306, doi:10.3390/ijms242417306 . . . . **66**

Oana Mirela Tiucă, Silviu Horia Morariu, Claudia Raluca Mariean, Robert Aurelian Tiucă, Alin Codrut Nicolescu and Ovidiu Simion Cotoi
Predictive Performances of Blood-Count-Derived Inflammatory Markers for Liver Fibrosis Severity in Psoriasis Vulgaris
Reprinted from: *Int. J. Mol. Sci.* **2023**, *24*, 16898, doi:10.3390/ijms242316898 . . . . **93**

Grisell Starita-Fajardo, David Lucena-López, María Asunción Ballester-Martínez, Montserrat Fernández-Guarino and Andrés González-García
Treatment Strategies in Neutrophilic Dermatoses: A Comprehensive Review
Reprinted from: *Int. J. Mol. Sci.* **2023**, *24*, 15622, doi:10.3390/ijms242115622 . . . . **106**

Basanth Babu Eedara, Bhagyashree Manivannan, Wafaa Alabsi, Bo Sun, Clara Curiel-Lewandrowski, Tianshun Zhang, et al.
Comprehensive Physicochemical Characterization, In Vitro Membrane Permeation, and In Vitro Human Skin Cell Culture of a Novel TOPK Inhibitor, HI-TOPK-032
Reprinted from: *Int. J. Mol. Sci.* **2023**, *24*, 15515, doi:10.3390/ijms242115515 . . . . **125**

Carlos Fernández-Lozano, Emilio Solano Solares, Isabel Elías-Sáenz, Isabel Pérez-Allegue, Monserrat Fernández-Guarino, Diego Fernández-Nieto, et al.
Value of the Lymphocyte Transformation Test for the Diagnosis of Drug-Induced Hypersensitivity Reactions in Hospitalized Patients with Severe COVID-19
Reprinted from: *Int. J. Mol. Sci.* **2023**, *24*, 11543, doi:10.3390/ijms241411543 . . . . **145**

Emilio Garcia-Mouronte, Emilio Berna-Rico, Belen de Nicolas-Ruanes, Carlos Azcarraga-Llobet, Luis Alonso-Martinez de Salinas and Sonia Bea-Ardebol
Imiquimod as Local Immunotherapy in the Management of Premalignant Cutaneous Conditions and Skin Cancer
Reprinted from: *Int. J. Mol. Sci.* **2023**, *24*, 10835, doi:10.3390/ijms241310835 . . . . **157**

About the Editors

Montserrat Fernández-Guarino

Professor Montserrat Fernández-Guarino has been a venerated dermatology specialist since 2008. Her comprehensive training at the Ramón y Cajal Dermatology Service culminated in a doctoral thesis that not only earned her Cum Laude distinction but also the esteemed "Extraordinary Thesis Award" for the best thesis of the year at the University of Alcalá. Her academic prowess extends into the field of psychology, in which she is certified, and she boasts four Masters degrees in diverse health service sectors, including nutrition, pharmacy, rehabilitation, and hospital management.

Recognized for her pedagogic contributions, Dr. Fernández-Guarino is accredited by the National Spanish Education Ministry as a University Professor in Medicine (ANECA), reflecting her commitment to medical education and academic rigor.

Currently, she is a staff dermatologist at Hospital Universitario Ramón y Cajal, Madrid (2008–present) and a mentor and tutor for dermatology residents and residents across other medical specialties (internal medicine, immunology, and allergy). She is also a coordinator of dermatology emergencies at the hospital and the lead of dermatology hospitalization services. She is a research consultant in photodynamic therapy and operates a part-time private practice in general dermatology at Madriderma, her own clinic.

Dr. Fernández-Guarino's expertise spans general and clinical dermatology, with a special interest in photobiology, phototherapy, and photodynamic therapy. She is adept at utilizing lasers and managing complex dermatological cases. Her work in inflammatory dermatology and emergency dermatological care positions her as a leading expert in her field.

Asunción Ballester-Martinez

Dr. Asunción Ballester Martínez is a distinguished dermatologist at Ramón y Cajal Hospital, renowned for her expertise in managing complex skin conditions. Specializing in psoriasis, inflammatory skin diseases, and bullous disorders, Dr. Ballester Martínez leads a dedicated clinic for these challenging conditions, providing her patients with advanced care and innovative treatments. Her commitment to dermatology extends beyond clinical practice, as she actively contributes to research in her fields of specialization, aiming to improve patient outcomes and quality of life. Dr. Ballester Martínez's dedication to her patients and her passion for advancing dermatological knowledge make her a respected figure in the medical community.

Andrés González-García

Dr. Andrés González García, MD, is a highly esteemed physician specializing in internal medicine with a profound commitment to managing systemic and rare diseases at Ramón y Cajal Hospital. His role extends to providing pivotal support to the Dermatology Department, particularly in the treatment of complex cases and the management of hospitalizations. Dr. González García's expertise is crucial in bridging the gap between internal medicine and dermatology, ensuring a comprehensive approach to patient care. His dedication to addressing challenging medical conditions and his collaborative efforts with dermatology highlight his integral role in the multidisciplinary healthcare team, significantly contributing to the hospital's reputation for excellence in patient care.

Preface

Welcome to this Special Issue of the *International Journal of Molecular Sciences*, dedicated to exploring the significant strides made in targeted therapies in dermatology. Over the last decade, the landscape of dermatological treatments has undergone a remarkable transformation, heralding a new era in the management and understanding of skin diseases.

The advent of novel treatments, such as biologics and small-molecule inhibitors, has revolutionized patient care, offering new hope to those suffering from conditions that were once untreatable or difficult to manage. The efficacy of these targeted therapies lies in their ability to home in on specific molecular pathways involved in the pathogenesis of dermatological conditions, thereby minimizing systemic side effects and optimizing therapeutic results.

One of the cornerstones of this advancement has been the deepening collaboration between clinicians and researchers in the basic sciences. This transnational approach has been instrumental in unraveling the molecular mechanisms underlying various skin diseases. By shedding light on the pathophysiology of these conditions, dermatologists have been able to identify novel therapeutic targets and prognostic factors that are crucial for the development of tailored treatments.

Understanding the basic mechanisms underlying disease pathology is not just an academic pursuit but also a step toward personalized medicine in dermatology. Personalized medicine enables dermatologists to predict disease progression, tailor treatments to individual patient profiles, and ultimately improve patient care and outcomes.

This Special Issue brings together a collection of articles that highlight the cutting-edge research and clinical applications of targeted therapies in dermatology. The work featured herein exemplifies the fruitful synergy between basic science and clinical practice, paving the way for the next generation of dermatological treatments.

We invite you to delve into these pages and explore the advancements that are shaping the future of dermatology. Through collaborative efforts and a deep commitment to understanding the fundamental aspects of skin diseases, we are moving toward a future where targeted therapies offer a beacon of hope for patients worldwide.

Montserrat Fernández-Guarino, Asunción Ballester-Martinez, and Andrés González-García
Editors

International Journal of *Molecular Sciences*

MDPI

Review

The Role of Physical Therapies in Wound Healing and Assisted Scarring

Montserrat Fernández-Guarino [1,*], Stefano Bacci [2], Luis Alfonso Pérez González [1], Mariano Bermejo-Martínez [3], Almudena Cecilia-Matilla [4] and Maria Luisa Hernández-Bule [5]

1 Dermatology Service, Instituto Ramón y Cajal de Investigación Sanitaria (IRYCIS), Hospital Ramón y Cajal, 28034 Madrid, Spain
2 Research Unit of Histology and Embryology, Department of Biology, University of Florence, 50121 Firenze, Italy
3 Specialist Nursing in Wound Healing, Angiology and Vascular Service, Instituto Ramón y Cajal de Investigación Sanitaria (IRYCIS), Hospital Ramón y Cajal, 28034 Madrid, Spain
4 Diabetic Foot Unit, Angiology and Vascular Service, Instituto Ramón y Cajal de Investigación Sanitaria (IRYCIS), Hospital Ramón y Cajal, 28034 Madrid, Spain
5 Bioelectromagnetic Lab, Instituto Ramón y Cajal de Investigación Sanitaria (IRYCIS), Hospital Ramón y Cajal, 28034 Madrid, Spain
* Correspondence: montserrat.fernandezg@salud.madrid.org; Tel.: +34-91-336-85-92

Abstract: Wound healing (WH) is a complex multistep process in which a failure could lead to a chronic wound (CW). CW is a major health problem and includes leg venous ulcers, diabetic foot ulcers, and pressure ulcers. CW is difficult to treat and affects vulnerable and pluripathological patients. On the other hand, excessive scarring leads to keloids and hypertrophic scars causing disfiguration and sometimes itchiness and pain. Treatment of WH includes the cleaning and careful handling of injured tissue, early treatment and prevention of infection, and promotion of healing. Treatment of underlying conditions and the use of special dressings promote healing. The patient at risk and risk areas should avoid injury as much as possible. This review aims to summarize the role of physical therapies as complementary treatments in WH and scarring. The article proposes a translational view, opening the opportunity to develop these therapies in an optimal way in clinical management, as many of them are emerging. The role of laser, photobiomodulation, photodynamic therapy, electrical stimulation, ultrasound therapy, and others are highlighted in a practical and comprehensive approach.

Keywords: chronic wound; electromagnetic fields; hypertrophic scar; keloid; laser; physical therapies; photobiomodulation; photodynamic therapy; radiofrequency; ultrasound therapy; wound healing

Citation: Fernández-Guarino, M.; Bacci, S.; Pérez González, L.A.; Bermejo-Martínez, M.; Cecilia-Matilla, A.; Hernández-Bule, M.L. The Role of Physical Therapies in Wound Healing and Assisted Scarring. *Int. J. Mol. Sci.* **2023**, *24*, 7487. https://doi.org/10.3390/ijms24087487

Academic Editor: Michael R. Hamblin

Received: 18 March 2023
Revised: 16 April 2023
Accepted: 17 April 2023
Published: 19 April 2023

1. Introduction

Wound healing (WH) is a main health problem in current society. Firstly, acute wounds could lead to scars and disfiguring lesions, and secondly, chronic wounds (CW) cause morbidity and high economic cost. AWs occur, in general, after surgery, trauma, or burns, whereas in CWs occur, in general, with an underlying systemic condition, such as diabetes, elderly, vascular alterations, or malnutrition.

Guidelines for care in wounds are useful, clear, and concise [1]. They represent the principal approach in clinical practice. The main CWs presented in clinical practice include leg ulcers (LU), diabetic foot ulcer (DFU), and pressure ulcer (PU). The main treatment of CWs include adequate dressing, debridement, and pressure control. Nevertheless, undoubtedly, there is an uncovered gap in this pathology, as scarring is sometimes unavoidable, and CWs could persist for months. The focus of this review is to provide a tool for clinicians, and a useful guide from the basic science, to develop and improve physical therapies in WH.

Lots of research works are nowadays focused on solving the problem of WH, most of them searching for very advanced therapies, such as cellular transplantation therapy [2,3], vascular enhancers [4], regenerative materials [5], or nanoparticles in hydrogels [6]. Despite the highly anticipated novel therapies in development, right now, they are very far from being used in real practice.

Physical therapy (PT) is present in daily clinical consultations and has demonstrated a certain utility in WH [7]. This review came across different techniques such as laser, low-level laser light therapy, photodynamic therapy, or electrical stimulation, among others, and their role in WH.

2. General Approach to Wounds

2.1. Epidemiology

The data in the literature referring to failure of WH show the seriousness of the problem.

WH failure, dermal fibrosis and scarring affect all ethnicities, while keloids or hypertrophic scars are more prevalent in American, African, and Asian populations, which can reach up to 16% of the population [8]. Factors associated with excessive scarring include genetic predisposition, hypertension, endocrine dysfunction, autoimmune diseases, and endocrine alterations [9]. The genetic factors described have been found to be associated with polymorphism alterations in genes such as TGF-beta, which evolved in fibrosis formation, opening, and interested therapeutic target [10]. The subsequent endothelial malfunction in hypertension has recently been associated with the risk of scarring and other diseases which have fibrosis and remodeling in their pathogenic [11].

On the other hand, the type of injury has also been associated with the risk of scarring and other factors often seen in clinical practice [12] (See Table 1). Two types of scars are described: keloids and hypertrophic scars (HS). HS are limited to the wound with an increase in cicatricial tissue, whereas keloids are invasive, going through the limit of the wound [12]. Table 1 summarized the differences between keloids and HS. The interaction between the environment of keloids and the scar is complex, and diet, smoking, stress, and physical exercise could influence the process [11].

Table 1. Clinical differences between keloids and hypertrophic scars.

Characteristic	Keloids	Hypertrophic Scars
Trauma	Non-severe (acne, folliculitis)	Burns, incision
Body sites	Chest, upper back, earlobe	Any
Symptoms	Erythema, itch, pain	Erythema, itch
Exploration	Beyond the limit of the trauma	Limited to the initial wound
Treatment	Combined therapies with frequent recurrence	Good response
Surgical excision	Contraindicated due to recurrence	Without recurrences, could be considered a treatment

Conversely, the failure of healing a wound also produces a high impact on the patients. A chronic wound (CW) is a wound that fails to repair and restore the skin in three months [13]. It is estimated that 1–2% of the population suffer from CWs [14], for example, in the United States more than 6.5 million patients are affected [15].

2.2. Process and Stages of Wound Healing

WH is a complex process evolving multiple biological pathways and mechanisms. Classically, it is divided into different phases, including hemostasis/inflammatory stage, proliferation, and remodeling (Figure 1) [2,16].

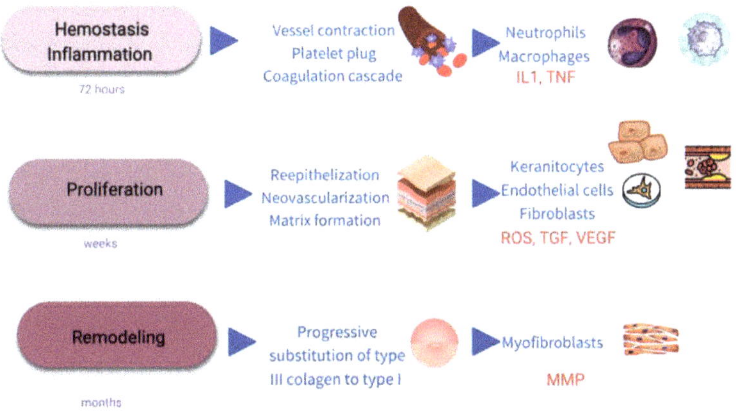

Figure 1. Scheme of the stages of wound healing. IL1: interkeukin1; TNF: Tumor necrosis factor; ROS: single oxygen radicals; TGF: transforming growth factor; VEGF: vascular endothelial growth factor; MMP: metalloproteinases.

2.2.1. Hemostasis/Inflammatory Stage

The first response to an injury is the constriction of the affected vessels and platelet activation to form a fibrin clot and stop the bleeding [3]. Platelets are activated for the exposure to collagen of the subendothelial matrix in the so-called primary hemostasis. Next, secondary hemostasis produces the activation of the coagulation cascade [17]. Local mast cell degranulation release occurs in the following minutes, and mediators such as histamine and TNF-alfa are released [18].

The next cells to appear in the wound scenario are the neutrophils which are not usually present on normal skin. Neutrophils represent an innate inflammation [19] and are recruited from damaged vessels and attracted by interleukin 1 (IL1), tumor necrosis factor alfa (TNFα) and bacterial toxins [20].

Activated neutrophils destroy bacteria and cell debris and provide a good environment for WH through the liberation of reactive oxygen species (ROS), antimicrobial peptides and proteolytic enzymes [16]. Clearance of neutrophils occurs by apoptosis or necrosis and ulterior phagocytosis by macrophages. Complete hemostasis and inflammatory phase in WH usually last 72 h [2].

2.2.2. Proliferation

The clot is substituted by connective tissue or granulation tissue, meanwhile neovascularization, re-epithelialization, and immunomodulation appear in parallel lasting days or weeks [16]. Many cytokines and growth-factors participate in this phase, such as the transforming growth factor-beta (TGF-β) family, and vascular epidermal growth-factors (VEGF) [2,16]. Most of these mediators support the mechanism of action of physical therapies in WH and are the focus to work in with. The duration of this phase is as follows: 3–21 days [21].

2.2.3. Maturation/Remodeling

Finally, a progressive substitution of the existing cells in the initial fibrin clot led to a wound contraction. This event is related to the maturation of type I collagen and the elimination of type III immature collagen, and by apoptosis of the myofibroblast during several weeks and months after the injury [22]. This change is regulated by metalloproteases (MMPs), collagenases express and secrete by macrophages, myofibroblasts, and keratinocytes [3,16]. The duration of this phase is as follows: 3 weeks–6 months [21].

2.3. Chronic Wounds

A chronic wound (CW) is described as a wound that fails to repair itself or remains unhealed after 12 weeks [1].

Most of the CW are classified as diabetic ulcers (DU), pressure ulcers (PU), or venous leg ulcers (VU), in relation to their clinical findings and cause.

2.3.1. Diabetic Ulcer

DU is a deleterious complication representing the first cause of amputation of the lower limb [23]. DU are located on the foot and are caused by neuropathy and vascular illness, which causes the inability to detect pain and injuries. In general, DUs are deep, similar to a crater and expose the tendon and the bone. A surrounded hyperkeratotic tissue is put in place, forming a callus-like ring. Imaging testing could be necessary to exclude osteomyelitis [1,13].

2.3.2. Pressure Ulcer

PU appears on areas under pressure, usually over a bony prominence such as the sacrum or the heels. The pression on the vessels decreases irrigation of the skin resulting in an initial dermatitis, which if prolonged leads to a loss of tissue. The cause is multifactorial, e.g., immobilization in bed, nutrition alteration, systemic diseases, or being elderly [1]. PUs varies in severity, and are classified in four different stages, IV being the more severe, which implies the loss of the full thickness of the skin. In those cases, the management of the PU should be surgical, and PT would not play a role.

2.3.3. Venous Ulcer

A VU typically appears in the lower limb over the medial supramalleolar area. The risk factors for VUs include obesity and venous insufficiency. About 75% of chronic ulcers are VU, being the most frequent, affecting 1–5% of the population [24]. VU are associated with more signs of venous malfunction in clinical exploration than oedema, hemosiderosis, cutaneous atrophy, lipodermatosclerosis or annexal absence. If necessary, further examination with a duplex ultrasonography confirms the diagnosis.

The management of a VU includes the general treatment of CW, adding compressive therapy and healing the venous system if possible, with surgery [13,25]. Adjuvant therapies include nutritional balance and supplementation, diet, physical exercise and improving blood circulation with drugs such as pentoxifylline. Despite using the correct treatment, a VU could take 6 to 12 months to heal, and relapsing is very frequent in the following year [13,24,25].

2.4. General Management of Chronic Wounds

WH and scarring is a complex process with multiple influencing and interacting factors. Additionally, some of those factors are not under the control of the dermatologist, such as age, vascular abnormalities, comorbidities, malnutrition, or smoking [1]. The management is challenging, and multiple approaches and visits are needed with the implication of different health care workers [1] and arisen important indirect costs.

All CW should be treated according to the TIME principles: tissue debridement, infection control, moisture balance and edges of the wound [13]. Debridement is the first step in the treatment of a CW, it must be carried out weekly and it increases the speed of healing by over 72% [26].

Biofilm is presented in the extracellular matrix and is considered the cause of 80% of the infections in CW [27]. Biofilm is invisible to the naked eye, and different techniques to assess its presence are being developed, apart from a cutaneous biopsy. Nevertheless, the biofilm must be removed because it maintains the CW in the inflammatory stage [28]. The risk of infection is usually controlled by topical antibiotics, silver dressing, or with other topical components.

The wound should not be exposed to air, and if the skin appears dry, moisturizer should be added to the dressing. On the other hand, if excessive drainage is present, it needs to be clean and dried. The wound edge, in case of overgrowth, must be excised for epithelization [29].

Table 2 describes the local cellular response alterations underlying a CW. CW are characterized by excessive inflammation, a decrease in growth factors secretion, and a disbalance in the proteolytic enzymes and cellular senescence which perpetuates the wound unhealed [25]. Therefore, a high number of mast cells, neutrophils and dendritic cells are found in CW with an increase in pro-inflammatory cytokines and proteases (see Figure 1). These inflammatory cells not only prolong the wound but also increase susceptibility to infections [22]. The alteration of the expression and activation of MMPs is strongly associated with CW, damaging the granulation tissue, and producing exudates in the wound [30]. Cells implicated in the remodeling and re-epithelization are dysfunctional too. Fibroblasts are senescent and the excess of wound proteases (MMPs, elastase, cathepsin G, and urokinase-type plasminogen activator (uPA)) activities degrade the extracellular matrix, the growth factors (VEGF, TGF-beta) and cytokines (TNF-alfa) [22]. Keratinocytes hyper proliferate at the edge of the wound, so hyperkeratosis appears, and the subsequent wound fails to close. The microbiome profiles of aged and diabetic patients with CW have been found to have a decrease in alfa-diversity [3,20,30].

Table 2. Mechanisms found in failure to heal wound (FHW).

Wound	Cellular Mechanisms	Mediators
Inflammation Exudates Infection	Neutrophils' excessive number and function Defective macrophages High number of mast cells Loss of microbiome diversity	Oxidative stress Wound proteases (MMPs, elastase, cathepsin G, and urokinase-type plasminogen activator (uPA)) Increase in inflammatory cytokines
Hyperkeratotic edge of the wound	Keratinocyte hyperproliferation and malfunction	Elevated b-catenin and c-myc
Failure to heal and close	Senescent fibroblasts	Degradation of VEGF, TGF-beta, and TNF-alfa

MMP: metalloproteinases; VEGF: vascular endothelial growth factor; TGF: transforming growth factor; TNF: tumoral necrosis factor.

2.5. General Prevention of Scarring

Excess WH or scarring is caused by an overproduction of extracellular matrix generated by myofibroblasts, which in this type of lesion are not replaced by fibroblasts during the proliferative phase. In this fibrosis, matrix proteins such as alpha-smooth muscle actin (alpha-SMA) are overexpressed, and the expression of MMP decreases, which induces an accumulation of collagen [12].

Keloid and HS are clinical expressions, and both can be considered successive stages of the same proliferative disorder. The initial common process is a purulent inflammatory skin lesion, the hyperfunction of the fibroblasts and excessive extracellular matrix deposition. HS consists of mainly type III collagen, whereas keloids contain type I and III [31].

The general strategy for the prevention of scarring is summarized in Table 3. The early recognition of the alteration is considered of cardinal importance for early treatment [32]. The healing process varies from one patient to another; thus, controlling the procedure, preventing the infection, and providing personalized wound care are the main prevention and treatment methods [33].

Table 3. Prevention and treatment of scarring, keloids, and hypertrophic scars (HS).

Prevention	Treatment	Alternative Therapies
Early diagnosis	Silicone gel or dressing Topical retinoids	Peelings
Careful wound care	Topical Imiquimod Topical 5-Fluorouracil Intralesional Bleomicin	Microneedling Dermabrasion Radiotherapy
Prevent infection		
Sun protection Avoid risk areas if possible Avoid risk patients if possible		

3. The Role of Physical Therapies in Hard-To-Heal Chronic Wounds

Principles and Basis

Once it is known what fails in WH, the possibility of understanding the role of physical therapies arises more clearly. Figure 2 shows a scheme of possible targets for increasing WH, and Figure 3 shows how to promote regeneration rather than scarring with physical therapies (PT). It is of notice that with their theoretical mechanisms, we can impact in all the phases completing and fostering traditional treatments with innocuity.

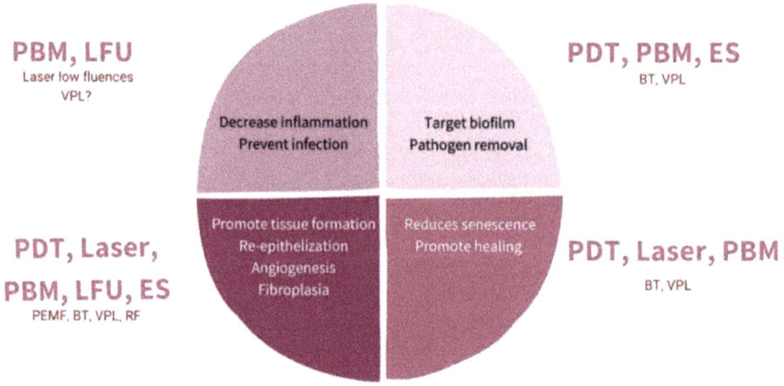

Figure 2. Diagram representing different targets with physical therapies (PT) for promoting wound healing (WH). PBM: photobiomodulation; LFU: low frequent ultrasound; PDT: photodynamic therapy; ES: electrostimulation; VPL: visible pulsed light; PEMF: pulsed electromagnetic fields; BT: biophotonic therapy; RF: radiofrequency.

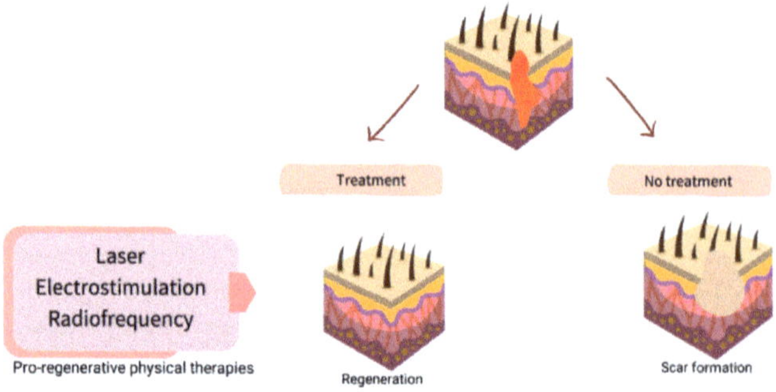

Figure 3. Scheme of strategies for physical therapies (PT) in assisted well-scaring.

The guidelines for the management of CW are extensive, but the pillars are promoting patient adherence to treatment, debridement control of the possible infection, covering with an appropriate dressing and effective compression if necessary [1].

Two options appear when PT are introduced in the treatment, either CW or scarring. One is proactive management, starting the treatment in the initial phases of the wound, as a prevention or adjuvant therapy. The other one is using those therapies when a CW, HS or keloid has appeared. Both situations not only depend on the physician but also the patient consultation.

4. Physical Therapies in Assisted Healing and Scar Prevention

4.1. Laser

The main target of laser therapy is the treatment and prevention of scarring, and there are few studies published in its assistance in WH. Among the different issues presented in an HS or keloids, different lasers could be used to target each objective [34] (Table 4). Laser treatment is flexible and allows for their combination in a single treatment session. The most widely applied are fractional lasers in combination with vascular lasers and lasers targeting melanin [35]. Basically, there are two different types of fractional laser: ablative (wavelengths of 2790–10,600 nm) and non-ablative (1320–1927 nm). Both ablative and non-ablative lasers have become the gold standard for the treatment of scarring, although ablative lasers are probably the most used [36].

Table 4. Targeting lasers according to clinical exploration in hypertrophic scars and keloids.

Skin Alteration	Type of Laser
Erythema	Pulsed dye laser Intense pulsed light Neodimio-Yag laser
Skin thickness/Hypertrophic	Erbio laser CO_2 laser Non-ablative laser
Hyperpigmentation	Alejandrita laser Intense pulsed light KTP 532 nm Q-switched laser

Erbio and CO_2 lasers are ablative lasers that target water, producing a selective burn in the skin. In a fractional mode, they work in separated columns, allowing for a better regeneration throughout the non-damage columns of skin. Both induce selective thermal necrosis in the skin, increasing in the first weeks of the inflammatory stage of the scar, but after three months, collagen remodeling in a thin bundle due to collagen III appears [37]. The clinical results show a decreasing dermis thickness and increasing skin flexibility [35]. On the other hand, vascular lasers target small vessels and are used for decreasing erythema in HS and keloids, causing excessive neovascularization. Pulsed dye laser (PDL) is probably the most used. PDL has been demonstrated to decrease connective tissue growth factor expression in keloids, despite targeting vessels [38] and inhibiting fibroblast proliferation in vitro [39]. After the vessel coagulation and subsequent hypoxia, PDL leads to an increase in collagen type III [40].

Apart from the treatment of scars, some studies of lasers in assisted WH and preventing scarring from the first day of surgery have been published showing different results. Curiously, the immediate application of lasers differs from other physical therapies, which need some healing days before they start to be applied. In a split-face study, no differences were found in the area treated with CO_2 laser immediately after surgery, but in other similar studies the scars treated exhibit better healing and cosmetic outcome [41–43]. PDL and non-ablative fractional laser have also been shown to improve scaring when used early; however, the differences with the untreated area were not statistically significant [44].

Different types of lasers could be applied in the same session, PDL plus ablative fractional CO_2 laser have been suggested to be the best combination [45].

An early start of the treatment is recommended in the literature reviewed when lasers are used to assist scarring. The optimal interval between sessions has been found to be 5 to 6 weeks during a period of months [46]. All the lasers applied in early treatment times have also been used under lower parameters [40]. Further clinical trials with long-term follow-up are needed to support the evidence of laser treatment in HS, keloids and WH alone or in combination with other options for treatment [47]; however, lasers are recommended for expert panels as a first-line therapy in scarring [48].

4.2. *Photobiomodulation (Low-Level Light Therapy-LLLT)*

LLLT has been intensely studied in WH, the near-infrared light (NIR) between 800 and 900 nm and red light (600–700 nm) being the most used. The use of light in a non-thermal effect is supported by the photon's absorption of the cells' receptors. The main three chromophores in the skin are melanin in the epidermis, hemoglobin in the dermis and water in all the skin [49] and longer wavelengths achieve deeper penetration (Figure 4).

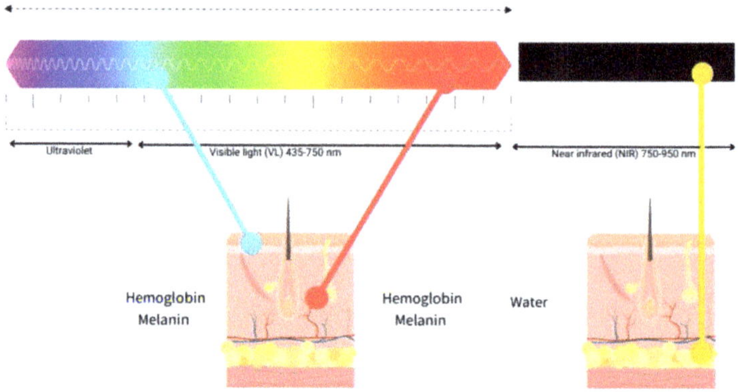

Figure 4. Diagram of the relationship between visible light (blue, red) and near-infrared (NIR), penetration and chromophores.

Hormesis responses occur in WH in response to low doses of light (LLLT) or photobiomodulation (PBM). Hormesis or biomodulation are terms used to describe a natural biological process in which low doses of an input, for example, light or energy, induce activation, but high doses produce an inhibition [50]. PBM induces the production of nitric oxide (NO), a vasodilator, and anti-inflammatory agent (Table 5) [51]. LLLT can trigger natural mechanisms involved in WH, including TGF-beta families of molecules, transforming growth platelet factor, interleukins (IL6, 13, 15), and matrix metalloproteinases (MMPs) associated with alterations in WH. TGF-beta is crucial in fibroblast proliferation [7,50,51]. Thus, PBM has been demonstrated to be useful in all the steps of WH.

Table 5. Summary of the beneficial effects of photobiomodulation (PBM) in wound healing (WH) and chronic wound (CW).

Effect	Mediator	Phase of WH/CW
Anti-inflammatory	ROS, NO, IL	Inflammation
Vasodilatation	NO	Proliferation
Matrix formation	TGF-beta and MMPs	Proliferation and remodeling
Promote epithelial cell function	Cyclin D1	Proliferation and remodeling

ROS: radical oxygen singlet; NO: nictric oxide; IL: interleukins; MMPs: metaloproteinases.

In animal models, LLLT increases collagen and reduces oxidative and nitroxidative stress in diabetic wounded mouse skin [51]. In vitro studies have also found an increased expression in keratinocytes after LLLT of cyclin D1 and cytokeratin, suggesting an increase in proliferation and maturation [52,53].

LLLT is not as widely used as laser despite being safer, without adverse reactions such as swelling, crusting or purpura. With respect to laser, LLLT is easy to apply, allows the treatment of bigger areas, a wearable device is available, self-treating is an opportunity and it is not as expensive. The main disadvantage of LLLT is the necessity of near-daily repeated sessions [54].

There are few studies of LLLT in WH with different results. In VU, red light did not demonstrate any additional benefit to conventional treatment [55]. Whereas in PU and DU, red light increases healing with better outcomes when compared with NIR [56]. A prophylactic treatment in the prevention of keloid in three patients was shown effective with NIR (LED 805 nm). In this small study, patients self-treated at home daily for one month [57].

LLLT improves inflammation, releases pain, and fosters healing in clinical practice. Even though it has been deeply investigated, further studies in the daily clinical application are necessary as no standard protocol has been developed [54].

Blue Light Emission Diode

LED technology greatly benefited from the pioneering research conducted during the gallium nitride crystal boom of the 1980s by Akasaki, Amano, and Nakamura, which led to the invention of the blue LED. This discovery was extremely important as it made it possible to obtain white light from LED sources, paving the way for revolutionary uses of radiation [58].

Blue-light PBM triggers a cascade of events attributable to the absorption of photons by intracellular photoreceptors. Among these effects, the impact of light on cytochrome-C oxidase can be observed: it induces an increase in cell proliferation, migration and differentiation, cytokine modulation, growth factor synthesis, and anti-inflammatory effects; thus, stimulating the improvement of the healing process [59,60].

In wounds treated with blue light, a faster healing process and better deposition and morphology of dermal collagen are observed when compared to wounds not treated with blue light. Furthermore, treated wounds show better modulation of the inflammatory response where mast cells assume a central role [50].

4.3. Photodynamic Therapy

Photodynamic therapy (PDT) is a safe and easy procedure to enhance WH, nevertheless, further studies are necessary to determine an exact protocol. Anyhow, PDT is versatile, with the limitation of pain during the treatment and repeat sessions.

PDT is indicated in dermatology for the treatment of actinic keratosis, basal cell carcinoma and Bowen disease [61]. PDT has been explored in WH and prevents scarring, whereas no results have been found in the treatment of keloids and HS. The main difference between PDT and other PT in WH is the ability to scope infections without resistance to antibiotics.

PDT consists of the combination of a photosensitizer (PS) in the target tissue and the subsequent illumination of an adequate light source for inducing necrosis and apoptosis of the tissue. Through the literature, a variety of lights and PS have been tested in WH. Nowadays, PS are preferred to be used topically, as they have lower side effects. A lot of optimal light sources could be used in the PpIX absorption spectrum; however, LEDs are mostly explored for their simplicity and lower side effects. Table 6 summarized which PS could be used in WH and different light devices [62,63]. Most of the light sources are in the red spectrum [63], although there are studies with green light. The protocols and doses for the use of PDT in WH are very different, which is a limitation when trying to come up with a conclusion [64].

Table 6. Summary of some of the photosensitizers (PS) and light sources used in photodynamic therapy (PDT) in wound healing (WH).

Group of Photosensitizers	Molecule	Light Sources (570–800 nm)	Protocol
Hematoporphyrin derivates	Photofrin®	LED (red and NIR)	37–100 J/cm^2/session
PpIX precursors	ALA, MAL	Laser (Vascular and Diode)	
Clorins	Foscan® (mTHPC)		1–2 sessions/week/1 month

PpIX: Protoporphyrin IX; ALA: aminolaevulinic acid; MAL: Methylaminolaevulinic acid; mTHPC: meso-tetrahydroyphenyl chlorin; LED: ligh emitting diodes; NIR: near infrared.

The PS increases the intracellular production of Protoporphyrin IX, which absorbs the light and produces the reaction. Destruction is mediated by the production of excessive intracellular ROS (radical oxygen singlet).

The mechanisms of action of PDT are well known; besides the necrosis of the tumors, a lot of parallel biological phenomena are produced, which lead to exploring other indications of WH (Table 7) [65].

Table 7. Summary of the mechanism of action revised of PDT in WH.

Effect	Mediator	Phase of Wound Healing
Activation/suppression of the immune system	TNF-alfa IL1, IL6, IL10	Inflammation
Antibacterial activity	ROS	Chronic inflammation
Reepithelization, matrix formation	MMPs	Regeneration and remodeling
Neovascularization	VEGF	Regeneration and remodeling

TNF: tumoral necrosis factor; IL: interleukins; ROS: radical oxygen singlet; MMPs: metalloproteinases; VEGF: vascular endothelial growth factor.

PDT produces the activation of acute inflammation in WH, fostering the natural process, and consequently, the neutrophils, TNF-alfa, and IL6 become increased [66]. PDT also induces neovascularization induced by VEGF needed for remodeling [30].

Additionally, studies have indicated that the early activation of fibroblasts and re-epithelization and increase in degranulation index by mast cells play a crucial role in the healing of chronic wounds. It is worth remembering how interactions of the immune system with the nervous system are important in the regulation of wound healing processes. Recent studies have demonstrated that MC interactions with neuronal cells containing neurotransmitters involved in wound healing processes, such as CGRP, NGF, NKA, NPY, SP, PGP 9.5, and VIP, are common in chronic wounds. This fact can be related to other facts such as the secretion of extracellular matrix by fibroblasts, as well as increases in TGF beta levels and the response of cellular infiltrates [18,30].

Afterwards, PDT a negative regulation of the inflammation appears with IL10 expression and down regulation of IL1 and IL6 [67]. It has been suggested that the modulatory effect of PDT in the immune system and the necrosis versus apoptosis induction depends on the intensity of the protocol [68], more specifically on the ROS levels. Therefore, high intracellular production of ROS could change the activation into destruction (hormesis) [69].

PDT increases the levels of MMPs after three weeks, and the histological improvement appears at nine months. On the other hand, PDT has antibacterial activity, targeting the biofilm, which is responsive to chronic inflammation [30,70].

4.4. Electrical Stimulation

Endogenous bioelectric fields (EBF) take place during WH, produced by the cells generated by the Na^+/K^+ ATPase of the epidermis. EBFs influence cell migration, proliferation, and function, but also gene and protein expression [71]. The underlying mechanisms presented in a CW could be targeted with electrical stimulation (ES) mimicking the natural process (Figure 2). Table 8 summarized the effects of ES in WH outlining in which part of the process this mechanism is working. Theoretically, ES offers benefits in WH after some days in the wound improving the proliferation and remodeling phase. Moreover, if a CW is established, ES could decrease inflammation and the risk of infection. In vitro studies have demonstrated a decrease in *Staphylococcus aureus*, *Pseudomonas aeruginosa* and *Escherichia coli* with ES [72]. Positive scattered results with ES have been reported in CW, VU, and LU, with a possible increase of 30–42% in the reduction in the wound area [72,73]. ES is a safe, simple, cheap, and easy procedure to use without adverse effects.

Table 8. Beneficial effects reported of electrical stimulation (ES) in wound healing (WH) and chronic wound (CW).

Effect	Mediator	Phase of WH/CW
Angiogenesis	VEGF	Proliferation
Fibroblast proliferation	FGF	Proliferation and remodeling
Reduces bacterial colonization	PH alteration	Persistent inflammation and risk of infection

EGF: vascular endothelial growth factor; FGF: fibroblast growth factor.

There are different forms of ES, including direct current, alternating current and pulsed current on mono or bipolar devices. That huge variability limits knowing the real exact beneficial protocol. Moreover, no comparative study between those modalities has been conducted, whereas it is supposed that the pulsed current is the most similar to the physiological(25) [25,71,72]. Theoretically, not all forms of ES are beneficial in all phases of WH, the alternative current only being useful in the first days [25]. There is also a lack of literature about standard protocols [73].

According to the mechanism of action of ES, it would be more effective in the proliferative and remodeling phase of WH, that implies, from days to months after the injury, either in acute wounds (AW) to prevent scarring or in CW to enhance healing [73].

If ES is applied, it should be added to the conventional treatment of the wound as a complementary treatment (Table 9). The ES devices are usually applied by setting electrodes around the wound. Repeated-weekly sessions are necessarily, lasting from 45 min to hours [25]. The therapy could last months, which is a great limitation due to time consumption and displacement. Therefore, ES might be used in selected patients with a risk of failure in WH. Novel devices are emerging, offering different possibilities such as home devices, electric dressings, or electric fields, providing a practical future [71].

Table 9. Summary of the practical initial application of electrical stimulation (ES) in wound healing (WH).

Modality	Type of Wound	Not yet Studied/Not Beneficial
Pulsed current Electrodes around the wound From 30 min to hours		Acute current in CW
From 5 to 7 days a week	DU	Scarring prevention or treatment
After 2–5 days of the injury	LU	

DU: diabetic ulcer; LU: Leg ulcer.

4.5. Others

4.5.1. Ultrasound Therapy

Ultrasound therapy (UT) consists of sound waves that cause thermal and non-thermal effects in tissues. When UT is strongly applied to the skin, the temperature will rise to 40 Celsius degrees and produces an increase in vessel flow, cell proliferation, collagen synthesis, and tissue regeneration. Moreover, UT has anti-inflammatory properties. The non-thermal effects comply with acoustic streaming with a displacement of the particles and cavitation with the generation of microenvironmental gases [74]. Cavitation cleans necrotic tissue preserving the healthy one [7].

UT accelerates the decrease in the wound area with respect to controls in LU, and it is approved as an adjuvant therapy in WH by the FDA [75,76].

Two types of therapeutic US exits are low frequency ultrasound (LFU) from 30 to 40 kHz and high-frequency ultrasound (HFU), ranging from 1 to 3 MHz. HFU has been used for decades for the treatment of muscular diseases in sports medicine. A variant of HFU, micro focused ultrasound in high intense mode (MFU, HIFU), is being widely studied because of its benefits in aesthetic medicine reducing wrinkles and laxity of the skin [75]. In contrast, LFU has demonstrated efficacy in WH and has been applied with good results in LU.

LFU is used directly on the skin, around the wound for 5 to 10 min (Table 10). A topical gel is usually needed between the skin surface and the applicator [74]. UT is contraindicated in a patient carrying a metal prosthesis in the leg, neuropathy, infection, or thrombophlebitis [75].

Table 10. Summary of the practical protocols reviewed in ultrasound therapy (UT) in wound healing (WH).

Modality	Type of Wound	Not yet Studied/Not Beneficial
LFU Around the wound	LU	HFU Contraindicated metal prosthesis, infection, or neuropathy
From 5 to 10 min Repeated sessions in a week		Prevent or treat keloids or HS
After 2–5 days of the injury		

LU: Leg ulcer; HFU: high-frequency ultrasound; HS: Hypertrophic scars.

UT has a possible application in WH; nevertheless, there are no clinical studies of the effects of UT in WH or scar prevention, most of the evidence is limited to LU and further randomized clinical essays and protocols are necessary [75,76].

4.5.2. Electromagnetic Fields

Low frequency pulsed electromagnetic fields (PEMF) can accelerate WH, generating connective tissue, enhancing the VEGF pathway and the production of collagen type I. There are some published studies with good results in PU, VLU and DU. PEMF are possible to apply at home on portable devices as multiple sessions are necessary [77,78].

4.5.3. Biophotonic Therapy

Biophotonic therapy (BT) consists of the application of the PBM applying a special gel over the CW containing the chromophores. Afterwards, an LED lamp with a hyper pulsed beam and low energy is used to activate the photoconverter gel. One concrete device known as "Lumihel®" was evaluated showing improvement in the healing of the CW, increasing the life quality of the patient without adverse events. The main limitations of the study were the simultaneous inclusion of VU, LU and PU and the weekly treatment sessions lasting 8 weeks [79].

4.5.4. Visible Polarized Light

Visible polarized light (VPL) has been used as a complementary therapy in WH. The device used emitted light like the sun but without ultraviolet radiation. Thus, the light used was safe, low energy light, polychromatic, incoherent, and polarized. The polarization allows it to work on flat surfaces and enhances light penetration. The molecular mechanism of action of VL is not well documented; however, some studies showing improvement in treated CW have been published [80,81]. PVL seems a promising possible treatment for WH but needs to be more deeply studied [82].

4.5.5. Radiofrequency

Radiofrequency therapies consist of the application of a high-frequency electromagnetic field (3 kHz and 300 GHz) that induces oscillation and friction in the molecules of the target tissue, which causes tissue hyperthermia. This electrically induced hyperthermia can degrade collagen, which stimulates neocollagenogenesis and tissue remodeling [83]. The main indicators of RF are skin tightening, the reduction of wrinkles and the treatment of scars. There are some studies assessing the efficacy of RF in WH with good results in releasing pain. Nevertheless, multiple sessions are necessary for 2–4 weeks. RF technology is rapidly developing, with new micro-needling devices and fractionated delivery, which shows good results in acne scars, HS, and keloids [21,84].

5. Summary of Clinical Trials of Physical Therapies in Wound Healing

Finally, it is important to take into consideration that there are few clinical trials published about interventions with PT in WH. When the term "Physical therapies skin wounds" is introduced in "Pubmed" and filters added as, "last 10 years", "clinical trials" a total of 66 results appeared. After having been selected, only 8 works were focused on skin and only 6 in CW (Figure S1).

PT are not included in clinical Guidelines of management of CW, and they are used as adjuvant therapies [1]. Polak treated with electrical stimulation (ES) areas of pressure injuries in patients with neurological damage. A total of 43 patients were divided into three groups, anodal, cathodal and placebo. A diminution of proinflammatory blood cytokines was found in the patients treated in correlation with an improvement in the clinical peripheric inflammation of the wound and a significant reduction in the size of the wound was assessed, in comparison to the placebo group. The same therapy was used for other authors [85] to explore the effect in CW in combination with silver dressing. Ten patients were treated only in one wound and the rest were used as controls, leading to significant differences. ES has also been proved to alleviate pain in CW, in addition to accelerating healing [86]. In a study of 10 patients treated with ES compared with 10 patients treated with placebo, ES improved in DU the blood levels of VEGF and NO [87].

In an interesting study, ultrasound (US) and electrical stimulation (ES) were compared in the treatment of PU. Both treatments improved WH in 27 patients treated without significant differences between them [88]. Another comparative study was carried out by Polak in 77 patients with PU using standard wound care, US, and ES. Patients treated with PT had a significant decrease in the ulcer area compared with placebo without differences between US and ES [89]. The main limitation of all those clinical trials is control over others factor that could influence the healing of the wound.

6. Conclusions and Future Perspectives

WH and pathological scars are important problems in daily practice causing pain and morbidity and are difficult to manage. PT arises as a possible safe complementary treatment that might improve the results of the traditional treatment. PT has been demonstrated to improve tissue healing with different grades or evidence; however, further studies are necessary to develop practical protocols in clinical practice based on the theoretical mechanism of action of the therapy. The main limitations of PT are the lack of clinical trials, the availability, the variability of the parameters used in different conditions and the lack of comparable results. Probably, electrical stimulation and ultrasound are the most studied. The scope of this review was to offer a complete view of PT for clinicians in WH so they can start working up new adjuvant protocols.

Supplementary Materials: The supporting information can be downloaded at: https://www.mdpi.com/article/10.3390/ijms24087487/s1.

Author Contributions: Conceptualization, M.F.-G. and M.L.H.-B.; methodology, S.B., M.F.-G. and M.L.H.-B.; software, M.F.-G.; investigation, M.B.-M. and A.C.-M.; resources, M.F.-G.; writing—original draft preparation, M.F.-G. and S.B.; writing—review and editing, M.F.-G., L.A.P.G. and S.B.; visualization, M.F.-G., M.L.H.-B. and S.B.; supervision, M.L.H.-B. and S.B. All authors have read and agreed to the published version of the manuscript.

Funding: This research received no external funding.

Institutional Review Board Statement: Not applicable.

Informed Consent Statement: Not applicable.

Data Availability Statement: All the data reviewed in the manuscript are published in the articles mentioned in the references and selected for being writing in English and indexed in PubMed.

Conflicts of Interest: The authors declare no conflict of interest.

Abbreviations

AU	Atypical ulcer
BT	Biophotonic therapy
CW	Chronic wound
DU	Diabetic ulcer
EBF	Endogenous bioelectric fields
ES	Electrical stimulation
FHW	Fail to heal wound
HS	Hypertrophic scar
LLLT	Low level laser light therapy
PDL	Pulsed dye laser
PEMF	Pulsed electromagnetic field
PT	Physical therapies
PU	Pressure ulcer
US	Ultrasound
UT	Ultrasound therapy
VU	Venous leg ulcer
WH	Wound healing

References

1. Gupta, S.; Andersen, C.; Black, J.; Fife, C.; Lantis, J.I.; Niezgoda, J.; Snyder, R.; Sumpio, B.; Tettelbach, W.; Treadwell, T.; et al. Management of Chronic Wounds: Diagnosis, Preparation, Treatment, and Follow-Up. *Wounds Compend. Clin. Res. Pract.* **2017**, *29*, S19–S36.
2. Wang, P.H.; Huang, B.S.; Horng, H.C.; Yeh, C.C.; Chen, Y.J. Wound healing. *J. Chin. Med. Assoc.* **2018**, *81*, 94–101. [CrossRef] [PubMed]
3. Rodrigues, M.; Kosaric, N.; Bonham, C.A.; Gurtner, G.C. Wound Healing: A Cellular Perspective. *Physiol. Rev.* **2019**, *99*, 665–706. [CrossRef] [PubMed]
4. Veith, A.P.; Henderson, K.; Spencer, A.; Sligar, A.D.; Baker, A.B. Therapeutic strategies for enhancing angiogenesis in wound healing. *Adv. Drug Deliv. Rev.* **2019**, *146*, 97–125. [CrossRef] [PubMed]
5. Monavarian, M.; Kader, S.; Moeinzadeh, S.; Jabbari, E. Regenerative Scar-Free Skin Wound Healing. *Tissue Eng. Part B Rev.* **2019**, *25*, 294–311. [CrossRef]
6. Bai, Q.; Han, K.; Dong, K.; Zheng, C.; Zhang, Y.; Long, Q.; Lu, T. Potential Applications of Nanomaterials and Technology for Diabetic Wound Healing. *Int. J. Nanomed.* **2020**, *15*, 9717–9743. [CrossRef]
7. Palmieri, B.; Vadalà, M.; Laurino, C. Electromedical devices in wound healing management: A narrative review. *J. Wound Care* **2020**, *29*, 408–418. [CrossRef]
8. Lu, W.-S.; Zheng, X.-D.; Yao, X.-H.; Zhang, L.-F. Clinical and epidemiological analysis of keloids in Chinese patients. *Arch. Dermatol. Res.* **2015**, *307*, 109–114. [CrossRef]
9. Berman, B.; Maderal, A.; Raphael, B. Keloids and Hypertrophic Scars: Pathophysiology, Classification, and Treatment. *Dermatol. Surg.* **2017**, *43*, S3–S18. [CrossRef]

10. He, Y.; Deng, Z.; Alghamdi, M.; Lu, L.; Fear, M.W.; He, L. From genetics to epigenetics: New insights into keloid scarring. *Cell Prolif.* **2017**, *50*, e12326. [CrossRef]
11. Huang, C.; Ogawa, R. Systemic factors that shape cutaneous pathological scarring. *FASEB J.* **2020**, *34*, 13171–13184. [CrossRef] [PubMed]
12. Huang, C.; Ogawa, R. Keloidal pathophysiology: Current notions. *Scars Burn. Health* **2021**, *7*. [CrossRef]
13. Bowers, S.; Franco, E. Chronic Wounds: Evaluation and Management. *Am. Fam. Physician* **2020**, *101*, 159–166.
14. Gottrup, F. A specialized wound-healing center concept: Importance of a multidisciplinary department structure and surgical treatment facilities in the treatment of chronic wounds. *Am. J. Surg.* **2004**, *187*, S38–S43. [CrossRef] [PubMed]
15. Fife, C.E.; Carter, M.J. Wound Care Outcomes and Associated Cost among Patients Treated in US Outpatient Wound Centers: Data from the US Wound Registry. *Wounds A Compend. Clin. Res. Pract.* **2012**, *24*, 10–17.
16. Gurtner, G.C.; Werner, S.; Barrandon, Y.; Longaker, M.T. Wound repair and regeneration. *Nature* **2008**, *453*, 314–321. [CrossRef]
17. Furie, B.; Furie, B.C. Mechanisms of thrombus formation. *N. Engl. J. Med.* **2008**, *359*, 938–949. [CrossRef]
18. Bacci, S. Fine Regulation during Wound Healing by Mast Cells, a Physiological Role Not Yet Clarified. *Int. J. Mol. Sci.* **2022**, *23*, 1820. [CrossRef]
19. Jorch, S.K.; Kubes, P. An emerging role for neutrophil extracellular traps in noninfectious disease. *Nat Med.* **2017**, *23*, 279–287. [CrossRef]
20. Kolaczkowska, E.; Kubes, P. Neutrophil recruitment and function in health and inflammation. *Nat. Rev. Immunol.* **2013**, *13*, 159–175. [CrossRef]
21. Akbik, D.; Ghadiri, M.; Chrzanowski, W.; Rohanizadeh, R. Curcumin as a wound healing agent. *Life Sci.* **2014**, *116*, 1–7. [CrossRef] [PubMed]
22. Wilkinson, H.N.; Hardman, M.J. Wound healing: Cellular mechanisms and pathological outcomes. *Open Biol.* **2020**, *10*, 200223. [CrossRef] [PubMed]
23. Jupiter, D.C.; Thorud, J.C.; Buckley, C.J.; Shibuya, N. The impact of foot ulceration and amputation on mortality in diabetic patients. I: From ulceration to death, a systematic review. *Int. Wound J.* **2016**, *13*, 892–903. [CrossRef] [PubMed]
24. Meulendijks, A.M.; de Vries, F.M.C.; van Dooren, A.A.; Schuurmans, M.J.; Neumann, H.A.M. A systematic review on risk factors in developing a first-time Venous Leg Ulcer. *J. Eur. Acad. Dermatol. Venereol.* **2019**, *33*, 1241–1248. [CrossRef] [PubMed]
25. Aleksandrowicz, H.; Owczarczyk-Saczonek, A.; Placek, W. Venous Leg Ulcers: Advanced Therapies and New Technologies. *Biomedicines* **2021**, *9*, 1569. [CrossRef]
26. Wilcox, J.R.; Carter, M.J.; Covington, S. Frequency of debridements and time to heal: A retrospective cohort study of 312 744 wounds. *JAMA Dermatol.* **2013**, *149*, 1050–1058. [CrossRef]
27. Azevedo, M.-M.; Lisboa, C.; Cobrado, L.; Pina-Vaz, C.; Rodrigues, A.G. Hard-to-heal wounds, biofilm and wound healing: An intricate interrelationship. *Br. J. Nurs.* **2020**, *29*, S6–S13. [CrossRef]
28. Sun, F.; Qu, F.; Ling, Y.; Mao, P.; Xia, P.; Chen, H.; Zhou, D. Biofilm-associated infections: Antibiotic resistance and novel therapeutic strategies. *Futur. Microbiol.* **2013**, *8*, 877–886. [CrossRef]
29. Pastar, I.; Stojadinovic, O.; Yin, N.C.; Ramirez, H.; Nusbaum, A.G.; Sawaya, A.; Patel, S.B.; Khalid, L.; Isseroff, R.R.; Tomic-Canic, M. Epithelialization in Wound Healing: A Comprehensive Review. *Adv. Wound Care* **2014**, *3*, 445–464. [CrossRef]
30. Grandi, V.; Corsi, A.; Pimpinelli, N.; Bacci, S. Cellular Mechanisms in Acute and Chronic Wounds after PDT Therapy: An Update. *Biomedicines* **2022**, *10*, 1624. [CrossRef]
31. Huang, C.; Akaishi, S.; Hyakusoku, H.; Ogawa, R. Are keloid and hypertrophic scar different forms of the same disorder? A fibroproliferative skin disorder hypothesis based on keloid findings. *Int. Wound J.* **2014**, *11*, 517–522. [CrossRef] [PubMed]
32. Khetarpal, S.; Kaw, U.; Dover, J.S.; Arndt, K.A. Laser advances in the treatment of burn and traumatic scars. *Semin. Cutan. Med. Surg.* **2017**, *36*, 185–191. [CrossRef] [PubMed]
33. Jourdan, M.; Madfes, D.C.; Lima, E.; Tian, Y.; Seité, S. Skin Care Management for Medical and Aesthetic Procedures to Prevent Scarring. *Clin. Cosmet. Investig. Dermatol.* **2019**, *12*, 799–804. [CrossRef] [PubMed]
34. Kauvar, A.N.B.; Kubicki, S.L.; Suggs, A.K.; Friedman, P.M. Laser Therapy of Traumatic and Surgical Scars and an Algorithm for Their Treatment. *Lasers Surg. Med.* **2020**, *52*, 125–136. [CrossRef]
35. Altemir, A.; Boixeda, P. Laser Treatment of Burn Scars. *Actas Dermosifiliogr.* **2022**, *113*, T938–T944. [CrossRef] [PubMed]
36. Clementoni, M.T.; Pedrelli, V.; Zaccaria, G.; Pontini, P.; Motta, L.R.; Azzopardi, E.A. New Developments for Fractional CO_2 Resurfacing for Skin Rejuvenation and Scar Reduction. *Facial Plast. Surg. Clin. N. Am.* **2020**, *28*, 17–28. [CrossRef]
37. Azzam, O.A.; Bassiouny, D.A.; El-Hawary, M.S.; El Maadawi, Z.M.; Sobhi, R.M.; El-Mesidy, M.S. Treatment of hypertrophic scars and keloids by fractional carbon dioxide laser: A clinical, histological, and immunohistochemical study. *Lasers Med. Sci.* **2016**, *31*, 9–18. [CrossRef]
38. Yang, Q.; Ma, Y.; Zhu, R.; Huang, G.; Guan, M.; Avram, M.M.; Lu, Z. The effect of flashlamp pulsed dye laser on the expression of connective tissue growth factor in keloids. *Lasers Surg. Med.* **2012**, *44*, 377–383. [CrossRef]
39. Zhibo, X.; Miaobo, Z. Molecular mechanism of pulsed-dye laser in treatment of keloids: An in vitro study. *Adv. Skin Wound Care* **2010**, *23*, 29–33. [CrossRef]
40. Lv, K.; Xia, Z.; Chinese Consensus Panel on the Prevention and Treatment of Scars. Chinese expert consensus on clinical prevention and treatment of scar+. *Burn. Trauma* **2018**, *6*, 27. [CrossRef]

41. Sobanko, J.F.; Vachiramon, V.; Rattanaumpawan, P.; Miller, C.J. Early postoperative single treatment ablative fractional lasing of Mohs micrographic surgery facial scars: A split-scar, evaluator-blinded study. *Lasers Surg. Med.* **2015**, *47*, 1–5. [CrossRef]
42. Shin, H.W.; Suk, S.; Chae, S.W.; Yoon, K.C.; Kim, J. Early postoperative treatment of mastectomy scars using a fractional carbon dioxide laser: A randomized, controlled, split-scar, blinded study. *Arch. Plast. Surg.* **2021**, *48*, 347–352. [CrossRef] [PubMed]
43. Lee, S.H.; Zheng, Z.; Roh, M.R. Early Postoperative Treatment of Surgical Scars Using a Fractional Carbon Dioxide Laser: A Split-Scar, Evaluator-Blinded Study. *Dermatol. Surg.* **2013**, *39*, 1190–1196. [CrossRef] [PubMed]
44. Kim, D.H.; Ryu, H.J.; Choi, J.E.; Ahn, H.H.; Kye, Y.C.; Seo, S.H. A Comparison of the Scar Prevention Effect between Carbon Dioxide Fractional Laser and Pulsed Dye Laser in Surgical Scars. *Dermatol. Surg.* **2014**, *40*, 973–978. [CrossRef] [PubMed]
45. Liu, X.-J.; Liu, W.-H.; Fang, S.-W.; Zhou, X.-L.; Xu, J.-X.; Li, G.-S. Lasers and Intense Pulsed Light for the Treatment of Pathological Scars: A Network Meta-Analysis. *Aesthetic Surg. J.* **2022**, *42*, NP675–NP687. [CrossRef]
46. Brewin, M.P.; Lister, T.S. Prevention or treatment of hypertrophic burn scarring: A review of when and how to treat with the Pulsed Dye Laser. *Burns* **2014**, *40*, 797–804. [CrossRef]
47. Leszczynski, R.; da Silva, C.A.; Pinto, A.; Kuczynski, U.; da Silva, E.M. Laser therapy for treating hypertrophic and keloid scars. *Cochrane Database Syst. Rev.* **2022**, *9*, CD011642. [CrossRef]
48. Seago, M.; Shumaker, P.R.; Spring, L.K.; Alam, M.; Al-Niaimi, F.; Anderson, R.R.; Artzi, O.; Bayat, A.; Cassuto, D.; Chan, H.H.; et al. Laser Treatment of Traumatic Scars and Contractures: 2020 International Consensus Recommendations. *Lasers Surg. Med.* **2020**, *52*, 96–116. [CrossRef]
49. Mosca, R.C.; Ong, A.A.; Albasha, O.; Bass, K.; Arany, P. Photobiomodulation Therapy for Wound Care: A Potent, Noninvasive, Photoceutical Approach. *Adv. Ski. Wound Care* **2019**, *32*, 157–167. [CrossRef]
50. Calabrese, E.J.; Dhawan, G.; Kapoor, R.; Agathokleous, E.; Calabrese, V. Hormesis: Wound healing and fibroblasts. *Pharmacol. Res.* **2022**, *184*, 106449. [CrossRef]
51. Tatmatsu-Rocha, J.C.; Ferraresi, C.; Hamblin, M.R.; Maia, F.D.; do Nascimento, N.R.; Driusso, P.; Parizotto, N. Low-level laser therapy (904 nm) can increase collagen and reduce oxidative and nitrosative stress in diabetic wounded mouse skin. *J. Photochem. Photobiol. B Biol.* **2016**, *164*, 96–102. [CrossRef] [PubMed]
52. Sperandio, F.F.; Simões, A.; Corrêa, L.; Aranha, A.C.C.; Giudice, F.S.; Hamblin, M.R.; Sousa, S.C. Low-level laser irradiation promotes the proliferation and maturation of keratinocytes during epithelial wound repair. *J. Biophotonics* **2014**, *8*, 795–803. [CrossRef] [PubMed]
53. Calabrese, E.J.; Dhawan, G.; Kapoor, R.; Agathokleous, E.; Calabrese, V. Hormesis: Wound healing and keratinocytes. *Pharmacol. Res.* **2022**, *183*, 106393. [CrossRef] [PubMed]
54. Heiskanen, V.; Hamblin, M.R. Photobiomodulation: Lasers vs. light emitting diodes? *Photochem. Photobiol. Sci.* **2018**, *17*, 1003–1017. [CrossRef] [PubMed]
55. Vitse, J.; Bekara, F.; Byun, S.; Herlin, C.; Teot, L. A Double-Blind, Placebo-Controlled Randomized Evaluation of the Effect of Low-Level Laser Therapy on Venous Leg Ulcers. *Int. J. Low. Extremity Wounds* **2017**, *16*, 29–35. [CrossRef]
56. Taradaj, J.; Halski, T.; Kucharzewski, M.; Urbanek, T.; Halska, U.; Kucio, C. Effect of Laser Irradiation at Different Wavelengths (940, 808, and 658 nm) on Pressure Ulcer Healing: Results from a Clinical Study. *Evid. Based Complement. Altern. Med.* **2013**, *2013*, 960240. [CrossRef]
57. Barolet, D.; Boucher, A. Prophylactic low-level light therapy for the treatment of hypertrophic scars and keloids: A case series. *Lasers Surg. Med.* **2010**, *42*, 597–601. [CrossRef]
58. Akasaki, I. Blue Light: A Fascinating Journey (Nobel Lecture). *Angew. Chem. Int. Ed. Engl.* **2015**, *54*, 7750–7763. [CrossRef]
59. Dini, V.; Romanelli, M.; Oranges, T.; Davini, G.; Janowska, A. Blue light emission in the management of hard-to-heal wounds. *G. Ital. Dermatol. E Venereol.* **2021**, *156*, 703–713. [CrossRef]
60. Ngoc, L.T.N.; Moon, J.Y.; Lee, Y.C. Utilization of light-emitting diodes for skin therapy: Systematic review and meta-analysis. *Photodermatol. Photoimmunol. Photomed.* **2022**. [CrossRef]
61. Morton, C.A.; Szeimies, R.M.; Basset-Seguin, N.; Calzavara-Pinton, P.; Gilaberte, Y.; Haedersdal, M.; Hofbauer, G.F.L.; Hunger, R.E.; Karrer, S.; Piaserico, S.; et al. European Dermatology Forum guidelines on topical photodynamic therapy 2019 Part 1: Treatment delivery and established indications—Actinic keratoses, Bowen's disease and basal cell carcinomas. *J. Eur. Acad. Dermatol. Venereol.* **2019**, *33*, 2225–2238. [CrossRef] [PubMed]
62. Oyama, J.; Ramos-Milaré, Á.C.F.H.; Lera-Nonose, D.S.S.L.; Nesi-Reis, V.; Demarchi, I.G.; Aristides, S.M.A.; Teixeira, J.J.V.; Silveira, T.G.V.; Lonardoni, M.V.C. Photodynamic therapy in wound healing in vivo: A systematic review. *Photodiagnosis Photodyn. Ther.* **2020**, *30*, 101682. [CrossRef]
63. Nesi-Reis, V.; Lera-Nonose, D.; Oyama, J.; Silva-Lalucci, M.P.P.; Demarchi, I.G.; Aristides, S.M.A.; Teixeira, J.J.V.; Silveira, T.G.V.; Lonardoni, M.V.C. Contribution of photodynamic therapy in wound healing: A systematic review. *Photodiagnosis Photodyn. Ther.* **2017**, *21*, 294–305. [CrossRef] [PubMed]
64. Kang, K.; Bacci, S. Photodynamic Therapy. *Biomedicines* **2022**, *10*, 2701. [CrossRef] [PubMed]
65. Fernández-Guarino, M.; García-Morales, I.; Harto, A.; Montull, C.; Pérez-García, B.; Jaén, P. Photodynamic Therapy: New Indications. *Actas Dermo-Sifiliográficas Engl. Ed.* **2007**, *98*, 377–395. [CrossRef]
66. Li, L.; Yang, Y.; Yang, Z.; Zheng, M.; Luo, G.; He, W.; Yin, R. Effects of ALA-PDT on the macrophages in wound healing and its related mechanisms in vivo and in vitro. *Photodiagnosis Photodyn. Ther.* **2022**, *38*, 102816. [CrossRef]

67. Choi, J.Y.; Park, G.T.; Na, E.Y.; Wi, H.S.; Lee, S.-C.; Lee, J.-B. Molecular changes following topical photodynamic therapy using methyl aminolaevulinate in mouse skin. *J. Dermatol. Sci.* **2010**, *58*, 198–203. [CrossRef]
68. Mroz, P.; Hamblin, M.R. The immunosuppressive side of PDT. *Photochem. Photobiol. Sci.* **2011**, *10*, 751–758. [CrossRef]
69. Khorsandi, K.; Hosseinzadeh, R.; Esfahani, H.; Zandsalimi, K.; Shahidi, F.K.; Abrahamse, H. Accelerating skin regeneration and wound healing by controlled ROS from photodynamic treatment. *Inflamm. Regen.* **2022**, *42*, 40. [CrossRef]
70. de Oliveira, A.B.; Ferrisse, T.M.; Fontana, C.R.; Basso, F.G.; Brighenti, F.L. Photodynamic therapy for treating infected skin wounds: A systematic review and meta-analysis from randomized clinical trials. *Photodiagnosis Photodyn Ther.* **2022**, *40*, 103118. [CrossRef]
71. Rajendran, S.B.; Challen, K.; Wright, K.L.; Hardy, J.G. Electrical Stimulation to Enhance Wound Healing. *J. Funct. Biomater.* **2021**, *12*, 40. [CrossRef] [PubMed]
72. Ud-Din, S.; Bayat, A. Electrical Stimulation and Cutaneous Wound Healing: A Review of Clinical Evidence. *Healthcare* **2014**, *2*, 445–467. [CrossRef] [PubMed]
73. Koel, G.; Houghton, P.E. Electrostimulation: Current Status, Strength of Evidence Guidelines, and Meta-Analysis. *Adv. Wound Care* **2014**, *3*, 118–126. [CrossRef] [PubMed]
74. Cullum, N.; Nelson, E.A.; Flemming, K.; Sheldon, T. Systematic reviews of wound care management: (5) beds; (6) compression; (7) laser therapy, therapeutic ultrasound, electrotherapy and electromagnetic therapy. *Health Technol. Assess.* **2001**, *5*, 9. [CrossRef] [PubMed]
75. Beheshti, A.; Shafigh, Y.; Parsa, H.; Zangivand, A.A. Comparison of High-Frequency and MIST Ultrasound Therapy for the Healing of Venous Leg Ulcers. *Adv. Clin. Exp. Med.* **2014**, *23*, 969–975. [CrossRef] [PubMed]
76. Cullum, N.; Liu, Z. Therapeutic ultrasound for venous leg ulcers. *Cochrane Database Syst. Rev.* **2017**, *5*, CD001180. [CrossRef]
77. Guerriero, F.; Botarelli, E.; Mele, G.; Polo, L.; Zoncu, D.; Renati, P.; Sgarlata, C.; Rollone, M.; Ricevuti, G.; Maurizi, N.; et al. Effectiveness of an Innovative Pulsed Electromagnetic Fields Stimulation in Healing of Untreatable Skin Ulcers in the Frail Elderly: Two Case Reports. *Case Rep. Dermatol. Med.* **2015**, *2015*, 576580. [CrossRef]
78. Kwan, R.L.; Wong, W.C.; Yip, S.L.; Chan, K.L.; Zheng, Y.P.; Cheing, G.L. Pulsed electromagnetic field therapy promotes healing and microcirculation of chronic diabetic foot ulcers: A pilot study. *Adv. Skin Wound Care* **2015**, *28*, 212–219. [CrossRef]
79. Romanelli, M.; Piaggesi, A.; Scapagnini, G.; Dini, V.; Janowska, A.; Iacopi, E.; Scarpa, C.; Fauverghe, S.; Bassetto, F.; EUREKA Study Group. Evaluation of fluorescence biomodulation in the real-life management of chronic wounds: The EUREKA trial. *J. Wound Care* **2018**, *27*, 744–753. [CrossRef]
80. Taha, M.M.; El-Nagar, M.M.; Elrefaey, B.H.; Elkholy, R.M.; Ali, O.I.; Alkhamees, N.; Felaya, E.-S.E.E.-S. Effect of Polarized Light Therapy (Bioptron) on Wound Healing and Microbiota in Diabetic Foot Ulcer: A Randomized Controlled Trial. *Photobiomodulation Photomed. Laser Surg.* **2022**, *40*, 792–799. [CrossRef]
81. M. Allam, N.; Eladl, H.M.; Eid, M.M. Polarized Light Therapy in the Treatment of Wounds: A Review. *Int. J. Low Extrem. Wounds* **2022**, 15347346221113991. [CrossRef] [PubMed]
82. Feehan, J.; Burrows, S.P.; Cornelius, L.; Cook, A.M.; Mikkelsen, K.; Apostolopoulos, V.; Husaric, M.; Kiatos, D. Therapeutic applications of polarized light: Tissue healing and immunomodulatory effects. *Maturitas* **2018**, *116*, 11–17. [CrossRef] [PubMed]
83. Ekelem, C.; Thomas, L.; Van Hal, M.; Valdebran, M.; Lotfizadeh, A.; Mlynek, K.; Mesinkovska, N.A. Radiofrequency Therapy and Noncosmetic Cutaneous Conditions. *Dermatol. Surg.* **2019**, *45*, 908–930. [CrossRef]
84. Cucu, C.; Butacu, A.; Niculae, B.D.; Tiplica, G.S. Benefits of fractional radiofrequency treatment in patients with atrophic acne scars—Literature review. *J. Cosmet. Dermatol.* **2021**, *20*, 381–385. [CrossRef] [PubMed]
85. Zhou, K.; Krug, K.; Stachura, J.; Niewczyk, P.; Ross, M.; Tutuska, J.; Ford, G. Silver-Collagen Dressing and High-voltage, Pulsed-current Therapy for the Treatment of Chronic Full-thickness Wounds: A Case Series. *J. Wound Ostomy Cont. Nurs.* **2016**, *62*, 36–44.
86. Fraccalvieri, M.; Salomone, M.; Zingarelli, E.M.; Rivarossa, F.; Bruschi, S. Electrical stimulation for difficult wounds: Only an alternative procedure? *Int. Wound J.* **2015**, *12*, 669–673. [CrossRef]
87. Mohajeri-Tehrani, M.R.; Nasiripoor, F.; Torkaman, G.; Hedayati, M.; Annabestani, Z.; Asadi, M.R. Effect of low-intensity direct current on expression of vascular endothelial growth factor and nitric oxide in diabetic foot ulcers. *J. Rehabil. Res. Dev.* **2014**, *51*, 815–824. [CrossRef]
88. Bora Karsli, P.; Gurcay, E.; Karaahmet, O.Z.; Cakci, A. High-Voltage Electrical Stimulation Versus Ultrasound in the Treatment of Pressure Ulcers. *Adv. Skin Wound Care* **2017**, *30*, 565–570. [CrossRef]
89. Polak, A.; Taradaj, J.; Nawrat-Szoltysik, A.; Stania, M.; Dolibog, P.; Blaszczak, E.; Zarzeczny, R.; Juras, G.; Franek, A.; Kucio, C. Reduction of pressure ulcer size with high-voltage pulsed current and high-frequency ultrasound: A randomised trial. *J. Wound Care* **2016**, *25*, 742–754. [CrossRef]

International Journal of
Molecular Sciences

MDPI

Review

From Molecular Insights to Clinical Perspectives in Drug-Associated Bullous Pemphigoid

Belen de Nicolas-Ruanes *, Asuncion Ballester-Martinez *, Emilio Garcia-Mouronte, Emilio Berna-Rico, Carlos Azcarraga-Llobet and Montserrat Fernandez-Guarino

Dermatology Department, Hospital Universitario Ramon y Cajal, 28034 Madrid, Spain; carlos.azcarraga95@gmail.com (C.A.-L.); montsefernandezguarino@gmail.com (M.F.-G.)
* Correspondence: mnicolas@salud.madrid.org (B.d.N.-R.); mariaasuncion.ballester@salud.madrid.org (A.B.-M.); Tel.: +34-913668582 (B.d.N.-R. & A.B.-M.)

Abstract: Bullous pemphigoid (BP), the most common autoimmune blistering disease, is characterized by the presence of autoantibodies targeting BP180 and BP230 in the basement membrane zone. This leads to the activation of complement-dependent and independent pathways, resulting in proteolytic cleavage at the dermoepidermal junction and an eosinophilic inflammatory response. While numerous drugs have been associated with BP in the literature, causality and pathogenic mechanisms remain elusive in most cases. Dipeptidyl peptidase 4 inhibitors (DPP4i), in particular, are the most frequently reported drugs related to BP and, therefore, have been extensively investigated. They can potentially trigger BP through the impaired proteolytic degradation of BP180, combined with immune dysregulation. DPP4i-associated BP can be categorized into true drug-induced BP and drug-triggered BP, with the latter resembling classic BP. Antineoplastic immunotherapy is increasingly associated with BP, with both B and T cells involved. Other drugs, including biologics, diuretics and cardiovascular and neuropsychiatric agents, present weaker evidence and poorly understood pathogenic mechanisms. Further research is needed due to the growing incidence of BP and the increasing identification of new potential triggers.

Keywords: autoimmune blistering diseases; bullous pemphigoid; drug-associated bullous pemphigoid; drug-induced bullous pemphigoid; dipeptidyl peptidase 4 inhibitors; gliptins; immunotherapy; immune checkpoint inhibitors; biologics; diuretics

Citation: de Nicolas-Ruanes, B.; Ballester-Martinez, A.; Garcia-Mouronte, E.; Berna-Rico, E.; Azcarraga-Llobet, C.; Fernandez-Guarino, M. From Molecular Insights to Clinical Perspectives in Drug-Associated Bullous Pemphigoid. *Int. J. Mol. Sci.* **2023**, *24*, 16786. https://doi.org/10.3390/ijms242316786

Academic Editors: Gian Marco Ghiggeri and Andrés González-García

Received: 21 October 2023
Revised: 19 November 2023
Accepted: 22 November 2023
Published: 26 November 2023

1. Introduction

Bullous pemphigoid (BP) stands as the most common autoimmune blistering disease, presenting an estimated incidence ranging from 10 to 43 cases per million individuals per year [1,2]. Remarkably, this disorder exhibits a distinct predilection for the elderly population, with escalating incidence beyond the age of 70 years old [1–5]. According to a retrospective study conducted in the United Kingdom, the median age of BP onset was 80 years, underscoring the advanced age at which BP commonly manifests [6].

The underlying mechanisms of BP remain largely unknown. However, it seems to rely upon the interaction between predisposing and triggering factors. Predisposing elements include genetic background, age and comorbidities such as neurological conditions. Eventually, the exposure to a specific trigger, such as drugs, physical factors, vaccines, infections or transplantations, holds the potential to induce or exacerbate BP [7].

The diagnosis of BP is established through a combination of criteria, including clinical features, histopathological findings, positive direct immunofluorescence (DIF) and the detection of circulating IgG anti-basement membrane zone (BMZ) autoantibodies [8].

The classical clinical manifestations of BP consist of tense bullae appearing on erythematous urticarial skin, primarily localized on the trunk and extremity flexures, as well as in the axillary and inguinal folds. Less frequently, bullae may appear on seemingly unaffected skin, a condition referred to as "non-inflammatory BP". Regardless of the inflammatory background, BP is characterized by its intense associated pruritus [1,8]. Mucosal involvement can be observed in up to 20% of BP patients, but is mild and predominantly affects the oral cavity [9]. Other bullous clinical variants include dyshidrosiform pemphioid, localized BP or lichen planus pemphigoides. Additionally, nonbullous presentations of BP encompass eczematous, urticarial and prurigo-like (pemphigoid nodularis) forms [5,8].

Histopathological examination usually reveals subepidermal detachment containing eosinophils, neutrophils and fibrin, alongside a dermal inflammatory infiltrate. In non-bullous forms, skin biopsy shows eosinophilic spongiosis with an eosinophilic dermal inflammatory infiltrate, although these findings might be non-specific [8]. Direct immunofluorescence (DIF) samples must be obtained from perilesional skin. The linear deposition of C3 and/or IgG along the BMZ in DIF displays the highest diagnostic sensitivity for BP (90.8%) [10].

Indirect immunofluorescence (IIF) displays a linear IgG deposition along the dermoepidermal junction, which is shown to occur on the epidermal side of the split while using salt-split human skin as a substrate. Enzyme linked immunosorbent assay (ELISA) testing can detect and quantify serum levels of anti-BP180 and anti-BP230 autoantibodies, which are usually positive in BP with ranging sensitivity [1]. A mosaic biochip designed to simultaneously detect multiple autoantibodies for the most common blistering diseases is commercially available. It has demonstrated high sensitivity and specificity, equivalent to each of its individual components, while streamlining the diagnostic process [8,11].

2. Pathogenesis of Bullous Pemphigoid (BP)

The pathogenesis initiates with the binding of autoantibodies against the hemidesmosomes in the basement membrane zone (BMZ) (Figure 1). This binding activates multiple pathways, both complement-mediated and non-mediated, leading to the release of cytokines and proteases and the chemotaxis of neutrophils and eosinophils. Proteolytic cleavage at the BMZ induces dermal–epidermal separation and blister formation, with the subsequent dispersion of hemidesmosome-associated protein fragments. These fragments may interact with autoreactive lymphocytes, intensifying the inflammatory response [1,5].

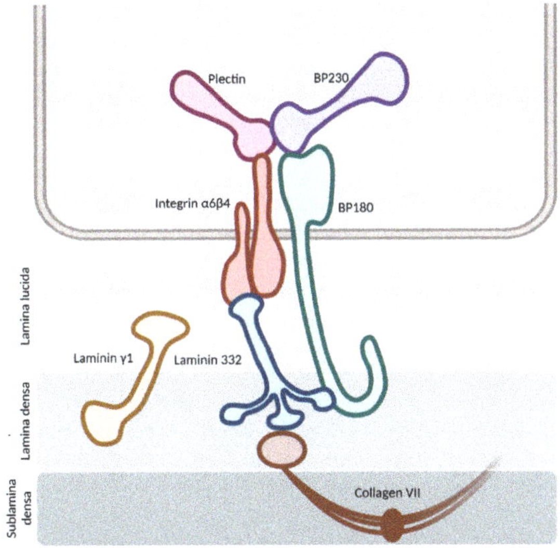

Figure 1. Schematic representation of hemidesmosomes in the basement membrane zone. The molecules of BP180 and BP230 stand as the main antigenic targets for autoantibody development in bullous pemphigoid.

2.1. Antigenic Targets

In bullous pemphigoid, we usually find autoantibodies against two principal hemidesmosomal proteins: bullous pemphigoid antigen 2 (BPAg2) and bullous pemphigoid antigen 1 (BPAg1). BPAg2 is a 180 kilodalton transmembrane protein, also known as bullous pemphigoid 180 (BP-180) or collagen XVII. BPAg1 is a 230 kilodalton intracellular hemidesmosomal protein, so it is also referred to as bullous pemphigoid antigen 230 (BP230) [12].

2.1.1. BP180

BP180 is a morphologically complex transmembrane protein (Figure 2). It is composed of a globular intracellular domain in the amino-terminal and a large extracellular segment (or ectodomain) in the carboxyl-terminal that encompass the lamina lucida in the dermoepidermal junction and expands into the lamina densa [13]. The ectodomain is composed of 15 collagenous domains interspersed with 16 non-collagenous (NC) domains, each designated in sequential order starting from the carboxyl-terminal (NC1, NC2 ... NC16) [14].

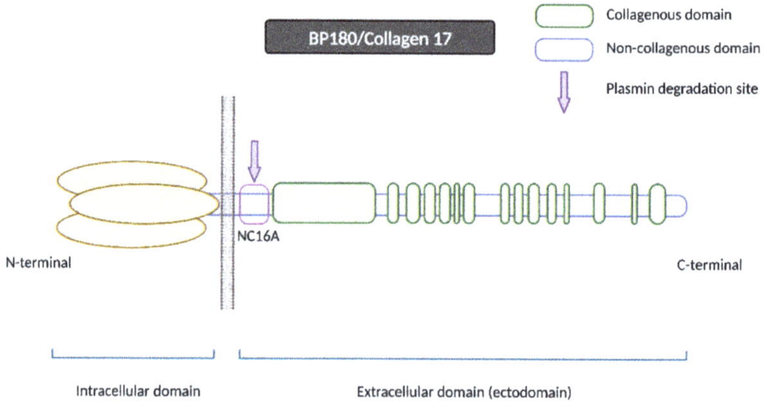

Figure 2. BP180/Collagen 17. BP180 is a transmembrane protein consisting of a globular intracellular domain at the amino-terminal and a large extracellular segment (or ectodomain) at the carboxyl-terminal. NC16A represents the juxtamembranous non-collagenous domain, and it contains the major pathogenic epitope for BP, in addition to being the primary site for plasmin and other serine proteases' degradation. N-terminal: amino-terminal; C-terminal: carboxyl-terminal.

The NC16A domain consists of an extracellular juxtamembranous region and contains the major pathogenic epitope for BP. Thus, most common commercialized ELISAs for BP diagnosis use a recombinant NC16A protein to detect and quantify BP autoantibodies [15] and 84–90% of BP sera react with the NC16A domain [16,17]. It is important to note that anti-BP180 antibodies can also recognize other epitopes on BP180 beyond the NC16A domain, extending into the midportion or carboxyl-terminal regions of the ectodomain [15]. Izumi et al. reported that these cases with non-NC16A anti-BP180 antibodies displayed a non-inflammatory phenotype with less erythema and a diminished eosinophilic infiltrate and were more likely to respond to corticosteroid treatment [18].

One of the hypotheses that has been put forth to explain the disease revolves around impaired proteolytic degradation. The physiological shedding of BP180 by serine proteases, including plasmin, exposes new antigens and generates neoepitopes, which could serve as targets for blister-inducing antibodies. The principal site of degradation for the BP180 molecule is the juxtamembranous domain NC16A, aligning with the major pathogenic epitope of BP [18,19]. Other proteinases, such as A Disintegrin and Metalloproteases (ADAMs) and Granzyme B (GzmB), might also contribute to the generation of neoepitopes and the onset of BP through BP180 cleavage. In fact, GzmB expression is upregulated with age, which could help to explain its role in this age-related autoimmune blistering disorder [20].

BP180 has also been demonstrated to be present in extracutaneous tissues, such as in various neuroanatomical regions in the brain [21], and as a component of the glomerular filtration barrier in the kidneys [22]. However, its precise function and potential role in neurodegenerative disorders or renal diseases remains to be elucidated [21–23].

2.1.2. BP230

BP230 is an intracellular component of hemidesmosomes and is part of the plakine family. Anti-BP230 antibodies mainly bind to the globular carboxyl-terminal domain and are detected in approximately 60–70% of BP serum samples [24]. Given the fully intracellular location of BP230, the accessibility of autoantibodies to this antigen is potentially limited. Consequently, it remains uncertain whether they exert a pathogenic role in BP or merely appear as a secondary event linked to keratinocyte injury (occurring as byproducts of epitope spreading associated with disease extension) [16].

Nonetheless, anti-BP230 antibodies have been associated with the appearance of non-bullous pemphigoid [25], whereas its absence may correlate with mucosal involvement in BP patients [9]. As a result, anti-BP230 antibodies might contribute to some extent in the development of BP; however, the precise mechanism and significance remain unclear.

2.2. *Hypothesis of Blister Formation*

It is well accepted that bullous pemphigoid arises from a loss of immune tolerance, resulting in the production of autoantibodies against BP180 and BP230. These antibodies trigger an inflammatory reaction, attracting numerous neutrophils, eosinophils and mast cells, which migrate to the dermis and release a wide range of cytokines and proteases, responsible for dermoepidermal cleavage and blister formation [26].

Until the last decade, a complement was believed to be a prerequisite for blister formation by autoantibodies. Complement components are present along the dermoepidermal junction in patients with BP, as demonstrated with direct immunofluorescence (DIF), which shows linear C3 deposition in 83–84% of BP cases [27,28]. Complement proteins are present also in the blister fluid of BP patients [29]. Furthermore, complement activation by autoantibodies may correlate with disease activity, as demonstrated in laboratory and clinical studies [28,30]. All this evidence suggests a potential pathogenic role of the complement system in BP development.

Nonetheless, more recent studies have questioned its major pathogenic role in bullous pemphigoid, proposing the existence of complement-independent mechanisms mediating blister formation [28,30]. In animal models, Ujiie et al. demonstrated that the passive transfer of BP autoantibodies induced blister formation in C3-deficient humanized mice, despite not being able to activate the complement cascade [31]. Furthermore, it should be noted that if DIF shows a C3 deposition in 83–84% of patients, then 16–17% of BP patients do not present this complement protein along the dermoepidermal junction and thus they might not be mediated by the complement system [27,28]. In these cases, IgG4 antibodies are the dominant IgG subclass, which are not able to activate the complement cascade [32].

2.2.1. Complement-Dependent Immune Response

The IgG1 and IgG3 antibodies bind to BP180, consequently initiating the activation of the complement cascade (Figure 3). The resulting anaphylatoxins C3a and C5a induce the chemotaxis and degranulation of neutrophils, eosinophils and mast cells. Neutrophils release proteolytic enzymes, including neutrophil elastase (NE) and matrix metalloproteinase 9 (MMP9), leading to the degradation of BP180 and subsequently weakening basal cells' adhesion to the basement membrane zone (BMZ). Simultaneously, mast cells secrete IL-8, which amplifies the neutrophilic infiltration, and numerous proinflammatory cytokines that recruit additional eosinophils. Upon reaching the BMZ, migrated eosinophils discharge their granule proteins, culminating in subepidermal blistering [12,33]. In addition to NE and MMP9, other proteases may potentially contribute to dermal–epidermal cleavage, as evidenced by studies detecting plasmin in BP blister fluid [29,34]. The binding of IgG to BP180 on keratinocytes could induce the liberation of tissue-type plasminogen activator (tPA), thereby catalyzing the conversion of plasminogen into active plasmin [18,34].

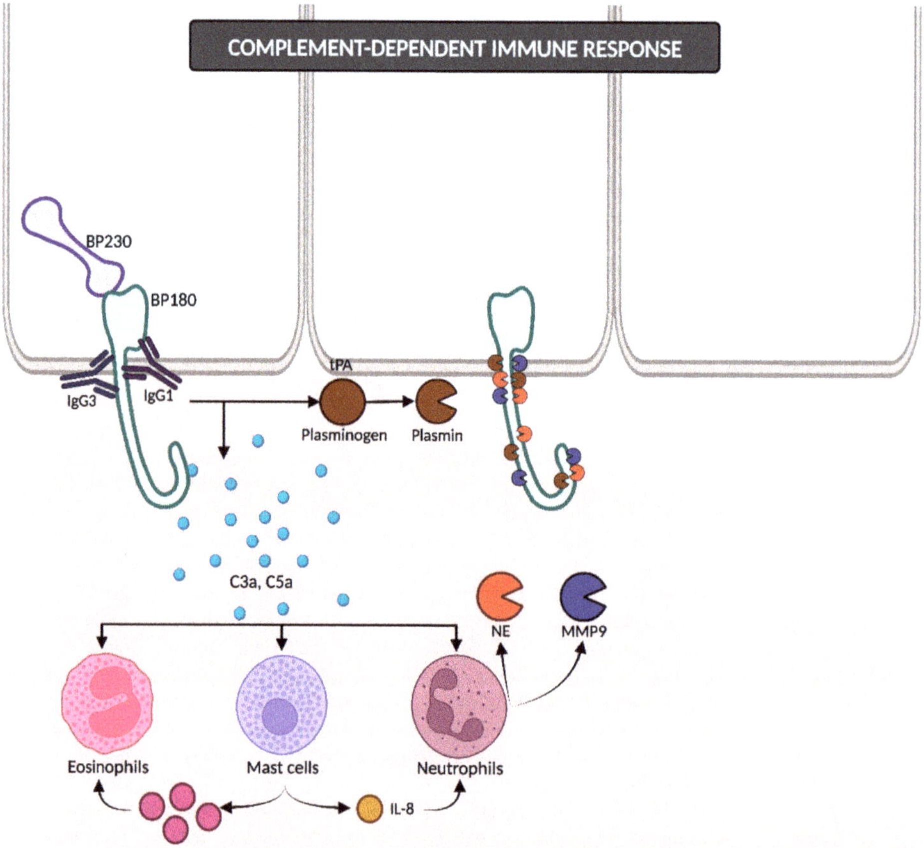

Figure 3. Complement-dependent immune response. IgG1 and IgG3 antibodies bind to BP180 and initiate the complement cascade, leading to eosinophils, mast cells and neutrophils' recruitment and subsequent degranulation. IgG binding on keratinocytes may also trigger tPA release, converting plasminogen into plasmin. Plasmin, along with NE and MMP9, promotes dermal–epidermal cleavage. tPA: tissue-type plasminogen activator; NE: neutrophil elastase; MMP9: matrix metalloproteinase 9.

2.2.2. Complement-Independent Immune Response

The binding of autoantibodies to BP180 in hemidesmosomes results in the internalization of BP180 into basal keratinocytes (Figure 4) [35], so the adhesive strength of the dermoepidermal junction decreases. This appears to be an early event in disease pathogenesis, followed by an inflammatory response that finally causes dermoepidermal separation [26,36]. BP180 internalization occurs through the micropinocytosis pathway [36]. Afterwards, it remains unclear whether they are degraded in lysosomes (as macropinosomes usually do) or if it is mediated by ubiquitylation and proteasomal degradation [14].

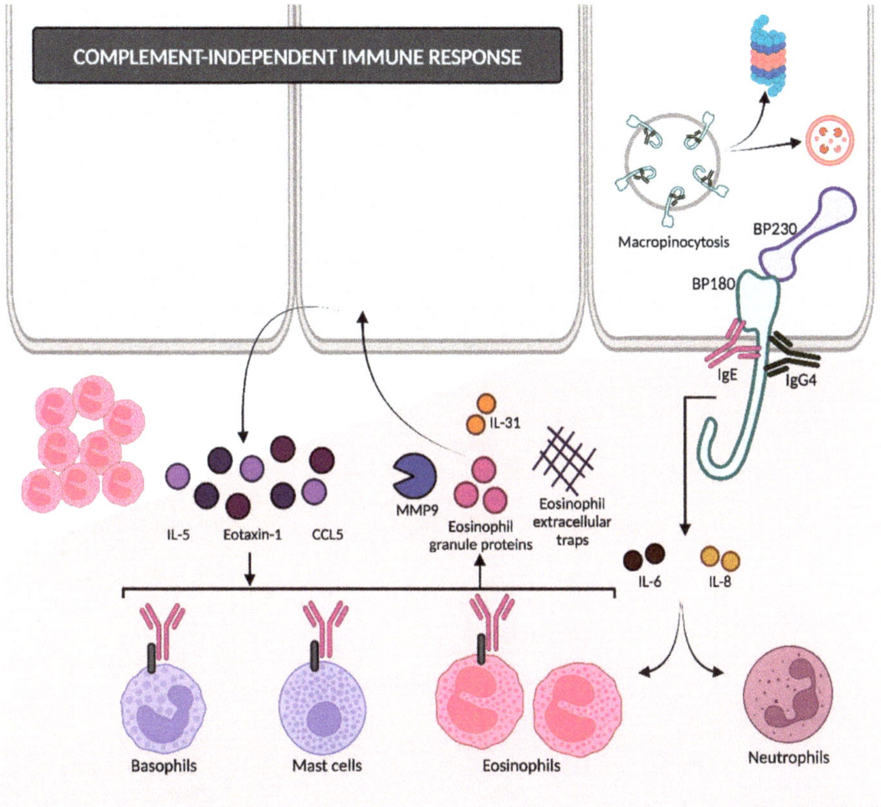

Figure 4. Complement-independent immune response. IgG4 and IgE are involved in BP pathogenesis through complement-independent mechanisms. Autoantibody binding to BP180 results in its internalization through the micropinocytosis pathway. The interaction between BP180 and autoantibodies triggers the release of several cytokines, ultimately attracting eosinophils and proteases that contribute to dermal–epidermal separation. MMP9: matrix metalloproteinase 9; CCL5: chemokine ligand 5.

Following the interaction between anti-BP180 antibodies and BP180 ectodomain, keratinocytes release proinflammatory cytokines such as IL-6 and IL-8 [37], possibly mediated by the upregulation of NF-kappa beta and STAT3 [38]. These cytokines and chemokines attract eosinophils and neutrophils, responsible for the inflammatory reaction [39].

IgG4 has a very limited ability to fix complements and has been reported by some studies as the predominant subclass of autoantibodies in BP, followed by IgG1 and IgG3 [40,41]. The dominance of IgG4 is more evident in the early stages of BP, suggesting that IgG4 may play a pathogenic role primarily in the initiation of the immune response [41].

The balance between the contributions of complement-dependent IgG1 and complement-independent IgG4 might explain the clinical diversity that we can find in BP. Certain authors support that C3-positive pemphigoids in DIF are mediated by IgG1/IgG3 and IgG4, and they would present as the classic BP with urticarial rash and worse clinical severity. On the other hand, C3-negative pemphigoids are IgG4-dominant and tend to have a non-inflammatory phenotype with milder severity [39].

Another immunoglobulin with little ability to activate complements is IgE, which is increasingly being linked to the pathogenesis of BP. Anti-BP180 IgE autoantibodies are detected in the majority of BP sera and are correlated with disease activity [42,43]. BP180–IgE complexes adhere to the keratinocyte basement membrane and bind with the FcεR1 receptors present on eosinophils, mast cells and basophils. This interaction triggers the release of proteases such as MMP9, eosinophil granule proteins and eosinophil extracellular traps. MMP9 degrades BP180, thereby contributing to dermal–epidermal separation. Eosinophils also secrete interleukin 31, which is directly related to pruritus in BP. In response to eosinophil granule proteins, keratinocytes release cytokines such as IL-5, eotaxin-1 and chemokine ligand 5 (CCL5). This cyclical process amplifies tissue eosinophilia and promotes eosinophilic spongiosis [26,27,44]. These facts support the relevance of complement-independent Th2-mediated pathways in the pathogenesis of BP.

Hence, it is plausible that both complement-dependent and independent mechanisms play a collaborative role in triggering and perpetuating bullous pemphigoid [45].

2.3. Breakdown of Self-Tolerance

The fundamental initial process in the development of bullous pemphigoid is the generation of autoantibodies targeting hemidesmosomal proteins. FoxP3+ regulatory T cells (FoxP3+ Treg) represent the pivotal cell population for self-tolerance maintenance, since they are responsible for suppressing excessive autoantibody production [16]. However, the scientific literature exhibits contradictory results in this regard. Some authors have documented decreased FoxP3+ Treg cells among BP patients [46,47], whereas other authors have identified a substantial increase [48]. These differences may stem from a selection bias associated with Treg markers. Specifically, Muramatsu et al. reported that total Treg cells are increased in classic BP patients before treatment, possibly secondary to the inflammatory background, but significantly decrease after corticosteroid treatment. This finding can be attributed to the inhibition of IL-2 by corticosteroids, which is required for the maintenance of Treg cells. Alternatively, corticosteroid treatment might suppress autoreactive T cells and therefore effector Treg cells would consequently decrease as they are no longer needed [49].

Nevertheless, the dysfunction of Treg cells has been identified in BP [50]. This malfunction can result in the suppression of self-tolerance and subsequently the formation of autoreactive T helper 2 (Th2) lymphocytes mediated by STAT6. Autoreactive Th2 cells are able to activate and sensitize B cells and generate antibodies against self-components [16].

2.4. Epitope Spreading

Epitope spreading (ES) is a phenomenon in which the immune responses of T and/or B cells extend from the original dominant epitope to other secondary epitopes as time progresses. These new epitopes may be located on the same autoantigen (intramolecular epitope spreading) or on different antigens within the same anatomical site [51].

It is widely recognized that ES is a frequent event in the development of BP. In vivo studies using murine models have demonstrated that IgG antibodies targeting BP180 initially react to epitopes situated within the ectodomain and, subsequently, they react to other extracellular and intracellular domains over time (Figure 5) [52,53]. However, this immunological reaction is not solely confined to antigens localized within BP180; rather, it progressively spreads over time to other molecules, including BP230 [53]. Furthermore, in a prospective multicenter study, ES was observed in 49% of patients following a 1-year observational period. These events exhibited a distinct propensity to occur during the early stages of the disease [54]. All these findings suggest that NC16A recognition in the BP180 ectodomain is an early event, succeeded by intra- and intermolecular ES events. These sequential occurrences collaboratively mold the individual course of each patient with BP [51].

The concept of epitope spreading has been suggested as an explanation for those cases in which BP develops in the setting of other diseases [53]. For example, the basement membrane zone disruption in oral lichen planus might expose hemidesmosome proteins and then trigger the autoimmune humoral response responsible for lichen planus pemphigoides [55]. BP may also develop after radiation therapy, possibly through the exposure of BMZ antigens during the course of the treatment [56]. Finally, ES from brain BP180 due to neurologic damage has also been proposed to partially explain the relationship between BP and certain neurocognitive diseases [57]. Although BP180 is diffusely expressed within the central nervous system, a recent study has revealed that it is not expressed in the hippocampus, which is the main area affected in neurocognitive disorders [23]. This underscores the need for future research to elucidate the intricate connection between neurological disorders and BP.

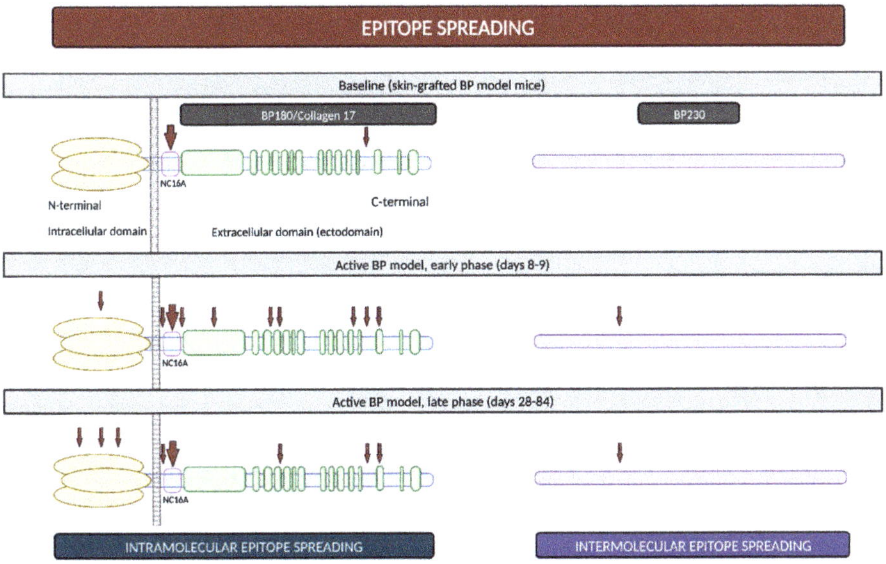

Figure 5. Epitope spreading. Epitope spreading in murine models according to the research conducted by Ujiie et al. Figure adapted from Ujiie et al. (2019) [53].

3. General Aspects of Drug-Associated Bullous Pemphigoid (DABP)

3.1. Drugs Related to DABP

The first case of drug-associated bullous pemphigoid (DABP) was reported in an 11-year-old patient receiving treatment with salicylazosulphapyridine [58]. Subsequently, a wide range of drugs have been linked to the pathogenesis of this disease.

According to the Naranjo Adverse Reaction Probability Scale [59] and the Karch–Lasagna algorithm [60], most bullous pemphigoid cases could be categorized as having a "probable" association with a drug regarding the temporal relationship, the available literature and the absence of alternative causes. However, while these scales are useful in assessing general drug reactions, their significance appears diminished when applied to the identification of potential triggers in drug-associated bullous pemphigoid. In contrast, Tan et al. proposed specific criteria to consider a drug as a potential trigger for BP. These criteria include the drug's initiation within the preceding year, a treatment duration of more than 2 weeks and drug continuation until at least 1 month before the diagnosis of BP [61].

Medications most frequently linked to BP include dipeptidyl peptidase 4 inhibitors (DPP4i), diuretics, neuroleptics, antibiotics, monoclonal antibodies against anti-tumor necrosis factor (TNF)-α, immune checkpoint inhibitors targeting programmed cell death protein 1 (PD-1) and its ligand (PD-L1), non-steroidal anti-inflammatory drugs (NSAID) and antihypertensive drugs. However, the list is exponentially growing (Table 1). BP has even been reported to develop after the application of certain topical drugs, inducing some form of "contact pemphigoid" [62]. However, the potential of topical agents to trigger BP remains controversial, as direct associations are not well established in most cases [63].

Table 1. List of drugs that have been linked to bullous pemphigoid development according to the scientific literature. Adapted from Verheyden et al. [4].

Drugs Associated with Bullous Pemphigoid Development			
Dipeptidyl peptidase 4 inhibitors	**Diuretics**	**Immune checkpoint inhibitors**	**Biologic agents**
Alogliptin Anagliptin Linagliptin Saxagliptin Sitagliptin Teneligliptin Vildagliptin	Acetazolamide Bumetanide Furosemide Hydrochlorothiazide Spironolactone Torsemide	Atezolizumab Cemiplimab Durvalumab Ipilimumab Nivolumab Pembrolizumab	Adalimumab Efalizumab Etanercept Guselkumab Infliximab Secukinumab Ustekinumab
Cardiovascular drugs	**Neurological drugs**	**Antimicrobial agents**	**Anti-inflammatory drugs and salicylates**
Amiodarone Amlodipine Atenolol Captopril Enalapril Lisinopril Losartan Nadolol Nifedipine Practolol Rosuvastatin Valsartan	Amantadine Doxepin Escitalopram Fluoxetin Flupenthixol Gabapentin Galantamine Levetiracetam Risperidone Teriflunomide	Actinomycin Amoxicilin Ampicilin Cephalexin Ciprofloxacin Chloroquine Dactinomycin Griseofulvin Levofloxacin Metronidazole Penicillin Rifampicin Sulfonamide Terbinafine	Aspirin Azapropazone Celecoxib Ibuprofen Mefenamic acid Mesalazine Metamizole Phenacetin Sulfasalazine Salicylazosulphapyridine
Other drugs		**Topical drugs**	
Aldesleukin Arsenic D-Penicillamine Dabrafenib Enoxaparin Erlotinib Everolimus Omeprazole	Palbociclib Potassium iodide Psoralens with ultraviolet A (PUVA) Serratiopeptidase Sirolimus Tiobutarit	5-Fluorouracil Anthralin Benzyl benzoate Coal tar Diclofenac Dorzolamide Iodophor adhesive band Timolol	

Verheyden et al. conducted a systematic review of drug-associated bullous pemphigoid and consequently developed a diagrammatic summary of the strength of supporting evidence for each drug. Within this framework, the evidence was stronger for DPP4i, followed by immune checkpoint inhibitors PD-1/PD-L1, loop diuretics, penicillins, NSAIDs, thiazides and psoralens with ultraviolet A phototherapy [4]. Additionally, Liu et al. recently published a meta-analysis of case–control studies, in which they found a significant association between BP and the prior use of DPP4i (odds ratio [OR] 1.92), aldosterone antagonists (OR 1.75), anticholinergics (OR 3.12) and dopaminergic medications (OR 2.03) [64].

Nonetheless, the majority of these associations are predominantly drawn from case reports, relying on factors such as temporal correlation or similarity to previously reported cases. As a result, the levels of evidence for most of the suspected medications are low due to the absence of controlled studies [64]. Furthermore, these clinical associations are subject to various confounding elements, including the prevalent polypharmacy among elderly individuals and the common use of over-the-counter drugs that are seldom reported to healthcare professionals. Unfortunately, ethical and safety concerns make it infeasible to rechallenge patients in order to definitively confirm the presumed link between BP and drug exposure [4,63].

As ongoing research continues to unravel the pathogenesis and natural history of DABP, clinicians should be aware of this association in order to identify and treat potential cases of DABP early on [4,63]. Drug discontinuation in DABP might lead to a reduction in the need for immunosuppression and a better prognosis when compared to missed DABP [65].

3.2. Pathogenic Mechanisms

Increasing interest is being directed towards the research of DABP pathogenesis, yet a precise understanding of the underlying mechanisms is still lacking. Drugs are thought to act as triggering factors in patients with an underlying genetic susceptibility. Various studies have suggested a potential correlation between DABP and specific major histocompatibility complex (MHC) class II alleles, since they could facilitate the presentation of BMZ autoantigens to T cells [4,7].

It has been hypothesized that the pathogenesis of DABP might be explained by the interaction of several mechanisms (Figure 6).

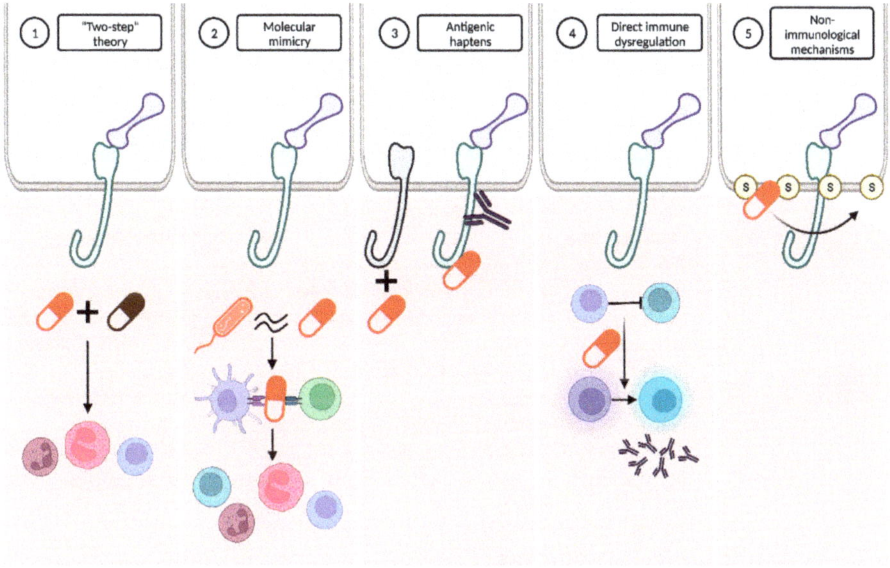

Figure 6. Proposed mechanisms to explain drug-associated bullous pemphigoid pathogenesis. (1) The "two-step" theory proposes that the interaction between two drugs may be necessary to initiate and amplify the immune response. (2) The molecular mimicry hypothesis suggests that the molecular similarity between certain drugs and microorganisms could trigger an immune response against the drugs. (3) Other drugs may act as antigenic haptens, modifying the antigenic properties of specific proteins. (4) Certain drugs may directly induce immune dysregulation. (5) Non-immunological mechanisms, involving interaction with sulfhydryl groups present in the dermoepidermal junction, are also plausible.

- "Two-step" theory: the interplay between two drugs with analogous molecular structures and their interaction with the immune system might represent the first and second "hits" required to initiate and amplify the immune response [4,7,63].
- Molecular mimicry: many drugs bind to RNA and proteins in a way that closely resembles the interaction pattern observed with viruses. This similarity raises the possibility that these drugs might be erroneously recognized as microbial antigens. The

immune system's misidentification of drugs in predisposed individuals could result in the activation of CD4+ T cells and the subsequent initiation of the autoimmune cascade [7,63].

- Antigenic haptens: some drugs may have the ability to function as antigenic haptens that can bind to and modify protein molecules within the lamina lucida of the BMZ. Such interactions might induce the modification of their antigenic properties, thereby acting as neoantigens. Alternatively, this phenomenon could lead to the exposure of a previously hidden antigenic site, supporting the drug-triggering epitope spreading theory [4,7,63,66].
- Direct immune dysregulation: drugs may cause immune reorganization, disrupting the endogenous regulatory processes that prevent the development of several diseases. Alterations in T-regulatory cell functions may suppress "forbidden" B cell clones and then result in the release of autoantibodies against the BMZ [63,66].
- Non-immunological mechanisms: thiol-containing drugs may directly interact with the sulfhydryl groups present in the BMZ proteins and subsequently disrupt the dermoepidermal junction without the involvement of immunological mechanisms. However, this dermoepidermal cleavage may also expose new, hidden antigenic sites [7,63].

Furthermore, Verheyden et al. [4] recently proposed that drugs related to BP may be categorized according to their chemical structure as thiol-based, phenol-based and non-thiol non-phenol-based drugs.

- Thiol-based drugs: they might induce BP acting as haptens or directly disrupting the dermoepidermal junction, as previously described. Moreover, penicillamine, a specific thiol-based drug, could decrease the activity of T-regulatory cells [62]. Many drugs, such as furosemide, hydrochlorothiazide, spironolactone, penicillins or sulfasalazine, contain sulfur atoms within their molecules, yet not as part of a thiol group. However, it is hypothesized that they may be able to form thiol groups during their metabolism, thereby inducing BP through a similar mechanism to thiol-based drugs [67].
- Phenol-based drugs: these medications incorporate a phenyl group in their molecular structure and are thought to interfere with the integrity of the BMZ, consequently revealing hidden epitopes. Examples of these phenol drugs are non-steroidal anti-inflammatory drugs (NSAID), cephalosporins, angiotensin II receptor blockers (ARB) and selective serotonin reuptake inhibitors (SSRI).
- Non-thiol non-phenol-based drugs: the number of these drugs is continuously growing, although the precise underlying mechanisms remain largely undefined.

3.3. General Differences between DABP and Idiopathic BP

3.3.1. Clinical Differences

Patients diagnosed with DABP are often younger than those affected by the idiopathic form [4,63]. In contrast to classic BP, the clinical manifestations of DABP may be more heterogenous, resembling other conditions like erythema multiforme or pemphigus, which often delays the diagnosis [4,68]. Lesions typically manifest as tense bullae on seemingly normal skin or, more infrequently, on an erythematous or urticarial base [63].

The natural course of DABP remains somewhat uncertain, although there have been recognized two variants based on their clinical history. The first is an acute, self-limited form characterized by definitive resolution upon discontinuation of the suspected drug. This form can be genuinely categorized as a drug reaction (true drug-induced bullous pemphigoid). Conversely, the second form presents a chronic and severe course, similar to classic bullous pemphigoid. It can persist even after the suspected drug is withdrawn and may require a prolonged treatment (drug-triggered bullous pemphigoid) [66].

3.3.2. Histological and Laboratory Differences

Despite all the extensive research conducted in bullous pemphigoid, no specific antigens for DABP have been identified. Therefore, it is believed that the autoantigens involved might align with those identified in idiopathic BP. Direct and indirect immunofluorescence typically exhibit similar patterns to those of idiopathic BP [4,63].

The typical histological findings in DABP encompass the presence of intraepidermal vesicles, necrotic keratinocytes and a prominent eosinophilic infiltrate, with occasional thrombus formation. However, idiopathic BP typically lacks intraepidermal vesicles, necrotic keratinocytes and thrombi, and the eosinophilic infiltrate is usually milder. Marked eosinophilia in serum is frequently observed in DABP cases [4,63].

4. Dipeptidyl Peptidase 4 Inhibitor-Associated Bullous Pemphigoid (DPP4i-BP)

Dipeptidyl peptidase 4 inhibitors (DPP4i), also known as gliptins, constitute a class of incretin-based drugs indicated for the treatment of type 2 diabetes mellitus. DPP4i suppress the enzyme dipeptidyl peptidase 4 (DPP4), which is responsible for the degradation of the incretin hormone glucagon-like peptide-1 (GLP-1). This inhibition results in the secretion of insulin and the reduction of glucagon [69]. Their favorable safety profile, even in patients with progressive renal insufficiency, the low risk of hypoglycemia and their oral administration have led to the frequent use of these agents among elderly patients [70]. Despite their good tolerability profile, in the last few years, they have been increasingly associated with the development of bullous pemphigoid.

4.1. *Epidemiology of DPP4i-BP*

4.1.1. General Risk of BP Development

The correlation between gliptin treatment and the development of BP initially emerged from anecdotal case reports. Subsequently, these associations underwent thorough examination through the analysis of two national pharmacovigilance databases [71,72], in addition to numerous observational controlled studies [73–78].

In a systematic review and meta-analysis published in 2018, the odds ratio for BP among patients receiving any DPP4i ranged from 1.27 to 3.45, with a pooled OR of 3.16 (95% CI 2.57–3.89; I2 = 36.09%; $p = 0.196$), so it can be concluded that gliptin intake might be associated with a threefold increased risk of developing BP [76]. However, this OR might have been overestimated, as some subsequent, large, nationwide case–control studies have reported milder associations following multivariant analysis (adjusted OR 1.58 [78]–1.86 [79], both statistically significant).

Notably, Kawaguchi et al. retrospectively analyzed the number of patients who had been first prescribed a DPP4i and all BP newly diagnosed cases at their medical facility for a study period of four years. They reported an incidence rate of BP among all patients taking DPP4i of 0.0859%. When stratified by specific DPP4i, BP was more incident in patients taking vildagliptin (0.292%), followed by linagliptin (0.076%), sitagliptin (0.059%) and alogliptin (0.052%) [75].

4.1.2. Risk of BP Development in Patients with Diabetes Mellitus in Absence of DPP4i

Even in the absence of DPP4i use, diabetes mellitus is found to be associated with bullous pemphigoid, exhibiting twofold higher incidence compared to the general population. The linkage between BP and diabetes might be attributed to the generation of autoantibodies due to the augmented skin fragility in diabetic patients, or as a consequence of the nonenzymatic glycosylation of dermal proteins [80].

Finnish nationwide studies have shown that the use of no other antidiabetic drugs, including metformin [73], thiazolidinediones, sulfonylureas and repaglinide [81], was associated with an increased risk of BP. This implies that, in BP cases diagnosed during metformin–DPP4i combination therapy, metformin treatment can be safely continued, while careful consideration should be given to the withdrawal of the gliptin component [73]. However, as these studies were conducted in 2018, new-generation diabetic medications were being taken by very few patients. In more recent studies, a possible association has been reported with previous exposure to a sodium glucose cotransporter 2 inhibitor and glucagon-like peptide 1 receptor agonist, suggesting the need for further large-scale epidemiological studies in the future [82,83].

4.1.3. Risk of BP Development in Patients with Diabetes Mellitus in Absence of DPP4i

Vildagliptin stands as the main DPP4i agent implicated in the development of BP across several studies that have included a subgroup analysis [71,72,76,78,79,84]. In a meta-analysis conducted by Kridin et al., the use of vildagliptin was reported to be associated with a ten-fold increased risk of BP, with a pooled OR of 10.16 (95% CI, 6.74–15.33; I2 = 0%; $p = 0.702$) [76]. In a more recent population-based, nested case–control study, also conducted by Kridin et al., vildagliptin again exhibited the strongest association, albeit with reduced odds (OR 3.40; 95% CI, 2.69–4.29; $p < 0.001$) [79]. Notably, vildagliptin displays relatively lower selectivity for the DPP4 enzyme when compared to other family members like DPP-8 and DPP-9 [85], which are recognized to retain procaspase-1. Consequently, it has been hypothesized that the off-target inhibition of DPP-8 and DPP-9 might trigger the activation of the inflammasome–caspase-1 pathway, potentially contributing to the pathogenesis of BP [78].

The sub-analysis of other individual DPP4i also revealed a significant association with BP development, suggesting the presence of a class effect [72]. Nevertheless, there exists greater variability in the results across them, ranging from some studies reporting a six-fold rise in the probability of BP with linagliptin [76] to others demonstrating a significant association with sitagliptin exposure [78,79].

The larger sample size offered by a retrospective population-based study conducted in Japan enabled a more comprehensive evaluation of the risk linked to each individual DPP4i. According to their findings, all daily DPP4i (alogliptin, anagliptin, linagliptin, saxagliptin, sitagliptin, teneligliptin and vildagliptin), as well as the available weekly DPP4i (omarigliptin and trelagliptin), exhibited a significant association with the risk of developing BP. Interestingly, both categories displayed roughly similar levels of risk [77].

4.1.4. Latency Period

Most studies agree on the long latency period that typically elapses between DPP4i initiation and the onset of BP. In the majority of these studies, the median latency time was approximately 6 to 8 months, ranging from as short as 10 days to more than 3 years [71–75]. However, a recent duration–response analysis conducted by Kridin et al. revealed that the highest probability of BP onset occurred 1–2 years following DPP4i initiation, with a median latency of 3.3 years and a continuous, statistically significant risk for BP development extending beyond 6 years from the beginning of the treatment [79]. The delayed onset of BP suggests that additional factors besides the drug itself are required to break the tolerance to BP180 and to trigger the autoimmune response.

Nevertheless, Kuwata et al. recently reported that the risk associated with DPP-4i use was restricted to a span of 3 months following the first use. The risk of developing BP was most pronounced within the initial 30 days after the first administration, with a gradual decline until no risk was observed after 90 days. They hypothesized that BP cases that develop within 3 months of initiating DPP4i might involve different pathogenic mechanisms compared to cases that emerge later [77].

4.2. Pathogenesis of DPP4i-BP

4.2.1. Genetic Predisposition

Ujiie et al. reported that 86% of their non-inflammatory DPP4i-BP Japanese patient cohort exhibited the HLA-DQB1*03:01 haplotype, compared to DPP4i-treated healthy controls, where this allele was found in only 31% of them [86]. Interestingly, this allele is also known to be associated with mucous membrane pemphigoid in Caucasian patients [87]. In a study conducted by Lindgren et al. in Finland, it was concluded that the HLA-DQB1*03:01 allele was more commonly present among BP patients when compared to the control population. However, this study failed to find significant differences in HLA haplotypes between DPP4i-associated and non-DPP4i-associated bullous pemphigoid cases [88].

4.2.2. DPP4 Functions

DPP4, also known as CD26, is widely expressed in various tissues, including keratinocytes and immune T CD4+ cells (Figure 7). It is therefore reasonable to hypothesize that the inhibition of CD26 on T cells could potentially dysregulate the immune system. CD26 expression is known to be increased in various immunomediated diseases, such as psoriasis and atopic dermatitis [89] Recently, it has been reported that the cutaneous expression of CD26 is also upregulated in BP patients, regardless of their previous gliptin exposure [88].

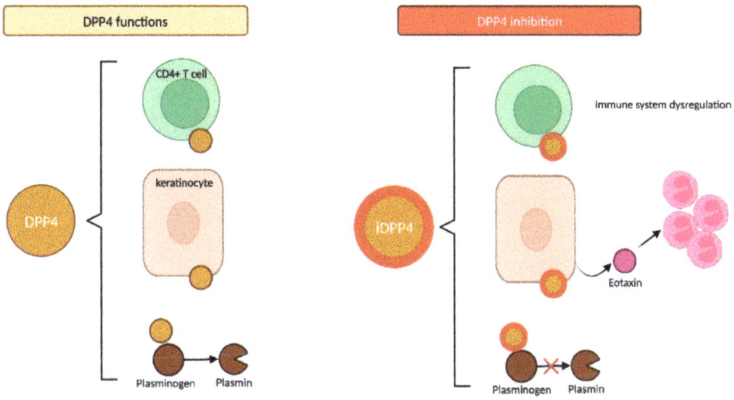

Figure 7. Schematic representation of DPP4 functions and, conversely, results following its inhibition. DPP4 is expressed in many tissues, such as CD4+ T cells and keratinocytes, and acts as a surface cell plasminogen that converts plasminogen into plasmin. As a result, DPP4 inhibition by gliptins may cause immune dysregulation, the release of eotaxin and other inflammatory mediators and the plasmin-independent cleavage of BP180.

The inhibition of DPP4 in keratinocytes may release eotaxin (CCL11) and other proinflammatory cytokines that promote dermal eosinophil recruitment, which is a common histopathologic feature of BP cases [90]. Conversely, Japanese studies have demonstrated that periblister eosinophil infiltration appears to be significantly lower in non-inflammatory DPP4i-BP than in inflammatory DPP4i-BP [18,86].

Furthermore, DPP4 acts as a surface cell plasminogen receptor that converts plasminogen into plasmin (Figure 7) [91]. Plasmin is a serine protease that can be detected in BP blister fluid that, in conjunction with other proteases, cleaves the BP180 molecule within the juxtamembranous NC16A domain. This initial N-terminal cleavage results in the production of the LAD-1 fragment (120 kDa), potentially followed by a further C-terminal deletion that would produce the LABD97 fragment (97 kDa) (Figure 8) [92,93]. Consequently, the inhibition of plasmin activation by gliptins may lead to the inappropriate plasmin-independent cleavage of BP180, resulting in the generation of neoepitopes along different domains [18].

4.2.3. DPP4i-BP Autoantibodies and Epitope Spreading

Izumi et al. first identified a subtype of BP patients characterized by the presence of anti-BP180 full-length (BP180fl) autoantibodies without anti-BP180 NC16A autoantibodies. This subtype exhibited a non-inflammatory phenotype with less pronounced eosinophilic infiltration. Additionally, these patients were more likely to have been treated with DPP4i before BP onset [18].

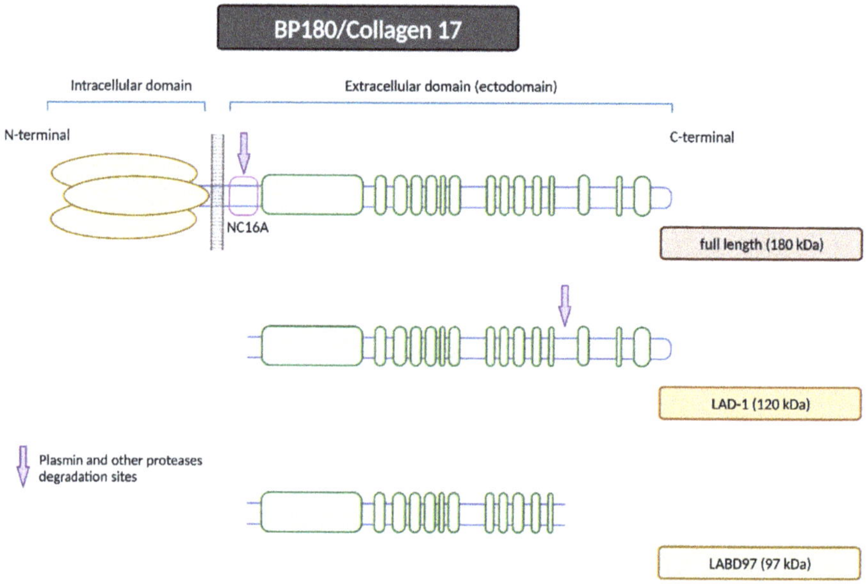

Figure 8. Plasmin and other proteases degrade the BP180 molecule within the juxtamembranous NC16A domain. The initial N-terminal cleavage results in the production of the LAD-1 fragment (120 kDa), which can be followed by a further C-terminal deletion that would result in the LABD97 fragment (97 kDa). Adapted from Mai et al. (2019) [92].

Subsequent studies further describe the immunological profile of gliptin-associated bullous pemphigoid. All DPP4i-BP patients included in most studies present positive anti-BP180fl, whereas the positivity rate of anti-BP180 NC16A is notably lower (29–58%) [94–96]. A significant percentage of patients (79–86%) also present IgG reactivity against the LAD-1 domain, situated in the mid-portion of the extracellular domain of BP180 [95,96]. In contrast, in a recent case series involving 18 patients, all DPP4i-BP sera showed reactivity against the extracellular domain of BP180, but with a preference for the LABD97 domain over full-length BP180 [92]. Although anti-BP230 autoantibodies are rarely detected in DPP4i-BP, one case has been reported in which the only positive autoantibody was targeted against BP230, while BP180 fl and NC16A were both negative [97]. Moreover, IgE antibodies against BP230 and not BP180 have also been identified in DPP4i-BP patients, while no IgA reactivity was detected against BP180 or BP230 [98]. Finally, a case of DPP4i-BP with autoantibodies against the extracellular domain of $\alpha6\beta4$ integrin, along with anti-BP180 NC16A antibodies, has been reported as well [99].

Although the presence of anti-BP180 NC16A autoantibodies is less common at the clinical onset of DPP4i-BP, several cases have been reported in the literature in which they become positive during the clinical follow-up. Mai et al. reported three cases of non-inflammatory DPP4i-BP with negative anti-BP180 NC16A that later evolved into an inflammatory phenotype, along with the appearance of positive anti-BP180 NC16A antibodies. It is notable that all these three patients had continued with the DPP4i treatment despite the BP diagnosis [100]. Takama et al. described the case of a patient who, even after discontinuing gliptin treatment, developed a positive response to anti-BP180 NC16A autoantibodies months after the diagnosis, coinciding with a clinical relapse [101]. In contrast, García-Díez et al. reported the case of a patient with an inflammatory subtype of DPP4i-BP and negative anti-BP180 NC16A autoantibodies who had discontinued gliptin treatment and was in clinical remission when anti-BP180 NC16A antibodies became positive [96]. These cases support the theory of epitope spreading in the pathogenesis of DPP4i-BP. It has been proposed that the discontinuation of DPP4i may lead to the restored cleavage of BP180 by plasmin within the NC16A domain, exposing the NC16A domain as an epitope for autoantibodies, as occurs in classic BP cases [101].

In classic BP, the initial autoantibody response commonly targets the NC16A domain on BP180. Subsequently, additional autoantibodies may emerge, typically directed towards other domains on BP180 or BP230. Conversely, in DPP4i-BP, the primary autoantibody response is directed against the extracellular domain of BP180, albeit in a distinct domain apart from NC16A, which likely involves the full-length molecule or the LAD-1/LABD97 domains. As a consequence of the phenomenon of epitope spreading, diverse additional autoantibodies may develop, even targeting the NC16A domain, despite the discontinuation of the drug and while the patient is in complete clinical remission (Figure 9) [102,103].

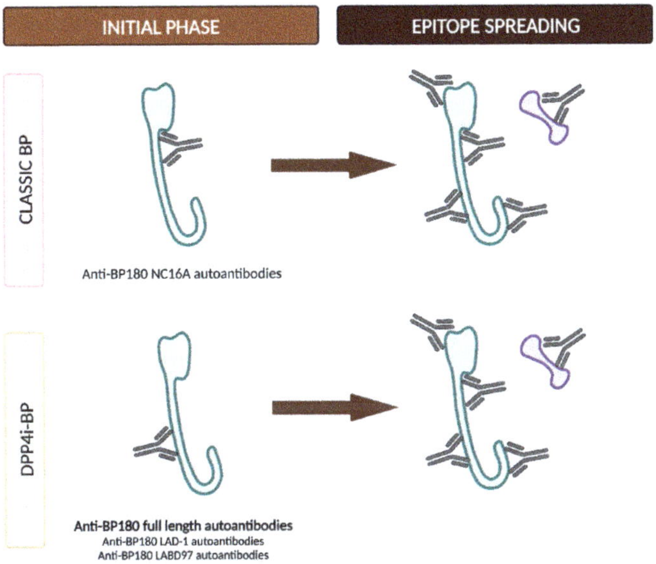

Figure 9. Presumed epitope spreading mechanisms in classic and DPP4i-associated BP.

4.2.4. Currently Described Immune and Pathogenic Mechanisms

While significant advancements have been achieved, the exact pathogenesis underlying the association of DPP4i and BP remains uncertain. However, recent research has demonstrated that DPP4i's inhibition of plasmin reduces the degradation of the NC16A BP180 domain and may trigger the breakdown of immune tolerance [103].

As previously stated, Muramatsu et al. described that total Treg cells and all Treg subsets are increased in classic BP, while, in DPP4i-BP, neither the total Treg cell count nor their subsets seem to be increased. These results suggest that effector Treg cells with suppressive functions may be expanded in response to the inflammation environment seen in active classic BP, as effector Treg cells restrain autoreactive T cells. Then, the authors hypothesized that effector Treg cells in DPP4i-BP may not expand sufficiently in response to the autoreactive T cells due to the influence of DPP-4i intake, leading to the development of bullous lesions even in a mild inflammatory background [49].

It is well known that both IgG1 and IgG4 are the predominant autoantibodies in BP. In a case series of DPP4i-BP patients, all of them presented IgG1 autoantibodies against BP180, in contrast to IgG4-subclass autoantibodies, which were observed in only 38.9% of patients. This finding might be surprising since it is widely recognized that IgG1, and not IgG4, antibodies are able to activate the complement system and consequently initiate the classic inflammatory cascade. The predominance of IgG1 in DPP4i-BP suggests the involvement of the complement system in BP development in these patients, despite their typical association with non- or less inflammatory phenotypes [92].

Interleukin 6 (IL-6) is involved in both the pathogenesis and maintenance of BP [104]. Interestingly, Hung et al. recently reported that vildagliptin can stimulate the expression of IL-6 by keratinocytes in vitro, subsequently increasing its levels through a positive feedback loop. As a result, keratinocytes treated with DPP4i may supply sufficient IL-6 in the skin of DPP4i-BP patients, even if eosinophils and other inflammatory cells are reduced [105].

A recent study has reported that DPP4i drugs such as saxagliptin and sitagliptin promote the migration and epithelial–mesenchymal transition (EMT) of keratinocytes in vitro [106]. In parallel, BP180 is known to be involved in keratinocyte migration [107], so it has been hypothesized that DPP4i might affect keratinocytes in an EMT-dependent manner [108].

In vitro experiments by Nozawa et al. have demonstrated that DPP4 inhibitors upregulate both MMP9 and angiotensin-converting enzyme 2 (ACE2) via the angiotensin 1–7/Mas receptor (MasR) axis, and they postulate that this pathway may play a pivotal role in the development of BP. Lisinopril and MasR inhibitors effectively suppress the DPP4i-induced upregulation of MMP9, suggesting that the modulation of the renin–angiotensin system could stand as a therapeutic approach for DPP4i-BP. This intriguing in vitro finding is sustained by research databases, which indicate that the concomitant use of lisinopril in patients taking DPP4i can significantly reduce the incidence of DPP4i-BP [109].

Despite the progress made in understanding the underlying pathogenic mechanisms of DPP4i-BP, a crucial question remains unresolved: whether mere DPP4i exposure alone can trigger BP or if additional contributing factors are required [103].

4.3. Clinical and Immunological Distinct Features in Classic and DPP4i-Associated BP

Most studies indicate that DPP4i-BP may exhibit a certain male preponderance [71,74,78,79]; nevertheless, this trend is not consistently observed [73,74,110] and it must be noted that, in healthy individuals, gender does not have an impact on the pharmacokinetics of vildagliptin [111]. However, further research is needed to validate any gender-related disparities in BP susceptibility during DPP4i therapy.

Notable differences are mainly observed among studies conducted in Japan, which show distinct features like a non-inflammatory phenotype and atypical epitopes along BP180, as opposed to studies reporting typical features in European patients.

A non-inflammatory phenotype has been defined as those BP cases in which the Bullous Pemphigoid Disease Area Index (BPDAI) for urticaria/erythema activity is less than 10 points [86]. This non-inflammatory phenotype was the prominent DPP4i-BP presentation in Japanese and Chinese studies, with an estimated prevalence of 50–70% among all cases and a significantly lower urticaria/erythema activity BPDAI score [18,86,94,105]. This non-inflammatory predilection was also observed in one European case series [112]. However, this finding was not reproduced in any other study involving Caucasian patients, where the authors failed to find differences in urticaria/erythema activity BPDAI scores between DPP41-BP- and non-DPP4i-associated BP [88,98,110].

In the same vein, Asiatic studies report that DPP4i-BP skin biopsies show a milder eosinophilic dermal infiltrate accompanying the non-inflammatory phenotype [18,94,105,113], while European studies describe similar eosinophil counts in the upper dermis when compared to non-DPP4i-associated BP [88,114]. However, in the context of circulating eosinophils, two Israeli and Hungarian studies reflect the Japanese findings, as they also reported lower eosinophil counts in DPP4i-BP cases [112,115].

Patients with DPP4i-BP may present with a more severe bullous component, according to their significantly higher blister/erosion BPDAI score [105,110] or to the larger body surface area affected [115]. Other studies have also observed a trend towards a more severe disease, albeit lacking statistical significance [94,114]. Furthermore, some authors have reported a higher likelihood of trunk [110,115] and head involvement [115] in DPP4i-BP patients, but these findings have not been consistently observed in other studies. Other reports suggest that mucous membrane involvement may be more common in DPP4i-BP than in patients without prior DPP4i exposure [113,116]. Despite the isolated clinical differences reported in some studies, most European studies have concluded that there are no major clinical differences between DPP4i-BP and non-DPP4i-BP [117,118].

From an immunological perspective, Japanese studies report lower seropositivity of the anti-BP180 NC16A autoantibodies, with preferential reactivity against anti-BP180 full-length instead [86,94,95]. In contrast, European studies have reported similar positivity rates of anti-BP180 NC16A autoantibodies between DPP4i-BP and non-DPP41-BP [88,98,110,118]. However, while the detection rate of anti-BP180 NC16A autoantibodies might be similar, the average titers were significantly lower in the DPP4i-BP group when compared to non-DPP4i-BP cases [110,112].

4.3.1. Effect of DPP4i Withdrawal

The available data regarding the effect of DPP4i withdrawal on the DPP4i-BP course present conflicting results.

A large multicentric, retrospective case–control study conducted by Benzaquen et al. clearly reported that DPP4i discontinuation led to partial or complete clinical remission in 95% of cases, with no further therapy needed to achieve and maintain this remission [74]. Other studies have also reported improved clinical outcomes, with most patients achieving remission after DPP4i withdrawal [72,116,119]. However, it is worth noting that most patients in these studies likewise received the standardized treatment protocol for BP, consisting of high-potency topical corticosteroids, with or without systemic corticosteroids. Since this standard treatment has consistently demonstrated high rates of complete remission in BP cases overall, it could mask the beneficial impact of gliptin withdrawal [8,118].

In contrast, other studies did not find significant differences in the prognosis or clinical response between patients who continued and discontinued DPP4i treatment [112,118]. Plaquevent et al. reported that the time required to achieve disease control (14–15 days) and the rate and timing of relapses were comparable in DPP4i-BP cases irrespective of gliptin discontinuation. Furthermore, they observed no differences in the incidence of relapses whether the DPP4i was stopped within the first month after BP diagnosis or at a later stage [118]. These findings do not support the previously suggested beneficial effect of gliptin withdrawal on the clinical outcomes of patients with BP.

It is currently unclear whether DPP4i-associated BP behaves as a true drug-induced BP, completely resolving upon drug discontinuation, or if it is indeed a drug-triggered or drug-aggravated BP, in which the drug acts as the immune response trigger, subsequently following an independent clinical course despite drug withdrawal. However, the long latency period between DPP4i initiation and BP development in most cases supports the drug-triggered hypothesis rather than the classical drug-induced cutaneous reaction [73].

As this issue continues to be a subject of debate, the most recent BP guidelines recommend, as a precautionary measure, at least considering gliptin withdrawal in patients with DPP4i-BP [8]. Given the potential severity of BP and the wide availability of alternative antidiabetic drugs, the current, safer approach is to replace gliptins with other diabetes medications. Combining gliptins with metformin has also been linked to an increased risk of BP, although such a risk has not been associated with metformin alone [81,116]. Therefore, as previously discussed in this review, in such cases, it is generally safe to continue metformin treatment, while careful consideration should be given to discontinuing the gliptin component [73].

4.3.2. DPP4i-BP Clinical Subtypes

Based on the comprehensive scientific literature reviewed in this study, it is postulated that DPP4i-BP patients could be categorized into two distinct subtypes (Table 2).

Table 2. Suggested clinical and immunological subtypes of DPP4i-associated bullous pemphigoid.

	Drug-Induced BP	Drug-Triggered BP
	Different clinical entity	Similar to classic BP
Clinical phenotype	Non-inflammatory BP	Inflammatory BP
Latency period after DPP4i initiation	Shorter; higher risk in the first 3 months	Longer; even more than 6 years after initiation
Autoantibody profile	Anti-BP180 full length, associated or not with anti-BP180 LAD-1 and LABD97	Anti-BP180 NC16A
Eosinophils in skin biopsies	Decreased	Moderate infiltrate
Eosinophils in serum	Decreased	Augmented
DPP4i withdrawal	Mandatory	Recommendable
Clinical course	Less likely to persist after drug withdrawal	More likely to persist after drug withdrawal

- **Drug-induced BP**. This subtype would represent the true drug-related BP and would appear de novo in patients with no prior genetic predisposition. Patients in this category exhibit distinctive features, including a non-inflammatory phenotype (Figure 10a), negative results for anti-BP180 NC16A autoantibodies and positivity for other epitopes within BP180, such as full-length autoantibodies, LAD-1 and LABD97. Additionally, they often display lower levels of tissue and peripheral eosinophilia. In these patients, discontinuation of DPP4i is considered mandatory to restrain the stimulus for the immune system and to ultimately achieve disease control.

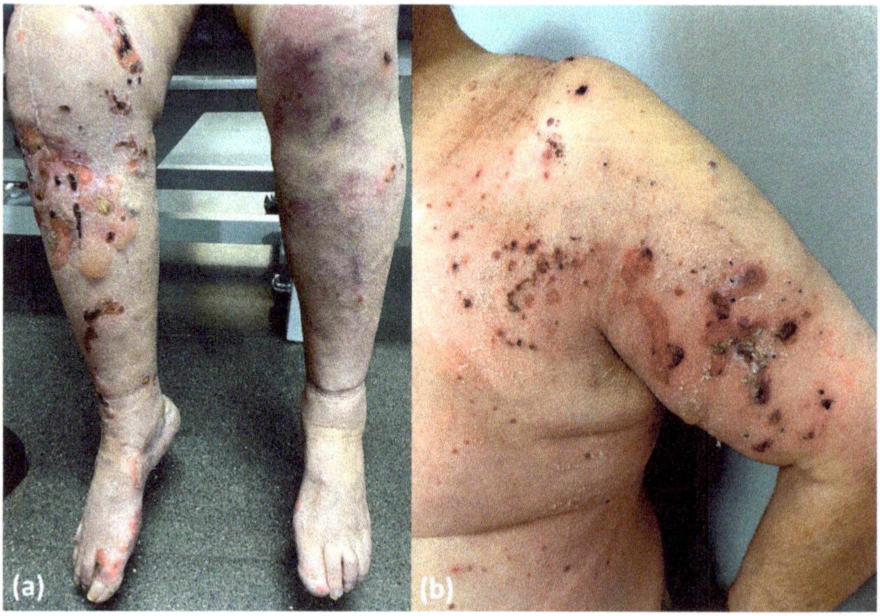

Figure 10. Clinical phenotypes in patients with DPP4i-BP: (**a**) Non-inflammatory phenotype, suggesting a drug-induced BP; (**b**) inflammatory phenotype, suggesting a drug-triggered BP. Commonly presumed epitope spreading mechanisms in classic and DPP4i-associated BP.

- **Drug-triggered BP**. This subtype would occur in patients already predisposed to developing BP, and the initiation of DPP4i treatment would merely precipitate the onset of the bullous disease. These patients typically display the characteristic features observed in classic BP, including an inflammatory phenotype (Figure 10b) and the positivity and high titers of anti-BP180 NC16A autoantibodies, along with higher levels of peripheral and tissue eosinophilia. In this subgroup of patients, discontinuing DPP4i is also advisable to eliminate at least one of the contributing factors to BP etiopathogenesis. However, it is important to note that BP may persist even after discontinuing gliptin treatment.

5. Bullous Pemphigoid Associated with Antineoplastic Drugs

5.1. Immune Checkpoint Inhibitor-Associated Bullous Pemphigoid (ICI-BP)

Immunotherapy with checkpoint inhibitors targeting programmed cell death protein 1 (PD-1), programmed cell death ligand 1 (PD-L1) and cytotoxic T-lymphocyte-associated protein 4 (CTLA-4) has emerged as a highly effective treatment, leading to improved overall survival rates in a growing spectrum of malignancies [120]. Immune checkpoint proteins prevent the immune system from recognizing and eliminating cancer cells. Consequently, the use of immune checkpoint inhibitors (ICI) disrupts the tumoral evasion mechanisms, resulting in the increased activation of the immune system against the tumor [121].

However, this heightened immune activation is non-specific and can affect various organs, leading to so-called immune-related adverse events (irAEs). Cutaneous toxicity is one of the most prevalent irAEs [122], affecting roughly 30% of patients treated with anti-PD-1/PD-L1 and 50% with anti-CTLA-4 [121]. The combination therapy of PD-1/PD-L1+CTLA-4 demonstrates the highest incidence of irAEs, reaching up to 70% [120]. Although maculopapular eruptions are the most common type of cutaneous irAE, immunobullous eruptions are being increasingly reported in the literature. Among these, bullous pemphigoid is the most frequently observed phenotype, although cases of lichen planus pemhigoides, mucous membrane pemphigoid and pemphigus vulgaris have also been documented [121].

5.1.1. Epidemiology of ICI-BP

The incidence of ICI-associated BP (ICI-BP) remains uncertain and varies across different studies, but it is estimated to occur in approximately 0.2 to 1% of patients undergoing treatment with PD-1/PD-L1 or CTLA-4 inhibitors [123–125]. Melanoma is the most frequently observed primary tumor associated with ICI-BP, followed by non-small-cell lung cancer (NSCLC) [121,123]. However, it must be noted that ICI have been approved and used for longer periods in melanoma patients compared to other tumor types, which could introduce potential confounding factors.

BP has been reported under treatment with both PD-1/PD-L1 and CTLA-4 drugs, including pembrolizumab, nivolumab, atezolizumab, durvalumab, cemiplimab, ipilimumab and combination therapies involving ipilumumab plus nivolumab or tremelimumab plus durvalumab. However, it is notably more prevalent in patients receiving anti-PD-1/PD-L1 agents (mainly pembrolizumab and nivolumab) than anti-CTLA-4 [121,123,126,127]. This discrepancy may be attributed to the distinct mode of action of each agent. PD-1 blockade is thought to operate during the effector phase of immune tolerance induction, aiming to restore the activity of quiescent T-regulatory cells. This reactivation in peripheral tissues may stimulate T cell cross-reactivity with self-antigens such as BP180 and BP230. In contrast, anti-CTLA-4 therapy is less likely associated with ICI-BP, possibly due to its preferential mechanism of action during the immune priming phase of tolerance induction, as well as its higher expression in lymphoid tissues compared to peripheral ones [128].

Unlike classic BP, which has a female predominance, ICI-BP is more frequent among male patients, accounting for approximately 71–77% of cases [121,124,129]. It has been reported that male patients with melanoma often display a higher tumor mutational burden and more immunogenic neoantigens, which can account for both the better survival outcomes and the increased susceptibility to irAEs including ICI-BP [130,131]. Similarly to general DABP, ICI-BP usually develops in younger patients compared to classic BP [121,129].

5.1.2. Pathogenesis of ICI-BP

The exact pathogenesis of ICI-BP remains unclear [7]. While immune checkpoint inhibitors primarily target T cells, the central role in the pathogenesis of BP is played by B cells via their autoantibody production [132]. Therefore, it is widely believed that the autoimmune phenomena induced by PD-1/PD-L1 inhibitors involve the dysregulation of both B and T cells [133].

In addition to the BMZ, BP180 has also been identified on the surfaces of malignant melanocytic tumors and NSCLC. Initially, this finding raised suspicion about the potential paraneoplastic nature of BP, but accumulating evidence showing BP resolution after immunotherapy discontinuation and relapse upon rechallenge strongly supports a causal relationship between PD-1/PD-L1 inhibitors and BP [133].

T-Cell-Independent B Cell Activation

Not only T cells but also B cells express PD-1 and PD-L1, suggesting that treatment with anti-PD-1/PD-L1 agents may potentially activate pathogenic B cells independently of T cells (Figure 11) [7].

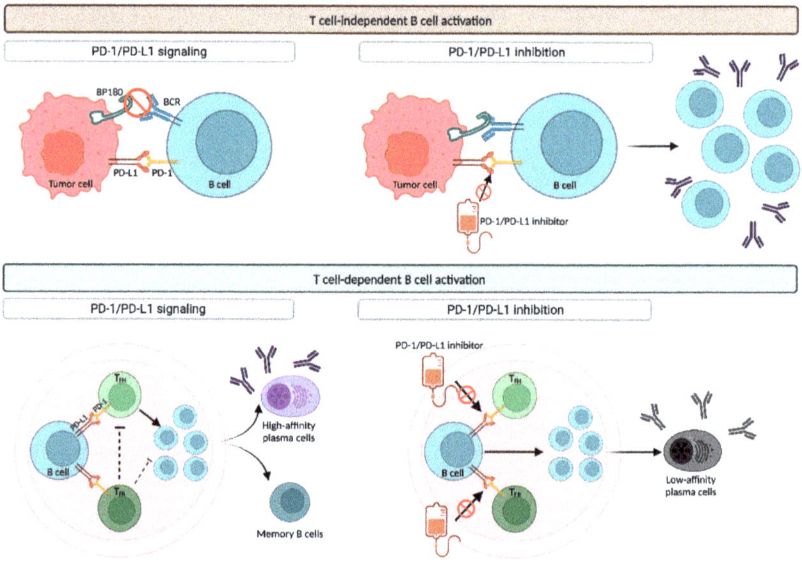

Figure 11. T-cell-independent and T-cell-dependent B cell activation in the pathogenesis of immune checkpoint inhibitor-associated bullous pemphigoid. Adapted from Tsiogka et al. (2021) [133].

The "same-antigen theory" suggests that targeting BP180 on tumor cells can trigger cross-reactivity against the BP180 present in the BMZ [121,133]. The PD-1/PD-L1 signaling pathway inhibits the binding of tumor antigens, including BP180, to their receptors on B cells (BCR), suppressing B cell expansion. Consequently, PD-1/PD-L1 blockade amplifies the BCR response to BP180, resulting in the expansion of B cells and subsequent antibody production, ultimately leading to subepidermal cleavage in the dermoepidermal junction [133].

T-Cell-Dependent B Cell Activation

Another proposed hypothesis to explain ICI-BP is that the blockade of PD-1/PD-L1 may lead to the dysregulation of B-cell-regulatory T cells, consequently promoting antibody production (Figure 11). PD-1/PD-L1 signaling stimulates both T follicular helper (TFH) and T follicular regulatory (TFR) cells within follicular germinal centers. TFH cells are responsible for the selection and survival of B cells, which subsequently differentiate into either high-affinity antibody-producing plasma cells or memory B cells. In contrast, TFR cells inhibit TFH and B cells, thereby controlling undesired T-cell-mediated autoimmune responses. Inhibiting PD-1/PD-L1 negatively impacts both TFH and TFR subpopulations, resulting in the increased production of low-affinity plasma cells. These plasma cells can contribute to antibody-mediated autoimmune phenomena, including BP [133].

Autoantigens and Epitope Spreading

In patients with ICI-BP, anti-BP180 NC16A autoantibodies have been detected more frequently (70–80%) than anti-BP230 autoantibodies (7–29%) [121,129,133]. However, other autoantibodies targeting various epitopes have also been reported, including LAD-1 or C-terminal regions in BP180, desmoglein 1/3 and demoplakin 1/2, while up to 16% of patients exhibit no detectable autoantibodies [133].

Beyond cross-reactivity, the presence of autoantibodies against different epitopes observed in ICI-BP may be attributed to the epitope spreading phenomena, as seen in DPP4i-BP [101]. It has been suggested that autoantibodies may develop as a secondary response to a lichenoid reaction, which is one of the most common cutaneous irAEs. The interface dermatitis in lichenoid reactions may potentially expose antigens at the BMZ, rendering them susceptible to autoantibody development. This could also explain why BP stands out as the most prevalent ICI-induced bullous dermatosis, since hemidesmosomes are more exposed and prone to autoantibody formation following interface damage compared to desmogleins or intracellular molecules [121,133].

5.1.3. Clinical Course and Management of ICI-BP

Unlike many cutaneous irAEs that occur shortly after ICI initiation, BP presents a longer latency period. According to a recent review by Merli et al., ICI-BP may develop after a median period of 26 weeks following the initiation of immunotherapy, ranging from 2 to a maximum of 209 weeks, and, in a small percentage, it can even develop after ICI treatment completion [121,123,129].

ICI-BP usually presents with a prolonged prodromal phase compared to classic BP, which is characterized by persistent pruritus and non-specific dermatitis [121]. Based on the existing literature, the median time between the initiation of ICI therapy and the onset of pruritus or a non-specific cutaneous eruption can be as short as 13–19 weeks. However, the development of bullae as in classic BP is frequently delayed, often occurring within the range of 28–39 weeks [134]. The fact that pruritus is one of the most common cutaneous irAEs makes the early diagnosis of ICI-BP during the pre-blistering phase quite challenging. To achieve this, a high awareness index is necessary, and any pruritic skin eruption that does not respond to topical corticosteroids should prompt consideration for a biopsy [127,135].

In terms of clinical presentation, ICI-BP typically displays a classic inflammatory phenotype, with tense blisters and erosions overlying erythematous plaques, commonly affecting more than 10% of the body surface area. The anatomical distribution of these lesions varies, but they most commonly appear on the trunk and extremities, with mucosal involvement in 17–20% of cases [121,129]. All these findings suggest that ICI-BP shares clinical features similar to classic BP. While most ICI-BP cases show histopathological findings similar to classic BP with eosinophil predominance, some neutrophil-predominant BP cases have also been reported in the literature [136]. No significant differences regarding DIF have been observed between classic and immunotherapy-associated BP [121].

Guidelines provided by oncologists for the management of irAEs recommend that the decision to stop immunotherapy should be based on the severity of BP. Given that the majority of ICI-BP cases can be classified as moderate to severe, a significant proportion of patients reported in the literature had to temporarily or permanently discontinue immunotherapy (58–75%) [123,125,127,129,133]. Notably, unlike traditional DABP, some cases of ICI-BP may develop or persist even after the cessation of immunotherapy, due to the prolonged immune activation associated with PD-1/PD-L1 inhibition or to the continual production of autoantibodies by activated B cells [125,129].

Lopez et al. suggest that immunotherapy could be reinitiated in patients whose BP can be effectively managed without systemic corticosteroids [137]. However, case series have reported relapse rates of approximately 50% following immunotherapy rechallenge, either with the same or alternative checkpoint inhibitors [123,133]. It is important to note that these case series involved only a limited number of patients who underwent rechallenge, making it difficult to draw definitive conclusions regarding the likelihood of recurrence after immunotherapy reinitiation.

Finally, while some retrospective studies have suggested a potential link between the onset of ICI-BP and an improved tumor response [138,139], the heterogeneity of the results and the small number of patients limit their potential applicability. Future prospective studies should be conducted to assess the tumor response in patients with ICI-BP to validate this hypothesis.

5.2. Other Antineoplastic Medications

Other antineoplastic medications have also been associated with the development of BP in single case reports.

- Recombinant interleukin-2 (IL-2). Aldesleukin's potential association with DABP is plausible due to the overexpression of IL-2 and its receptor in BP [140].
- Epidermal growth factor receptor (EGFR) inhibitors. Erlotinib has been associated with BP development in a patient with lung adenocarcinoma, possibly linked to the expression of EGFR in basal keratinocytes [141].
- Mammalian target of rapamycin (mTOR) inhibitors. Three cases of sirolimus- and everolimus-related BP in kidney transplant recipients have been reported in the literature. The pathogenic mechanisms could be attributed to the role of mTOR in the cell cycle or to the imbalance between cell-mediated and humoral immunity induced by mTOR inhibitors. Additionally, it might also be associated with factors related to the renal graft itself [142,143].
- BRAF inhibitors. Dabrafenib might induce a pemphigoid-like reaction with typical clinical and histological features, despite negative DIF [144].
- Cyclin-dependent kinase 4/6 (CDK4/6) inhibitors. BP has recently been linked with novel targeted antineoplastic therapies such as palbociclib, but the underlying pathogenic mechanisms remain unknown [145].

6. Bullous Pemphigoid Associated with Biologic Agents (BIBP)

Several biologic agents used to treat immune-related diseases have been identified as potential triggers of biologic-induced bullous pemphigoid (BIBP). These agents include TNF-α inhibitors like adalimumab, etanercept, efalizumab and infliximab; the anti-IL-12/IL-23 agent ustekinumab; and the anti-IL-17 and -23 inhibitors secukinumab and guselkumab [146,147]. As biologics are being more extensively used in the treatment of a wider range of immune-related disorders, there has been an increasing incidence of BIBP reported in recent years [147].

6.1. Pathogenesis of BIBP

6.1.1. TNF-α Pathway

The pathogenesis of anti-TNF-α BIBP remains unclear, but three hypotheses have been suggested to explain the underlying mechanisms. Firstly, patients undergoing anti-TNF-α therapy may exhibit increased cell apoptosis, exposing novel autoantigens and subsequently triggering autoantibody formation [147]. In addition, anti-TNF-α agents may imbalance the cytotoxic T cell response, relieving the suppression of autoreactive B cells, resulting equally in the increased production of autoantibodies [148]. Lastly, TNF-α inhibitors may act as haptens, binding to and modifying the antigenic properties of BMZ components, which would be more susceptible to an immune attack [63].

Adding further complexity, anti-TNF-α agents have also been described as effective therapies for BP patients, in a somewhat paradoxical phenomenon [147]. This paradoxical phenomenon has been reported also in other immune-mediated dermatological conditions, such as pyoderma gangrenosum [149]. In BP, mast cells release TNF-α alongside various other mediators upon degranulation, which are responsible for recruiting neutrophils and eosinophils to the surrounding tissue [33]. Additionally, TNF-α is found in higher concentrations in BP blister fluid compared to non-inflammatory blisters [150], and its circulating levels have been correlated with the severity and number of lesions in BP patients [151].

Liu et al. studied the impact of TNF-α on eosinophils and described that they can release both Th1 and Th2 chemokines depending on the surrounding microenvironment, particularly influenced by the presence of interferon (INF)-γ or IL-4 [152]. Consequently, it has been proposed that anti-TNF-α agents may have a dual role, as they can either treat or induce Th2-mediated diseases like BP according to the underlying immune profile [147].

6.1.2. IL-17/23 Pathway

The IL-17/23 pathway is activated by several proinflammatory cytokines, including TNF-α. Therefore, IL-17, IL-12/IL-23 or IL-23 inhibitors may present a similar mechanism in the development of BIBP as with TNF-α blockers, which includes dysregulation in the Th1/Th2 immune response and the disinhibition of autoreactive B cells [147]. These findings suggest that the immunological state may shift from Th1 to Th2 dominance, leading to the release of Th2 chemokines like eotaxin, known in the pathogenesis of BP [153]. Notably, all reported cases of BP induced by IL-12/IL-23 or IL-23 inhibitors had a previous history of anti-TNF-α treatment [147] and the only anti-IL-17-related case had been previously treated with ustekinumab [154], thereby increasing the susceptibility to BP.

Conversely, the IL-17/IL-23 axis plays an essential role in the pathogenesis of BP, confirmed by the increased levels of both IL-17 and IL-23 in the sera and blister fluid of BP patients [45]. IL-17 induces neutrophils to release NE and MMP9, which can degrade BP180 and ultimately lead to dermal–epidermal cleavage [155]. This could explain the paradoxical phenomenon wherein there are cases of BP successfully treated by IL-17 and IL-12/IL-23 inhibitors [147].

6.2. Clinical Features of BIBP

The relationship between BP and biologic agents might be controversial due to the higher incidence of BP among psoriatic patients [156]. However, all reported cases of BIBP in patients with psoriasis were assessed as "probable" or "possible" according to the Naranjo scale and Karch–Lasagna algorithm [146].

Classic and biologic-induced BP usually present similar clinical features but, interestingly, BIBP itself may exhibit distinct features depending on the specific biologic agent involved. Husein-Elahmed et al. recently reviewed all BIBP cases in psoriatic patients and found that the mean latency time for BIBP to develop was shorter in individuals treated with anti-TNF-α agents (5 weeks) compared to those receiving ustekinumab (28 weeks). As a result, it is suggested that TNF-α inhibitors may cause a true drug-induced BP with rapid and widespread bullous eruption early in treatment, while IL-12/IL-23 blockers might cause a "drug-triggered BP", characterized by a slower onset and sometimes a refractory course even after drug withdrawal and systemic treatment [146].

7. Bullous Pemphigoid Associated with Other Drugs

7.1. Bullous Pemphigoid Associated with Diuretics

Diuretics are commonly associated with BP development in the scientific literature. Multiple case reports and case–control studies have linked various diuretics with BP, including loop diuretics, thiazides and aldosterone antagonists. These three groups of diuretics contain sulfur groups within their molecular structures, thus suggesting a potential non-immunological mechanism for BP development involving interaction with the sulfhydryl groups present in the basement membrane zone [4]. An additional immunologic mechanism where these drugs act as haptens has also been suggested [157].

- Loop diuretics (furosemide, bumetanide, torsemide). Some case–control and database studies suggest a link between furosemide and DABP development (OR 3.3–3.8) [72,158,159], while other studies do not find this association with loop diuretics [3,64]. Interestingly, furosemide-induced BP may primarily affects sun-exposed areas due to the drug's well-known photosensitivity [160]. In one case report, switching from furosemide to bumetanide resulted in the complete clinical remission of BP [161], although bumetanide itself has also been associated with BP development in some patients [162,163]. Finally, torsemide has been linked to DABP in one case report due to its temporal relationship and structural similarity to furosemide [164].
- Aldosterone antagonists (spironolactone). Similar to furosemide, studies on the association between spironolactone and BP exhibit conflicting results [3,61,78,159]. However, a meta-analysis conducted by Liu et al., which included all previous case–control studies, reported a significant association between the use of aldosterone antagonists and BP, with a pooled OR of 1.75 (95% CI, 1.28–2.40; I2 = 4%) [64].
- Thiazides (hydrochlorothiazide). While some case reports suggest a clinical relationship between hydrochlorothiazide and DABP [157,165], larger case–control studies have not found a significant association [64].
- Acetazolamide. A single case report highlights a patient who experienced a relapse of well-controlled BP lesions one month after initiating acetazolamide. The authors suggest that this diuretic, commonly used in ophthalmology, may have triggered the BP's recurrence due to its structural similarity to other diuretics like furosemide [166].

7.2. Bullous Pemphigoid Associated with Neurological Drugs

Multiple neurological drugs have been linked to BP development according to numerous clinical case reports, although only a limited number of case–control studies have been conducted. These neurological medications encompass neuroleptics (risperidone and flupenthixol), anti-depressants (escitalopram, fluoxetine and doxepin), antiepileptics (levetiracetam), dopaminergic drugs (amantadine) and anticholinergic agents (biperiden), as well as other medications, such as galantamine, gabapentin or teriflunomide [3,4,167,168]. In their meta-analysis, Liu et al. identified a significant association solely with anticholinergic and dopaminergic drugs [64].

Nevertheless, the main challenge when discussing neurological drug-related BP stems from the well-established association between neurologic and psychiatric disorders and the etiopathogenesis of BP itself. Although the studies referenced here employed multivariate analysis to mitigate their impact, the possibility of residual confounding factors persisting should be acknowledged [169]. Consequently, studies that further minimize the influence of concomitant neuropsychiatric disorders and that focus on understanding the responsible pathogenic mechanisms are needed before definitively establishing the risk between BP and the use of neurological drugs.

7.3. Bullous Pemphigoid Associated with Cardiovascular Drugs

Angiotensin-converting enzyme (ACE) inhibitors, angiotensin II receptor blockers (ARB) and calcium channel blockers (CCB) have been associated with the development or exacerbation of BP in several case reports, but these findings have not been consistently supported by larger case–control studies [4].

ACE inhibitors may induce BP through various mechanisms. Firstly, it has been proposed that ACE inhibition could activate the pro-inflammatory kinin system, potentially triggering BP. Secondly, ACE inhibitors might bind to lamina lucida proteins and modify their antigenic properties, acting as haptens [170]. Additionally, certain ACE inhibitors have shown acantholysis properties in vitro, suggesting that the subsequent exposure of BMZ antigens may contribute to BP development [171]. Specifically, captopril contains a thiol group within its molecular structure, so it can directly interact with sulfhydryl groups in the BMZ [172]. These proposed pathogenic mechanisms contrast with in vitro and population-based studies that show the decreased incidence of DPP4i-BP when lisinopril is used concomitantly with DPP4i [109].

DABP has also been reported in association with ARBs such as valsartan and losartan. It is hypothesized that they may induce BP in a similar way to ACE inhibitors through their acantholytic properties [173,174]. Moreover, since they present phenyl groups in their molecules, ARBs might be able to expose hidden epitopes following interaction with the BMZ [4].

Regarding CCB, DABP has been reported during treatment with dihydropyridines such as amlodipine and nifedipine [175,176]. Nifedipine has been demonstrated to induce acantholysis and subepidermal cleavage in skin models in vitro [177].

Finally, some case–control studies have suggested an inverse relationship between the use of lipid-lowering agents and the development of BP, pointing out that statins might have a protective role against BP due to their anti-inflammatory properties [3,178]. However, the prescription of statins is associated with cerebrovascular accidents, which are in turn involved in the etiopathogenesis of BP. Indeed, a larger recent study found no significant association between BP and statin use after adjusting for potential confounding factors [179].

7.4. *Bullous Pemphigoid Associated with Antimicrobial Agents*

Establishing a causal relationship between antimicrobial agents and BP is even more challenging compared to other drugs, since they are not chronically administered and obtaining a complete drug history can be especially difficult when latency periods are prolonged. There is only one case–control study that has reported the significantly higher use of antibiotics in general in BP patients compared to the control population [159], while other studies have failed to find such differences [3,61]. The remaining evidence regarding antibiotics-associated BP is largely based on single case reports, which may reflect casual rather than causal associations.

Several groups of antibiotics have been linked to BP, including penicillins, cephalosporins, quinolones, metronidazole, rifampicin and actinomycin, as well as antifungal agents such as terbinafine and griseofulvin. Penicillins and cephalosporins are sulfur-containing drugs, so they could induce BP through immune dysregulation affecting T-regulatory cells, or through a non-immunological mechanism by directly interacting with sulfhydryl groups in the dermoepidermal junction [4,7,67]. On the other hand, levofloxacin and ciprofloxacin are believed to act as haptens, binding to the proteins in the lamina lucida and modifying their antigenic properties [180,181].

8. Conclusions

Drug-associated bullous pemphigoid has been linked to nearly a hundred medications, with various mechanisms proposed for their potential role, including the two-step theory, molecular mimicry, hapten-like properties, immune dysregulation and direct non-immunologic actions. However, the majority of these associations are primarily based on temporal relationships, which do not necessarily establish causality. Confirming drug reactions through rechallenge is, in most cases, infeasible due to ethic concerns, except for immunotherapy agents, which can be often reintroduced and frequently result in the relapse of the skin lesions.

Larger and stronger evidence is available for gliptin-associated BP, as DPP4i are the most-frequently reported drugs associated with DABP. Consequently, their underlying pathogenic mechanisms have been extensively studied. Two DPP4i-BP phenotypes have been described: the true drug-induced one, with its own distinct features, and the drug-triggered one, resembling classic BP. Although not well defined, several pathogenic mechanisms have been suggested to explain DPP4i's role in BP development, including impaired BP180 cleavage along with immune dysregulation mediated by distinct autoantibody profiles and the involvement of T-regulatory cells.

Immunotherapy-induced BP is gaining relevance due to the paradigm shift in antineoplastic treatment in oncology. While their exact pathogenic mechanisms remain unclear, it is widely believed that BP induced by PD-1/PD-L1 involves both B and T cell dysregulation. Biologic agents including anti-TNF-α and anti-IL17/23 have been described as both triggers and potential treatments for BP, in what appears to be a paradoxical phenomenon. Other medications associated with DABP, although with weaker evidence, include diuretics, antibiotics and neuropsychiatric and cardiovascular drugs (Table 3). In most cases, they are presumed to act as haptens, inducing an immunological response, or to directly disrupt the hemidesmosomal proteins along the dermoepidermal junction.

Table 3. Summary of the drugs that are more and less likely associated with BP development according to the current scientific evidence.

Summary of Drugs Associated with Bullous Pemphigoid Development	
Strongly associated	Anecdotally associated
Dipeptidyl peptidase 4 inhibitors Immune checkpoint inhibitors Biologic agents (anti-TNF-α, anti-IL17/23)	Diuretics Neurological drugs Cardiovascular drugs Antimicrobial agents Anti-inflammatory drugs and salicylates Other drugs (D-Penicillamine, antineoplastic agents, topical drugs)

Future studies investigating genetic predisposition and molecular mechanisms should help us to better understand the clinical course of DABP, identify at-risk individuals and improve their prognosis and quality of life.

9. Future Directions

Future research on drug-associated bullous pemphigoid should depart from uncovering the pathogenic mechanisms that explain why such a diverse range of medications can trigger the same cutaneous disease. DABP presents a compelling etiopathogenesis, as its clinical course differs significantly from what is typically expected from drug reactions. Understanding why drug exposure can modulate the immune system, triggering a persistent immune reaction that remains even after discontinuing the culprit drug, presents a formidable challenge. Additionally, investigating HLA phenotypes and specific gene expression patterns among DABP patients could shed light on whether genetic predisposition plays a leading role in individual susceptibility to BP development following exposure to certain drugs. Finally, larger population-based observational studies are necessary to strengthen the link between DABP and other drugs beyond DPP4i and immunotherapy, as existing studies and reports lack robust evidence on this topic.

Author Contributions: Conceptualization, B.d.N.-R., A.B.-M. and M.F.-G.; methodology, B.d.N.-R. and A.B.-M.; formal analysis, B.d.N.-R. and M.F.-G.; investigation, B.d.N.-R.; resources, B.d.N.-R., E.G.-M. and E.B.-R.; data curation, B.d.N.-R.; writing—original draft preparation, B.d.N.-R., E.G.-M. and E.B.-R.; writing—review and editing, B.d.N.-R., A.B.-M., E.G.-M., E.B.-R., C.A.-L. and M.F.-G.; supervision, M.F.-G. All authors have read and agreed to the published version of the manuscript.

Funding: This research received no external funding.

Institutional Review Board Statement: Not applicable.

Informed Consent Statement: Not applicable.

Data Availability Statement: The data presented in this study are available on request from the corresponding author.

Conflicts of Interest: The authors declare no conflict of interest.

References

1. Montagnon, C.M.; Tolkachjov, S.N.; Murrell, D.F.; Camilleri, M.J.; Lehman, J.S. Subepithelial Autoimmune Blistering Dermatoses: Clinical Features and Diagnosis. *J. Am. Acad. Dermatol.* **2021**, *85*, 1–14. [CrossRef]
2. Aoki, V.; Miyamoto, D. Unfolding the Worldwide Incidence of Bullous Pemphigoid: What Are We Missing? *Br. J. Dermatol.* **2022**, *186*, 386–387. [CrossRef]
3. Bastuji-Garin, S.; Joly, P.; Lemordant, P.; Sparsa, A.; Bedane, C.; Delaporte, E.; Roujeau, J.-C.; Bernard, P.; Guillaume, J.-C.; Ingen-Housz-Oro, S.; et al. Risk Factors for Bullous Pemphigoid in the Elderly: A Prospective Case–Control Study. *J. Investig. Dermatol.* **2011**, *131*, 637–643. [CrossRef] [PubMed]
4. Verheyden, M.; Bilgic, A.; Murrell, D. A Systematic Review of Drug-Induced Pemphigoid. *Acta Derm. Venereol.* **2020**, *100*, 1–9. [CrossRef] [PubMed]
5. Miyamoto, D.; Santi, C.G.; Aoki, V.; Maruta, C.W. Bullous Pemphigoid. *An. Bras. Dermatol.* **2019**, *94*, 133–146. [CrossRef] [PubMed]
6. Langan, S.M.; Smeeth, L.; Hubbard, R.; Fleming, K.M.; Smith, C.J.P.; West, J. Bullous Pemphigoid and Pemphigus Vulgaris—Incidence and Mortality in the UK: Population Based Cohort Study. *BMJ* **2008**, *337*, a180. [CrossRef] [PubMed]
7. Moro, F.; Fania, L.; Sinagra, J.L.M.; Salemme, A.; Di Zenzo, G. Bullous Pemphigoid: Trigger and Predisposing Factors. *Biomolecules* **2020**, *10*, 1432. [CrossRef] [PubMed]
8. Borradori, L.; Van Beek, N.; Feliciani, C.; Tedbirt, B.; Antiga, E.; Bergman, R.; Böckle, B.C.; Caproni, M.; Caux, F.; Chandran, N.S.; et al. Updated S2 K Guidelines for the Management of Bullous Pemphigoid Initiated by the European Academy of Dermatology and Venereology (EADV). *J. Eur. Acad. Dermatol. Venereol.* **2022**, *36*, 1689–1704. [CrossRef] [PubMed]
9. Clapé, A.; Muller, C.; Gatouillat, G.; Le Jan, S.; Barbe, C.; Pham, B.-N.; Antonicelli, F.; Bernard, P. Mucosal Involvement in Bullous Pemphigoid Is Mostly Associated with Disease Severity and to Absence of Anti-BP230 Autoantibody. *Front. Immunol.* **2018**, *9*, 479. [CrossRef]
10. Sárdy, M.; Kostaki, D.; Varga, R.; Peris, K.; Ruzicka, T. Comparative Study of Direct and Indirect Immunofluorescence and of Bullous Pemphigoid 180 and 230 Enzyme-Linked Immunosorbent Assays for Diagnosis of Bullous Pemphigoid. *J. Am. Acad. Dermatol.* **2013**, *69*, 748–753. [CrossRef]
11. Yang, A.; Xuan, R.; Murrell, D.F. A New Indirect Immunofluorescence BIOCHIP Method for the Serological Diagnosis of Bullous Pemphigoid: A Review of Literature. *Australas. J. Dermatol.* **2019**, *60*, e173–e177. [CrossRef]
12. Yang, M.; Wu, H.; Zhao, M.; Chang, C.; Lu, Q. The Pathogenesis of Bullous Skin Diseases. *J. Transl. Autoimmun.* **2019**, *2*, 100014. [CrossRef] [PubMed]
13. Hirako, Y.; Usukura, J.; Nishizawa, Y.; Owaribe, K. Demonstration of the Molecular Shape of BP180, a 180-kDa Bullous Pemphigoid Antigen and Its Potential for Trimer Formation. *J. Biol. Chem.* **1996**, *271*, 13739–13745. [CrossRef] [PubMed]
14. Tuusa, J.; Kokkonen, N.; Tasanen, K. BP180/Collagen XVII: A Molecular View. *Int. J. Mol. Sci.* **2021**, *22*, 12233. [CrossRef] [PubMed]
15. Liu, Y.; Li, L.; Xia, Y. BP180 Is Critical in the Autoimmunity of Bullous Pemphigoid. *Front. Immunol.* **2017**, *8*, 1752. [CrossRef] [PubMed]
16. Ujiie, H. What's New in the Pathogeneses and Triggering Factors of Bullous Pemphigoid. *J. Dermatol.* **2023**, *50*, 140–149. [CrossRef] [PubMed]
17. Kobayashi, M.; Amagai, M.; Kuroda-Kinoshita, K.; Hashimoto, T.; Shirakata, Y.; Hashimoto, K.; Nishikawa, T. BP180 ELISA Using Bacterial Recombinant NC16a Protein as a Diagnostic and Monitoring Tool for Bullous Pemphigoid. *J. Dermatol. Sci.* **2002**, *30*, 224–232. [CrossRef] [PubMed]
18. Izumi, K.; Nishie, W.; Mai, Y.; Wada, M.; Natsuga, K.; Ujiie, H.; Iwata, H.; Yamagami, J.; Shimizu, H. Autoantibody Profile Differentiates between Inflammatory and Noninflammatory Bullous Pemphigoid. *J. Investig. Dermatol.* **2016**, *136*, 2201–2210. [CrossRef]
19. Nishie, W.; Lamer, S.; Schlosser, A.; Licarete, E.; Franzke, C.-W.; Hofmann, S.C.; Jackow, J.; Sitaru, C.; Bruckner-Tuderman, L. Ectodomain Shedding Generates Neoepitopes on Collagen XVII, the Major Autoantigen for Bullous Pemphigoid. *J. Immunol.* **2010**, *185*, 4938–4947. [CrossRef]
20. Hiroyasu, S.; Turner, C.T.; Richardson, K.C.; Granville, D.J. Proteases in Pemphigoid Diseases. *Front. Immunol.* **2019**, *10*, 1454. [CrossRef]
21. Seppänen, A.; Suuronen, T.; Hofmann, S.C.; Majamaa, K.; Alafuzoff, I. Distribution of Collagen XVII in the Human Brain. *Brain Res.* **2007**, *1158*, 50–56. [CrossRef] [PubMed]
22. Hurskainen, T.; Moilanen, J.; Sormunen, R.; Franzke, C.-W.; Soininen, R.; Loeffek, S.; Huilaja, L.; Nuutinen, M.; Bruckner-Tuderman, L.; Autio-Harmainen, H.; et al. Transmembrane Collagen XVII Is a Novel Component of the Glomerular Filtration Barrier. *Cell Tissue Res.* **2012**, *348*, 579–588. [CrossRef]
23. Barrick, B.J.; Ida, C.M.; Laniosz, V.; Jentoft, M.E.; Sominidi-Damodaran, S.; Wieland, C.N.; Meves, A.; Lehman, J.S. Bullous Pemphigoid, Neurodegenerative Disease, and Hippocampal BP180 Expression: A Retrospective Postmortem Neuropathologic Study. *J. Investig. Dermatol.* **2016**, *136*, 2090–2092. [CrossRef] [PubMed]
24. Kasperkiewicz, M.; Zillikens, D.; Schmidt, E. Pemphigoid Diseases: Pathogenesis, Diagnosis, and Treatment. *Autoimmunity* **2012**, *45*, 55–70. [CrossRef] [PubMed]

25. Meijer, J.M.; Diercks, G.F.H.; De Lang, E.W.G.; Pas, H.H.; Jonkman, M.F. Assessment of Diagnostic Strategy for Early Recognition of Bullous and Nonbullous Variants of Pemphigoid. *JAMA Dermatol.* **2019**, *155*, 158. [CrossRef] [PubMed]
26. Cole, C.; Vinay, K.; Borradori, L.; Amber, K.T. Insights into the Pathogenesis of Bullous Pemphigoid: The Role of Complement-Independent Mechanisms. *Front. Immunol.* **2022**, *13*, 912876. [CrossRef]
27. Romeijn, T.R.; Jonkman, M.F.; Knoppers, C.; Pas, H.H.; Diercks, G.F.H. Complement in Bullous Pemphigoid: Results from a Large Observational Study. *Br. J. Dermatol.* **2017**, *176*, 517–519. [CrossRef]
28. Ständer, S.; Holtsche, M.M.; Schmidt, E.; Hammers, C.M.; Zillikens, D.; Ludwig, R.J.; Kridin, K. Presence of Cutaneous Complement Deposition Distinguishes between Immunological and Histological Features of Bullous Pemphigoid—Insights from a Retrospective Cohort Study. *J. Clin. Med.* **2020**, *9*, 3928. [CrossRef]
29. Solimani, F.; Didona, D.; Li, J.; Bao, L.; Patel, P.M.; Gasparini, G.; Kridin, K.; Cozzani, E.; Hertl, M.; Amber, K.T. Characterizing the Proteome of Bullous Pemphigoid Blister Fluid Utilizing Tandem Mass Tag Labeling Coupled with LC–MS/MS. *Arch. Dermatol. Res.* **2021**, *314*, 921–928. [CrossRef]
30. Chiorean, R.M.; Baican, A.; Mustafa, M.B.; Lischka, A.; Leucuta, D.-C.; Feldrihan, V.; Hertl, M.; Sitaru, C. Complement-Activating Capacity of Autoantibodies Correlates with Disease Activity in Bullous Pemphigoid Patients. *Front. Immunol.* **2018**, *9*, 2687. [CrossRef]
31. Ujiie, H.; Sasaoka, T.; Izumi, K.; Nishie, W.; Shinkuma, S.; Natsuga, K.; Nakamura, H.; Shibaki, A.; Shimizu, H. Bullous Pemphigoid Autoantibodies Directly Induce Blister Formation without Complement Activation. *J. Immunol.* **2014**, *193*, 4415–4428. [CrossRef] [PubMed]
32. Dainichi, T.; Nishie, W.; Yamagami, Y.; Sonobe, H.; Ujiie, H.; Kaku, Y.; Kabashima, K. Bullous Pemphigoid Suggestive of Complement-independent Blister Formation with Anti- BP 180 IgG4 Autoantibodies. *Br. J. Dermatol.* **2016**, *175*, 187–190. [CrossRef] [PubMed]
33. Fang, H.; Zhang, Y.; Li, N.; Wang, G.; Liu, Z. The Autoimmune Skin Disease Bullous Pemphigoid: The Role of Mast Cells in Autoantibody-Induced Tissue Injury. *Front. Immunol.* **2018**, *9*, 407. [CrossRef]
34. Schmidt, E.; Wehr, B.; Tabengwa, E.M.; Reimer, S.; Bröcker, E.-B.; Zillikens, D. Elevated Expression and Release of Tissue-Type, but Not Urokinase-Type, Plasminogen Activator after Binding of Autoantibodies to Bullous Pemphigoid Antigen 180 in Cultured Human Keratinocytes. *Clin. Exp. Immunol.* **2004**, *135*, 497–504. [CrossRef] [PubMed]
35. Iwata, H.; Kamio, N.; Aoyama, Y.; Yamamoto, Y.; Hirako, Y.; Owaribe, K.; Kitajima, Y. IgG from Patients with Bullous Pemphigoid Depletes Cultured Keratinocytes of the 180-kDa Bullous Pemphigoid Antigen (Type XVII Collagen) and Weakens Cell Attachment. *J. Investig. Dermatol.* **2009**, *129*, 919–926. [CrossRef]
36. Hiroyasu, S.; Ozawa, T.; Kobayashi, H.; Ishii, M.; Aoyama, Y.; Kitajima, Y.; Hashimoto, T.; Jones, J.C.R.; Tsuruta, D. Bullous Pemphigoid IgG Induces BP180 Internalization via a Macropinocytic Pathway. *Am. J. Pathol.* **2013**, *182*, 828–840. [CrossRef] [PubMed]
37. Schmidt, E.; Reimer, S.; Jainta, S.; Bröcker, E.-B.; Zillikens, D.; Kruse, N.; Marinkovich, M.P.; Marinkovich, M.P.; Giudice, G.J. Autoantibodies to BP180 Associated with Bullous Pemphigoid Release Interleukin-6 and Interleukin-8 from Cultured Human Keratinocytes. *J. Investig. Dermatol.* **2000**, *115*, 842–848. [CrossRef]
38. Tukaj, S.; Grüner, D.; Tukaj, C.; Zillikens, D.; Kasperkiewicz, M. Calcitriol Exerts Anti-Inflammatory Effects in Keratinocytes Treated with Autoantibodies from a Patient with Bullous Pemphigoid. *J. Eur. Acad. Dermatol. Venereol.* **2016**, *30*, 288–292. [CrossRef]
39. Dainichi, T.; Chow, Z.; Kabashima, K. IgG4, Complement, and the Mechanisms of Blister Formation in Pemphigus and Bullous Pemphigoid. *J. Dermatol. Sci.* **2017**, *88*, 265–270. [CrossRef]
40. Sitaru, C.; Mihai, S.; Zillikens, D. The Relevance of the IgG Subclass of Autoantibodies for Blister Induction in Autoimmune Bullous Skin Diseases. *Arch. Dermatol. Res.* **2007**, *299*, 1–8. [CrossRef]
41. Lamb, P.M.; Patton, T.; Deng, J.-S. The Predominance of IgG4 in Prodromal Bullous Pemphigoid. *Int. J. Dermatol.* **2008**, *47*, 150–153. [CrossRef] [PubMed]
42. Hashimoto, T.; Ohzono, A.; Teye, K.; Numata, S.; Hiroyasu, S.; Tsuruta, D.; Hachiya, T.; Kuroda, K.; Hashiguchi, M.; Kawakami, T.; et al. Detection of IgE Autoantibodies to BP180 and BP230 and Their Relationship to Clinical Features in Bullous Pemphigoid. *Br. J. Dermatol.* **2017**, *177*, 141–151. [CrossRef] [PubMed]
43. Van Beek, N.; Lüttmann, N.; Huebner, F.; Recke, A.; Karl, I.; Schulze, F.S.; Zillikens, D.; Schmidt, E. Correlation of Serum Levels of IgE Autoantibodies Against BP180 with Bullous Pemphigoid Disease Activity. *JAMA Dermatol.* **2017**, *153*, 30. [CrossRef] [PubMed]
44. Messingham, K.N.; Crowe, T.P.; Fairley, J.A. The Intersection of IgE Autoantibodies and Eosinophilia in the Pathogenesis of Bullous Pemphigoid. *Front. Immunol.* **2019**, *10*, 2331. [CrossRef]
45. Maglie, R.; Solimani, F.; Didona, D.; Pipitò, C.; Antiga, E.; Di Zenzo, G. The Cytokine Milieu of Bullous Pemphigoid: Current and Novel Therapeutic Targets. *Front. Med.* **2023**, *10*, 1128154. [CrossRef]
46. Quaglino, P.; Antiga, E.; Comessatti, A.; Caproni, M.; Nardò, T.; Ponti, R.; Novelli, M.; Osella-Abate, S.; Fabbri, P.; Bernengo, M.G. Circulating CD4+ CD25brightFOXP3+ Regulatory T-Cells Are Significantly Reduced in Bullous Pemphigoid Patients. *Arch. Dermatol. Res.* **2012**, *304*, 639–645. [CrossRef]

47. Antiga, E.; Quaglino, P.; Volpi, W.; Pierini, I.; Del Bianco, E.; Bianchi, B.; Novelli, M.; Savoia, P.; Bernengo, M.G.; Fabbri, P.; et al. Regulatory T Cells in Skin Lesions and Blood of Patients with Bullous Pemphigoid. *J. Eur. Acad. Dermatol. Venereol.* **2014**, *28*, 222–230. [CrossRef]
48. Gambichler, T.; Tsitlakidon, A.; Skrygan, M.; Höxtermann, S.; Susok, L.; Hessam, S. T Regulatory Cells and Other Lymphocyte Subsets in Patients with Bullous Pemphigoid. *Clin. Exp. Dermatol.* **2017**, *42*, 632–637. [CrossRef]
49. Muramatsu, K.; Zheng, M.; Yoshimoto, N.; Ito, T.; Ujiie, I.; Iwata, H.; Shimizu, H.; Ujiie, H. Regulatory T Cell Subsets in Bullous Pemphigoid and Dipeptidyl Peptidase-4 Inhibitor-Associated Bullous Pemphigoid. *J. Dermatol. Sci.* **2020**, *100*, 23–30. [CrossRef]
50. Cao, T.; Shao, S.; Fang, H.; Li, B.; Wang, G. Role of Regulatory Immune Cells and Molecules in Autoimmune Bullous Dermatoses. *Front. Immunol.* **2019**, *10*, 1746. [CrossRef]
51. Didona, D.; Di Zenzo, G. Humoral Epitope Spreading in Autoimmune Bullous Diseases. *Front. Immunol.* **2018**, *9*, 779. [CrossRef] [PubMed]
52. Di Zenzo, G.; Calabresi, V.; Olasz, E.B.; Zambruno, G.; Yancey, K.B. Sequential Intramolecular Epitope Spreading of Humoral Responses to Human BPAG2 in a Transgenic Model. *J. Investig. Dermatol.* **2010**, *130*, 1040–1047. [CrossRef] [PubMed]
53. Ujiie, H.; Yoshimoto, N.; Natsuga, K.; Muramatsu, K.; Iwata, H.; Nishie, W.; Shimizu, H. Immune Reaction to Type XVII Collagen Induces Intramolecular and Intermolecular Epitope Spreading in Experimental Bullous Pemphigoid Models. *Front. Immunol.* **2019**, *10*, 1410. [CrossRef] [PubMed]
54. Di Zenzo, G.; Thoma-Uszynski, S.; Calabresi, V.; Fontao, L.; Hofmann, S.C.; Lacour, J.-P.; Sera, F.; Bruckner-Tuderman, L.; Zambruno, G.; Borradori, L.; et al. Demonstration of Epitope-Spreading Phenomena in Bullous Pemphigoid: Results of a Prospective Multicenter Study. *J. Investig. Dermatol.* **2011**, *131*, 2271–2280. [CrossRef] [PubMed]
55. Mignogna, M.D.; Fortuna, G.; Leuci, S.; Stasio, L.; Mezza, E.; Ruoppo, E. Lichen Planus Pemphigoides, a Possible Example of Epitope Spreading. *Oral Surg. Oral Med. Oral Pathol. Oral Radiol. Endodontology* **2010**, *109*, 837–843. [CrossRef] [PubMed]
56. Nguyen, T.; Kwan, J.M.; Ahmed, A.R. Relationship between Radiation Therapy and Bullous Pemphigoid. *Dermatology* **2014**, *229*, 88–96. [CrossRef] [PubMed]
57. Amber, K.T.; Zikry, J.; Hertl, M. A Multi-Hit Hypothesis of Bullous Pemphigoid and Associated Neurological Disease: Is HLA-DQB1*03:01, a Potential Link between Immune Privileged Antigen Exposure and Epitope Spreading? *HLA* **2017**, *89*, 127–134. [CrossRef]
58. Bean, S.F.; Good, R.A.; Windhorst, D.B. Bullous Pemphigoid in an 11-Year-Old Boy. *Arch. Dermatol.* **1970**, *102*, 205–208. [CrossRef]
59. Naranjo, C.A.; Busto, U.; Sellers, E.M.; Sandor, P.; Ruiz, I.; Roberts, E.A.; Janecek, E.; Domecq, C.; Greenblatt, D.J. A Method for Estimating the Probability of Adverse Drug Reactions. *Clin. Pharmacol. Ther.* **1981**, *30*, 239–245. [CrossRef]
60. Karch, F.E.; Lasagna, L. Toward the Operational Identification of Adverse Drug Reactions. *Clin. Pharmacol. Ther.* **1977**, *21*, 247–254. [CrossRef]
61. Tan, C.W.X.; Pang, Y.; Sim, B.; Thirumoorthy, T.; Pang, S.M.; Lee, H.Y. The Association between Drugs and Bullous Pemphigoid. *Br. J. Dermatol.* **2017**, *176*, 549–551. [CrossRef]
62. Vassileva, S. Drug-Induced Pemphigoid: Bullous and Cicatricial. *Clin. Dermatol.* **1998**, *16*, 379–387. [CrossRef]
63. Stavropoulos, P.G.; Soura, E.; Antoniou, C. Drug-Induced Pemphigoid: A Review of the Literature. *J. Eur. Acad. Dermatol. Venereol.* **2014**, *28*, 1133–1140. [CrossRef] [PubMed]
64. Liu, S.-D.; Chen, W.-T.; Chi, C.-C. Association Between Medication Use and Bullous Pemphigoid: A Systematic Review and Meta-Analysis. *JAMA Dermatol.* **2020**, *156*, 891. [CrossRef]
65. Molina, G.E.; Yanovsky, R.L.; Wei, E.X.; Chen, S.T. Missed Drug-Induced Bullous Pemphigoid Leads to Longer Immunosuppression than Recognized Cases: A 9-Year Retrospective Review. *J. Am. Acad. Dermatol.* **2020**, *82*, 1255–1258. [CrossRef] [PubMed]
66. Ruocco, V.; Sacerdoti, G. Pemphigus and Bullous Pemphigoid Due to Drugs. *Int. J. Dermatol.* **1991**, *30*, 307–312. [CrossRef]
67. Borch, J.E.; Andersen, K.E.; Clemmensen, O.; Bindslev-Jensen, C. Drug-Induced Bullous Pemphigoid with Positive Patch Test and in Vitro IgE Sensitization. *Acta Derm. Venereol.* **2005**, *85*, 171–172. [CrossRef] [PubMed]
68. Alcalay, J.; Hazaz, B.; Sandbank, M. Bullous Pemphigoid Mimicking Bullous Erythema Multiforme: An Untoward Side Effect of Penicillins. *J. Am. Acad. Dermatol.* **1988**, *18*, 345–349. [CrossRef]
69. Drucker, D.J.; Nauck, M.A. The Incretin System: Glucagon-like Peptide-1 Receptor Agonists and Dipeptidyl Peptidase-4 Inhibitors in Type 2 Diabetes. *Lancet* **2006**, *368*, 1696–1705. [CrossRef]
70. Bellary, S.; Kyrou, I.; Brown, J.E.; Bailey, C.J. Type 2 Diabetes Mellitus in Older Adults: Clinical Considerations and Management. *Nat. Rev. Endocrinol.* **2021**, *17*, 534–548. [CrossRef]
71. García, M.; Aranburu, M.A.; Palacios-Zabalza, I.; Lertxundi, U.; Aguirre, C. Dipeptidyl Peptidase-IV Inhibitors Induced Bullous Pemphigoid: A Case Report and Analysis of Cases Reported in the European Pharmacovigilance Database. *J. Clin. Pharm. Ther.* **2016**, *41*, 368–370. [CrossRef] [PubMed]
72. Béné, J.; Moulis, G.; Bennani, I.; Auffret, M.; Coupe, P.; Babai, S.; Hillaire-Buys, D.; Micallef, J.; Gautier, S.; the French Association of Regional Pharmaco Vigilance Centres. Bullous Pemphigoid and Dipeptidyl Peptidase IV Inhibitors: A Case-Noncase Study in the French Pharmacovigilance Database. *Br. J. Dermatol.* **2016**, *175*, 296–301. [CrossRef] [PubMed]
73. Varpuluoma, O.; Försti, A.-K.; Jokelainen, J.; Turpeinen, M.; Timonen, M.; Huilaja, L.; Tasanen, K. Vildagliptin Significantly Increases the Risk of Bullous Pemphigoid: A Finnish Nationwide Registry Study. *J. Investig. Dermatol.* **2018**, *138*, 1659–1661. [CrossRef]

74. Benzaquen, M.; Borradori, L.; Berbis, P.; Cazzaniga, S.; Valero, R.; Richard, M.-A.; Feldmeyer, L. Dipeptidyl Peptidase IV Inhibitors, a Risk Factor for Bullous Pemphigoid: Retrospective Multicenter Case-Control Study from France and Switzerland. *J. Am. Acad. Dermatol.* **2018**, *78*, 1090–1096. [CrossRef] [PubMed]
75. Kawaguchi, Y.; Shimauchi, R.; Nishibori, N.; Kawashima, K.; Oshitani, S.; Fujiya, A.; Shibata, T.; Ohashi, N.; Izumi, K.; Nishie, W.; et al. Dipeptidyl Peptidase-4 Inhibitors-Associated Bullous Pemphigoid: A Retrospective Study of 168 Pemphigoid and 9,304 Diabetes Mellitus Patients. *J. Diabetes Investig.* **2019**, *10*, 392–398. [CrossRef] [PubMed]
76. Kridin, K.; Cohen, A.D. Dipeptidyl-Peptidase IV Inhibitor–Associated Bullous Pemphigoid: A Systematic Review and Meta-Analysis. *J. Am. Acad. Dermatol.* **2021**, *85*, 501–503. [CrossRef]
77. Kuwata, H.; Nishioka, Y.; Noda, T.; Kubo, S.; Myojin, T.; Higashino, T.; Takahashi, Y.; Ishii, H.; Imamura, T. Association between Dipeptidyl Peptidase-4 Inhibitors and Increased Risk for Bullous Pemphigoid within 3 Months from First Use: A 5-year Population-based Cohort Study Using the Japanese National Database. *J. Diabetes Investig.* **2022**, *13*, 460–467. [CrossRef]
78. Lee, S.G.; Lee, H.J.; Yoon, M.S.; Kim, D.H. Association of Dipeptidyl Peptidase 4 Inhibitor Use with Risk of Bullous Pemphigoid in Patients with Diabetes. *JAMA Dermatol.* **2019**, *155*, 172. [CrossRef]
79. Kridin, K.; Avni, O.; Damiani, G.; Tzur Bitan, D.; Onn, E.; Weinstein, O.; Cohen, A.D. Dipeptidyl-Peptidase IV Inhibitor (DPP4i) Confers Increased Odds of Bullous Pemphigoid Even Years after Drug Initiation. *Arch. Dermatol. Res.* **2022**, *315*, 33–39. [CrossRef]
80. Guo, W.; Rathi, S.; Marquez, J.; Smith, H.; Kuruvilla, A.; Tonnesen, M.G.; Salvemini, J.N. Prevalence of Diabetes Mellitus in Bullous Pemphigoid Patients in the Absence of Dipeptidyl Peptidase-4 Inhibitors: A Systematic Review and Meta-Analysis. *Arch. Dermatol. Res.* **2023**, *315*, 2207–2213. [CrossRef]
81. Varpuluoma, O.; Försti, A.-K.; Jokelainen, J.; Turpeinen, M.; Timonen, M.; Tasanen, K.; Huilaja, L. Oral Diabetes Medications Other than Dipeptidyl Peptidase 4 Inhibitors Are Not Associated with Bullous Pemphigoid: A Finnish Nationwide Case-Control Study. *J. Am. Acad. Dermatol.* **2018**, *79*, 1034–1038.e5. [CrossRef]
82. Kridin, K. Comment on "Oral Diabetes Medications Other than Dipeptidyl Peptidase-4 Inhibitors Are Not Associated with Bullous Pemphigoid: A Finnish Nationwide Case Control Study". *J. Am. Acad. Dermatol.* **2018**, *79*, e111–e112. [CrossRef] [PubMed]
83. Schwager, Z.; Mikailov, A.; Lipworth, A.D. Comment on "Oral Diabetes Medications Other than Dipeptidyl Peptidase-4 Inhibitors Are Not Associated with Bullous Pemphigoid: A Finnish Nationwide Case-Control Study" and a Case Report of Glucagon-like Peptide-1 Receptor Agonist–Induced Bullous Pemphigoid. *J. Am. Acad. Dermatol.* **2019**, *80*, e189–e190. [CrossRef] [PubMed]
84. Lambadiari, V.; Kountouri, A.; Kousathana, F.; Korakas, E.; Kokkalis, G.; Theotokoglou, S.; Palaiodimou, L.; Katsimbri, P.; Ikonomidis, I.; Theodoropoulos, K.; et al. The Association of Bullous Pemphigoid with Dipeptidyl-Peptidase 4 Inhibitors: A Ten-Year Prospective Observational Study. *BMC Endocr. Disord.* **2021**, *21*, 23. [CrossRef]
85. Baetta, R.; Corsini, A. Pharmacology of Dipeptidyl Peptidase-4 Inhibitors: Similarities and Differences. *Drugs* **2011**, *71*, 1441–1467. [CrossRef] [PubMed]
86. Ujiie, H.; Muramatsu, K.; Mushiroda, T.; Ozeki, T.; Miyoshi, H.; Iwata, H.; Nakamura, A.; Nomoto, H.; Cho, K.Y.; Sato, N.; et al. HLA-DQB1*03:01 as a Biomarker for Genetic Susceptibility to Bullous Pemphigoid Induced by DPP-4 Inhibitors. *J. Investig. Dermatol.* **2018**, *138*, 1201–1204. [CrossRef]
87. Oyama, N.; Setterfield, J.F.; Powell, A.M.; Sakuma-Oyama, Y.; Albert, S.; Bhogal, B.S.; Vaughan, R.W.; Kaneko, F.; Challacombe, S.J.; Black, M.M. Bullous Pemphigoid Antigen II (BP180) and Its Soluble Extracellular Domains Are Major Autoantigens in Mucous Membrane Pemphigoid: The Pathogenic Relevance to HLA Class II Alleles and Disease Severity: Circulating Autoantibody Profile of MMP. *Br. J. Dermatol.* **2006**, *154*, 90–98. [CrossRef]
88. Lindgren, O.; Varpuluoma, O.; Tuusa, J.; Ilonen, J.; Huilaja, L.; Kokkonen, N.; Tasanen, K. Gliptin-Associated Bullous Pemphigoid and the Expression of Dipeptidyl Peptidase-4/CD26 in Bullous Pemphigoid. *Acta Derm. Venereol.* **2019**, *99*, 602–609. [CrossRef]
89. Klemann, C.; Wagner, L.; Stephan, M.; Von Hörsten, S. Cut to the Chase: A Review of CD26/Dipeptidyl Peptidase-4's (DPP4) Entanglement in the Immune System. *Clin. Exp. Immunol.* **2016**, *185*, 1–21. [CrossRef]
90. Forssmann, U.; Stoetzer, C.; Stephan, M.; Kruschinski, C.; Skripuletz, T.; Schade, J.; Schmiedl, A.; Pabst, R.; Wagner, L.; Hoffmann, T.; et al. Inhibition of CD26/Dipeptidyl Peptidase IV Enhances CCL11/Eotaxin-Mediated Recruitment of Eosinophils In Vivo. *J. Immunol.* **2008**, *181*, 1120–1127. [CrossRef]
91. Gonzalez-Gronow, M. Dipeptidyl Peptidase IV (DPP IV/CD26) Is a Cell-Surface Plasminogen Receptor. *Front. Biosci.* **2008**, *13*, 1610. [CrossRef] [PubMed]
92. Mai, Y.; Nishie, W.; Izumi, K.; Shimizu, H. Preferential Reactivity of Dipeptidyl Peptidase-IV Inhibitor-Associated Bullous Pemphigoid Autoantibodies to the Processed Extracellular Domains of BP180. *Front. Immunol.* **2019**, *10*, 1224. [CrossRef] [PubMed]
93. Hofmann, S.C.; Voith, U.; Schönau, V.; Sorokin, L.; Bruckner-Tuderman, L.; Franzke, C.-W. Plasmin Plays a Role in the In Vitro Generation of the Linear IgA Dermatosis Antigen LADB97. *J. Investig. Dermatol.* **2009**, *129*, 1730–1739. [CrossRef] [PubMed]
94. Horikawa, H.; Kurihara, Y.; Funakoshi, T.; Umegaki-Arao, N.; Takahashi, H.; Kubo, A.; Tanikawa, A.; Kodani, N.; Minami, Y.; Meguro, S.; et al. Unique Clinical and Serological Features of Bullous Pemphigoid Associated with Dipeptidyl Peptidase-4 Inhibitors. *Br. J. Dermatol.* **2018**, *178*, 1462–1463. [CrossRef] [PubMed]
95. Hayashi, M.; Tsunoda, T.; Sato, F.; Yaguchi, Y.; Igarashi, M.; Izumi, K.; Nishie, W.; Ishii, N.; Okamura, K.; Suzuki, T.; et al. Clinical and Immunological Characterization of 14 Cases of Dipeptidyl Peptidase-4 Inhibitor-associated Bullous Pemphigoid: A Single-centre Study. *Br. J. Dermatol.* **2020**, *182*, 806–807. [CrossRef]

96. García-Díez, I.; Ivars-Lleó, M.; López-Aventín, D.; Ishii, N.; Hashimoto, T.; Iranzo, P.; Pujol, R.M.; España, A.; Herrero-Gonzalez, J.E. Bullous Pemphigoid Induced by Dipeptidyl Peptidase-4 Inhibitors. Eight Cases with Clinical and Immunological Characterization. *Int. J. Dermatol.* **2018**, *57*, 810–816. [CrossRef]
97. Sawada, K.; Sawada, T.; Kobayashi, T.; Fujiki, A.; Matsushita, T.; Kawara, S.; Izumi, K.; Nishie, W.; Shimizu, H.; Takehara, K.; et al. A Case of Anti-BP230 Antibody-Positive Bullous Pemphigoid Receiving DPP-4 Inhibitor. *Immunol. Med.* **2021**, *44*, 53–55. [CrossRef]
98. Fania, L.; Salemme, A.; Provini, A.; Pagnanelli, G.; Collina, M.C.; Abeni, D.; Didona, B.; Di Zenzo, G.; Mazzanti, C. Detection and Characterization of IgG, IgE, and IgA Autoantibodies in Patients with Bullous Pemphigoid Associated with Dipeptidyl Peptidase-4 Inhibitors. *J. Am. Acad. Dermatol.* **2018**, *78*, 592–595. [CrossRef]
99. Yamashita, C.; Arase, N.; Higuchi, S.; Arase, H.; Takagi, J.; Nojima, S.; Tanemura, A.; Fujimoto, M. Serum Autoantibodies against the Extracellular Region of A6β4 Integrin in a Patient with Dipeptidyl Peptidase-4 Inhibitor–Induced Bullous Pemphigoid. *JAAD Case Rep.* **2022**, *20*, 65–68. [CrossRef]
100. Mai, Y.; Nishie, W.; Izumi, K.; Yoshimoto, N.; Morita, Y.; Watanabe, M.; Toyonaga, E.; Ujiie, H.; Iwata, H.; Fujita, Y.; et al. Detection of Anti-BP180 NC16A Autoantibodies after the Onset of Dipeptidyl Peptidase-IV Inhibitor-Associated Bullous Pemphigoid: A Report of Three Patients. *Br. J. Dermatol.* **2018**, *179*, 790–791. [CrossRef]
101. Takama, H.; Yoshida, M.; Izumi, K.; Yanagishita, T.; Muto, J.; Ohshima, Y.; Nishie, W.; Shimizu, H.; Akiyama, M.; Watanabe, D. Dipeptidyl Peptidase-4 Inhibitor-Associated Bullous Pemphigoid: Recurrence with Epitope Spreading. *Acta Derm. Venereol.* **2018**, *98*, 983–984. [CrossRef]
102. García-Díez, I.; España, A.; Iranzo, P. Epitope-spreading Phenomena in Dipeptidyl Peptidase-4 Inhibitor-associated Bullous Pemphigoid. *Br. J. Dermatol.* **2019**, *180*, 1267–1268. [CrossRef] [PubMed]
103. Tasanen, K. Dipeptidyl Peptidase-4 Inhibitor-Associated Bullous Pemphigoid. *Front. Immunol.* **2019**, *10*, 1238. [CrossRef] [PubMed]
104. Giusti, D.; Le Jan, S.; Gatouillat, G.; Bernard, P.; Pham, B.N.; Antonicelli, F. Biomarkers Related to Bullous Pemphigoid Activity and Outcome. *Exp. Dermatol.* **2017**, *26*, 1240–1247. [CrossRef]
105. Hung, C.-T.; Chang, Y.-L.; Wang, W.-M. Dipeptidyl Peptidase-4 Inhibitor-Related Bullous Pemphigoid: Clinical, Laboratory, and Histological Features, and Possible Pathogenesis. *Int. J. Mol. Sci.* **2022**, *23*, 14101. [CrossRef] [PubMed]
106. Long, M.; Cai, L.; Li, W.; Zhang, L.; Guo, S.; Zhang, R.; Zheng, Y.; Liu, X.; Wang, M.; Zhou, X.; et al. DPP-4 Inhibitors Improve Diabetic Wound Healing via Direct and Indirect Promotion of Epithelial-Mesenchymal Transition and Reduction of Scarring. *Diabetes* **2018**, *67*, 518–531. [CrossRef]
107. Tasanen, K.; Tunggal, L.; Chometon, G.; Bruckner-Tuderman, L.; Aumailley, M. Keratinocytes from Patients Lacking Collagen XVII Display a Migratory Phenotype. *Am. J. Pathol.* **2004**, *164*, 2027–2038. [CrossRef]
108. Nishie, W. Dipeptidyl Peptidase IV Inhibitor-Associated Bullous Pemphigoid: A Recently Recognized Autoimmune Blistering Disease with Unique Clinical, Immunological and Genetic Characteristics. *Immunol. Med.* **2019**, *42*, 22–28. [CrossRef]
109. Nozawa, K.; Suzuki, T.; Kayanuma, G.; Yamamoto, H.; Nagayasu, K.; Shirakawa, H.; Kaneko, S. Lisinopril Prevents Bullous Pemphigoid Induced by Dipeptidyl Peptidase 4 Inhibitors via the Mas Receptor Pathway. *Front. Immunol.* **2023**, *13*, 1084960. [CrossRef]
110. Ständer, S.; Schmidt, E.; Zillikens, D.; Ludwig, R.J.; Kridin, K. More Severe Erosive Phenotype Despite Lower Circulating Autoantibody Levels in Dipeptidyl Peptidase-4 Inhibitor (DPP4i)-Associated Bullous Pemphigoid: A Retrospective Cohort Study. *Am. J. Clin. Dermatol.* **2021**, *22*, 117–127. [CrossRef]
111. He, Y.-L.; Sabo, R.; Campestrini, J.; Wang, Y.; Riviere, G.-J.; Nielsen, J.C.; Rosenberg, M.; Ligueros-Saylan, M.; Howard, D.; Dole, W.P. The Effect of Age, Gender, and Body Mass Index on the Pharmacokinetics and Pharmacodynamics of Vildagliptin in Healthy Volunteers. *Br. J. Clin. Pharmacol.* **2008**, *65*, 338–346. [CrossRef]
112. Kinyó, Á.; Hanyecz, A.; Lengyel, Z.; Várszegi, D.; Oláh, P.; Gyömörei, C.; Kálmán, E.; Berki, T.; Gyulai, R. Clinical, Laboratory and Histological Features of Dipeptidyl Peptidase-4 Inhibitor Related Noninflammatory Bullous Pemphigoid. *J. Clin. Med.* **2021**, *10*, 1916. [CrossRef] [PubMed]
113. Chijiwa, C.; Takeoka, S.; Kamata, M.; Tateishi, M.; Fukaya, S.; Hayashi, K.; Fukuyasu, A.; Tanaka, T.; Ishikawa, T.; Ohnishi, T.; et al. Decrease in Eosinophils Infiltrating into the Skin of Patients with Dipeptidyl Peptidase-4 Inhibitor-Related Bullous Pemphigoid. *J. Dermatol.* **2018**, *45*, 596–599. [CrossRef] [PubMed]
114. Patsatsi, A.; Kyriakou, A.; Meltzanidou, P.; Trigoni, A.; Lamprou, F.; Kokolios, M.; Giannakou, A. Bullous Pemphigoid in Patients with DPP-4 Inhibitors at the Onset of Disease: Does This Differ from Common Bullous Pemphigoid? *Eur. J. Dermatol. EJD* **2018**, *28*, 711–713. [CrossRef] [PubMed]
115. Kridin, K. Dipeptidyl-peptidase IV Inhibitors (DPP4i)-associated Bullous Pemphigoid: Estimating the Clinical Profile and Exploring Intraclass Differences. *Dermatol. Ther.* **2020**, *33*, e13790. [CrossRef] [PubMed]
116. Kridin, K.; Bergman, R. Association of Bullous Pemphigoid with Dipeptidyl-Peptidase 4 Inhibitors in Patients with Diabetes: Estimating the Risk of the New Agents and Characterizing the Patients. *JAMA Dermatol.* **2018**, *154*, 1152–1158. [CrossRef]
117. Patsatsi, A.; Vyzantiadis, T.-A.; Chrysomallis, F.; Devliotou-Panagiotidou, D.; Sotiriadis, D. Medication History of a Series of Patients with Bullous Pemphigoid from Northern Greece—Observations and Discussion. *Int. J. Dermatol.* **2009**, *48*, 132–135. [CrossRef] [PubMed]

118. Plaquevent, M.; Tétart, F.; Fardet, L.; Ingen-Housz-Oro, S.; Valeyrie-Allanore, L.; Bernard, P.; Hebert, V.; Roussel, A.; Avenel-Audran, M.; Chaby, G.; et al. Higher Frequency of Dipeptidyl Peptidase-4 Inhibitor Intake in Bullous Pemphigoid Patients than in the French General Population. *J. Investig. Dermatol.* **2019**, *139*, 835–841. [CrossRef]
119. Armanious, M.; AbuHilal, M. Gliptin-Induced Bullous Pemphigoid: Canadian Case Series of 10 Patients. *J. Cutan. Med. Surg.* **2021**, *25*, 163–168. [CrossRef]
120. Quach, H.T.; Johnson, D.B.; LeBoeuf, N.R.; Zwerner, J.P.; Dewan, A.K. Cutaneous Adverse Events Caused by Immune Checkpoint Inhibitors. *J. Am. Acad. Dermatol.* **2021**, *85*, 956–966. [CrossRef]
121. Merli, M.; Accorinti, M.; Romagnuolo, M.; Marzano, A.; Di Zenzo, G.; Moro, F.; Antiga, E.; Maglie, R.; Cozzani, E.; Parodi, A.; et al. Autoimmune Bullous Dermatoses in Cancer Patients Treated by Immunotherapy: A Literature Review and Italian Multicentric Experience. *Front. Med.* **2023**, *10*, 1208418. [CrossRef]
122. Bhardwaj, M.; Chiu, M.N.; Pilkhwal Sah, S. Adverse Cutaneous Toxicities by PD-1/PD-L1 Immune Checkpoint Inhibitors: Pathogenesis, Treatment, and Surveillance. *Cutan. Ocul. Toxicol.* **2022**, *41*, 73–90. [CrossRef] [PubMed]
123. Kawsar, A.; Edwards, C.; Patel, P.; Heywood, R.M.; Gupta, A.; Mann, J.; Harland, C.; Heelan, K.; Larkin, J.; Lorigan, P.; et al. Checkpoint Inhibitor-Associated Bullous Cutaneous Immune-Related Adverse Events: A Multicentre Observational Study. *Br. J. Dermatol.* **2022**, *187*, 981–987. [CrossRef]
124. Said, J.T.; Liu, M.; Talia, J.; Singer, S.B.; Semenov, Y.R.; Wei, E.X.; Mostaghimi, A.; Nelson, C.A.; Giobbie-Hurder, A.; LeBoeuf, N.R. Risk Factors for the Development of Bullous Pemphigoid in US Patients Receiving Immune Checkpoint Inhibitors. *JAMA Dermatol.* **2022**, *158*, 552. [CrossRef]
125. Siegel, J.; Totonchy, M.; Damsky, W.; Berk-Krauss, J.; Castiglione, F.; Sznol, M.; Petrylak, D.P.; Fischbach, N.; Goldberg, S.B.; Decker, R.H.; et al. Bullous Disorders Associated with Anti–PD-1 and Anti–PD-L1 Therapy: A Retrospective Analysis Evaluating the Clinical and Histopathologic Features, Frequency, and Impact on Cancer Therapy. *J. Am. Acad. Dermatol.* **2018**, *79*, 1081–1088. [CrossRef] [PubMed]
126. Molle, M.F.; Capurro, N.; Herzum, A.; Micalizzi, C.; Cozzani, E.; Parodi, A. Self-resolving Bullous Pemphigoid Induced by Cemiplimab. *Dermatol. Ther.* **2022**, *35*, e15466. [CrossRef]
127. Mazumder, A.; Darji, K.; Smith, K.; Guo, M. Two Rare Cases of Bullous Pemphigoid Associated with Immune Checkpoint Inhibitors. *BMJ Case Rep.* **2022**, *15*, e253059. [CrossRef] [PubMed]
128. Buchbinder, E.I.; Desai, A. CTLA-4 and PD-1 Pathways: Similarities, Differences, and Implications of Their Inhibition. *Am. J. Clin. Oncol.* **2016**, *39*, 98–106. [CrossRef]
129. Asdourian, M.S.; Shah, N.; Jacoby, T.V.; Reynolds, K.L.; Chen, S.T. Association of Bullous Pemphigoid with Immune Checkpoint Inhibitor Therapy in Patients with Cancer: A Systematic Review. *JAMA Dermatol.* **2022**, *158*, 933. [CrossRef]
130. Ye, Y.; Jing, Y.; Li, L.; Mills, G.B.; Diao, L.; Liu, H.; Han, L. Sex-Associated Molecular Differences for Cancer Immunotherapy. *Nat. Commun.* **2020**, *11*, 1779. [CrossRef]
131. Jang, S.R.; Nikita, N.; Banks, J.; Keith, S.W.; Johnson, J.M.; Wilson, M.; Lu-Yao, G. Association Between Sex and Immune Checkpoint Inhibitor Outcomes for Patients with Melanoma. *JAMA Netw. Open* **2021**, *4*, e2136823. [CrossRef] [PubMed]
132. Lee, H.; Chung, J.H.; Jo, S.J. Pruritic Bullous Skin Eruption in a Male Patient Receiving Immunotherapy for Oropharyngeal Cancer. *Int. J. Dermatol.* **2020**, *59*, 685–686. [CrossRef] [PubMed]
133. Tsiogka, A.; Bauer, J.; Patsatsi, A. Bullous Pemphigoid Associated with Anti-Programmed Cell Death Protein 1 and Anti-Programmed Cell Death Ligand 1 Therapy: A Review of the Literature. *Acta Derm. Venereol.* **2021**, *101*, adv00377. [CrossRef]
134. Gresham, L.M.; Kirchhof, M.G. A Case of Drug-Induced Bullous Pemphigoid Secondary to Immunotherapy Treated with Upadacitinib: A Case Report. SAGE Open Med. *Case Rep.* **2023**, *11*, 2050313X2311609. [CrossRef] [PubMed]
135. Muntyanu, A.; Netchiporouk, E.; Gerstein, W.; Gniadecki, R.; Litvinov, I.V. Cutaneous Immune-Related Adverse Events (irAEs) to Immune Checkpoint Inhibitors: A Dermatology Perspective on Management. *J. Cutan. Med. Surg.* **2021**, *25*, 59–76. [CrossRef]
136. Morris, L.M.; Lewis, H.A.; Cornelius, L.A.; Chen, D.Y.; Rosman, I.S. Neutrophil-predominant Bullous Pemphigoid Induced by Checkpoint Inhibitors: A Case Series. *J. Cutan. Pathol.* **2020**, *47*, 742–746. [CrossRef] [PubMed]
137. Lopez, A.T.; Geskin, L. A Case of Nivolumab-Induced Bullous Pemphigoid: Review of Dermatologic Toxicity Associated with Programmed Cell Death Protein-1/Programmed Death Ligand-1 Inhibitors and Recommendations for Diagnosis and Management. *Oncologist* **2018**, *23*, 1119–1126. [CrossRef]
138. Nelson, C.A.; Singer, S.; Chen, T.; Puleo, A.E.; Lian, C.G.; Wei, E.X.; Giobbie-Hurder, A.; Mostaghimi, A.; LeBoeuf, N.R. Bullous Pemphigoid after Anti–Programmed Death-1 Therapy: A Retrospective Case-Control Study Evaluating Impact on Tumor Response and Survival Outcomes. *J. Am. Acad. Dermatol.* **2022**, *87*, 1400–1402. [CrossRef]
139. Tang, K.; Seo, J.; Tiu, B.C.; Le, T.K.; Pahalyants, V.; Raval, N.S.; Ugwu-Dike, P.O.; Zubiri, L.; Naranbhai, V.; Carrington, M.; et al. Association of Cutaneous Immune-Related Adverse Events with Increased Survival in Patients Treated with Anti–Programmed Cell Death 1 and Anti–Programmed Cell Death Ligand 1 Therapy. *JAMA Dermatol.* **2022**, *158*, 189. [CrossRef]
140. Hofmann, M.; Audring, H.; Sterry, W.; Trefzer, U. Interleukin-2-Associated Bullous Drug Dermatosis. *Dermatology* **2005**, *210*, 74–75. [CrossRef]
141. Stingeni, L.; Bianchi, L.; Minotti, V.; Lisi, P. Erlotinib-Induced Bullous Pemphigoid. *J. Am. Acad. Dermatol.* **2012**, *67*, e199–e201. [CrossRef]
142. Atzori, L.; Conti, B.; Zucca, M.; Pau, M. Bullous Pemphigoid Induced by M-TOR Inhibitors in Renal Transplant Recipients. *J. Eur. Acad. Dermatol. Venereol.* **2015**, *29*, 1626–1630. [CrossRef] [PubMed]

143. De Simone, C.; Caldarola, G.; Castriota, M.; Salerno, M.P.; Citterio, F. Bullous Pemphigoid in a Transplant Recipient: Is This a Sign of Allograft Rejection? *Eur. J. Dermatol.* **2012**, *22*, 280–281. [CrossRef] [PubMed]
144. Satta, R.; Onnis, G.; Gunnella, S.; Montesu, M.A.; Agnoletti, A.F.; Cozzani, E. Dabrafenib-Induced Pemphigoid-like Reaction. *Clin. Exp. Dermatol.* **2018**, *43*, 222–224. [CrossRef] [PubMed]
145. Chawla, S.; Hill, A.; Fearfield, L.; Johnston, S.; Parton, M.; Heelan, K. Cutaneous Toxicities Occurring during Palbociclib (CDK4/6 Inhibitor) and Endocrine Therapy in Patients with Advanced Breast Cancer: A Single-Centre Experience. *Breast Cancer Res. Treat.* **2021**, *188*, 535–545. [CrossRef] [PubMed]
146. Husein-ElAhmed, H.; Steinhoff, M. Bullous Pemphigoid Induced by Biologic Drugs in Psoriasis: A Systematic Review. *J. Dermatol. Treat.* **2022**, *33*, 2886–2893. [CrossRef] [PubMed]
147. Zhang, J.; Wang, S.-H.; Zuo, Y.-G. Paradoxical Phenomena of Bullous Pemphigoid Induced and Treated by Identical Biologics. *Front. Immunol.* **2023**, *13*, 1050373. [CrossRef]
148. Genovese, G.; Di Zenzo, G.; Cozzani, E.; Berti, E.; Cugno, M.; Marzano, A.V. New Insights into the Pathogenesis of Bullous Pemphigoid: 2019 Update. *Front. Immunol.* **2019**, *10*, 1506. [CrossRef]
149. Rhodes, L.E.; Hashim, A.; McLaughlin, P.J.; Friedmann, P.S. Blister Fluid Cytokines in Cutaneous Inflammatory Bullous Disorders. *Acta Derm Venereol.* **1999**, *79*, 288–290. [CrossRef]
150. Ameglio, F.; D'Auria, L.; Cordiali-Fei, P.; Mussi, A.; Valenzano, L.; D'Agosto, G.; Ferraro, C.; Bonifati, C.; Giacalone, B. Bullous Pemphigoid and Pemphigus Vulgaris: Correlated Behaviour of Serum VEGF, sE-Selectin and TNF-Alpha Levels. *J. Biol. Regul. Homeost. Agents* **1997**, *11*, 148–153.
151. Liu, L.Y.; Bates, M.E.; Jarjour, N.N.; Busse, W.W.; Bertics, P.J.; Kelly, E.A.B. Generation of Th1 and Th2 Chemokines by Human Eosinophils: Evidence for a Critical Role of TNF-α. *J. Immunol.* **2007**, *179*, 4840–4848. [CrossRef] [PubMed]
152. Romagnuolo, M.; Moltrasio, C.; Iannone, C.; Gattinara, M.; Cambiaghi, S.; Marzano, A.V. Pyoderma Gangrenosum Following Anti-TNF Therapy in Chronic Recurrent Multifocal Osteomyelitis: Drug Reaction or Cutaneous Manifestation of the Disease? A Critical Review on the Topic with an Emblematic Case Report. *Front. Med.* **2023**, *10*, 1197273. [CrossRef] [PubMed]
153. Gounni Abdelilah, S.; Wellemans, V.; Agouli, M.; Guenounou, M.; Hamid, Q.; Beck, L.A.; Lamkhioued, B. Increased Expression of Th2-Associated Chemokines in Bullous Pemphigoid Disease. Role of Eosinophils in the Production and Release of These Chemokines. *Clin. Immunol.* **2006**, *120*, 220–231. [CrossRef] [PubMed]
154. Ho, P.-H.; Tsai, T.-F. Development of Bullous Pemphigoid during Secukinumab Treatment for Psoriasis. *J. Dermatol.* **2017**, *44*, e220–e221. [CrossRef]
155. Giusti, D.; Bini, E.; Terryn, C.; Didier, K.; Le Jan, S.; Gatouillat, G.; Durlach, A.; Nesmond, S.; Muller, C.; Bernard, P.; et al. NET Formation in Bullous Pemphigoid Patients with Relapse Is Modulated by IL-17 and IL-23 Interplay. *Front. Immunol.* **2019**, *10*, 701. [CrossRef]
156. Maronese, C.A.; Cassano, N.; Genovese, G.; Foti, C.; Vena, G.A.; Marzano, A.V. The Intriguing Links between Psoriasis and Bullous Pemphigoid. *J. Clin. Med.* **2022**, *12*, 328. [CrossRef] [PubMed]
157. Warner, C.; Kwak, Y.; Glover, M.H.B.; Davis, L.S. Bullous Pemphigoid Induced by Hydrochlorothiazide Therapy. *J. Drugs Dermatol. JDD* **2014**, *13*, 360–362.
158. Tanaka, H.; Ishii, T. Analysis of Patients with Drug-induced Pemphigoid Using the Japanese Adverse Drug Event Report Database. *J. Dermatol.* **2019**, *46*, 240–244. [CrossRef]
159. Lloyd-Lavery, A.; Chi, C.-C.; Wojnarowska, F.; Taghipour, K. The Associations Between Bullous Pemphigoid and Drug Use: A UK Case-Control Study. *JAMA Dermatol.* **2013**, *149*, 58. [CrossRef]
160. Takeichi, S.; Kubo, Y.; Arase, S.; Hashimoto, T.; Ansai, S. Brunsting-Perry Type Localized Bullous Pemphigoid, Possibly Induced by Furosemide Administration and Sun Exposure. *Eur. J. Dermatol.* **2009**, *19*, 500–503. [CrossRef]
161. Lee, J.J.; Downham, T.F. Furosemide-Induced Bullous Pemphigoid: Case Report and Review of Literature. *J. Drugs Dermatol. JDD* **2006**, *5*, 562–564. [PubMed]
162. Ambur, A.B.; Nathoo, R.; Saeed, S. A Case of Drug-Induced Bullous Pemphigoid with an Isomorphic Response and Updated Review of Koebnerization in Bullous Diseases. *Cureus* **2021**, *13*, e20647. [CrossRef] [PubMed]
163. Boulinguez, B.; Bernard, B.; Bedane, B.; Le Brun, L.B.; Bonnetblanc, B. Bonnetblanc Bullous Pemphigoid Induced by Bumetanide. *Br. J. Dermatol.* **1998**, *138*, 548–549. [CrossRef]
164. Wurtz, P.; Borucki, R.; Georgesen, C. A Case of Bullous Pemphigoid Induced by Torsemide. *JAAD Case Rep.* **2022**, *26*, 95–97. [CrossRef] [PubMed]
165. García Sanchez, V.C.; Calle Romero, Y.; De La Peña Parra, E.; Lorenzo Borda, S. Penfigoide ampolloso inducido por hidroclorotiazida. *SEMERGEN—Med. Fam.* **2013**, *39*, 214–217. [CrossRef] [PubMed]
166. Cozzani, E.; Muracchioli, A.; Russo, R.; Burlando, M.; Parodi, A. Acetazolamide: A New Trigger for Bullous Pemphigoid? *Eur. J. Dermatol.* **2020**, *30*, 321–322. [CrossRef]
167. Varpuluoma, O.; Jokelainen, J.; Försti, A.-K.; Turpeinen, M.; Timonen, M.; Huilaja, L.; Tasanen, K. Drugs Used for Neurologic and Psychiatric Conditions Increase the Risk for Bullous Pemphigoid: A Case–Control Study. *J. Am. Acad. Dermatol.* **2019**, *81*, 250–253. [CrossRef]
168. Arslan, D.; Aksakal, A.B.; Erdem, Ö.; Tuncer, M.A. A Case of Drug-Induced Bullous Pemphigoid Associated with Teriflunomide: A Patient with Relapsing Multiple Sclerosis. *Mult. Scler. Relat. Disord.* **2020**, *43*, 102157. [CrossRef]

169. Kridin, K.; Zelber-Sagi, S.; Kridin, M.; Cohen, A.D. Bullous Pemphigoid and Neuropsychiatric Medications: An Influence of Drugs or of Underlying Conditions? *J. Am. Acad. Dermatol.* **2023**, *88*, e137. [CrossRef]
170. Ballout, R.A.; Musharrafieh, U.; Khattar, J. Lisinopril-associated Bullous Pemphigoid in an Elderly Woman: A Case Report of a Rare Adverse Drug Reaction. *Br. J. Clin. Pharmacol.* **2018**, *84*, 2678–2682. [CrossRef]
171. Angelis, E.; Lombardi, M.L.; Grassi, M.; Ruocco, V. Enalapril: A Powerful in Vitro Non-Thiol Acantholytic Agent. *Int. J. Dermatol.* **1992**, *31*, 722–724. [CrossRef] [PubMed]
172. Mallet, L.; Cooper, J.W.; Thomas, J. Bullous Pemphigoid Associated with Captopril. *DICP* **1989**, *23*, 63. [CrossRef]
173. Saraceno, R.; Citarella, L.; Spallone, G.; Chimenti, S. A Biological Approach in a Patient with Psoriasis and Bullous Pemphigoid Associated with Losartan Therapy. *Clin. Exp. Dermatol.* **2008**, *33*, 154–155. [CrossRef] [PubMed]
174. Gao, Z.; Cao, Y.; Zeng, X.; Song, X. Valsartan-associated Bullous Pemphigoid Initially Presenting as Erythema Multiforme. *Health Sci. Rep.* **2021**, *4*, e452. [CrossRef] [PubMed]
175. Park, K.Y.; Kim, B.J.; Kim, M.N. Amlodipine-Associated Bullous Pemphigoid with Erythema Multiforme-like Clinical Features: Correspondence. *Int. J. Dermatol.* **2011**, *50*, 637–639. [CrossRef] [PubMed]
176. Ameen, M.; Harman, K.E.; Black, M.M. Pemphigoid Nodularis Associated with Nifedipine. *Br. J. Dermatol.* **2000**, *142*, 575–577. [CrossRef]
177. Brenner, S.; Ruocco, V.; Bialy-Golan, A.; Tur, E.; Flaminio, C.; Ruocco, E.; Lombardi, M.L. Pemphigus and Pemphigoid-like Effects of Nifedipine on in Vitro Cultured Normal Human Skin Explants: Pemphigus and Pemphigoid-like Effects of Nifedipine. *Int. J. Dermatol.* **1999**, *38*, 36–40. [CrossRef]
178. Papadopoulou, A.; Zafiriou, E.; Koukoulis, G.K.; Roussaki-Schulze, A.V. Drugs Associated with Bullous Pemphigoid: Role of HMG- CO a Reductase Inhibitors. *J. Eur. Acad. Dermatol. Venereol.* **2020**, *34*, e269–e270. [CrossRef]
179. Chang, T.-H.; Wu, C.-Y.; Chang, Y.-T.; Lin, Y.-H.; Wu, C.-Y. The Association between Statins and Subsequent Risk of Bullous Pemphigoid: A Population-Based Cohort Study. *JAAD Int.* **2021**, *3*, 23–25. [CrossRef]
180. Ma, H.-J.; Hu, R.; Jia, C.-Y.; Yang, Y.; Song, L.-J. Case of Drug-Induced Bullous Pemphigoid by Levofloxacin. *J. Dermatol.* **2012**, *39*, 1086–1087. [CrossRef]
181. Cozzani, E.; Chinazzo, C.; Burlando, M.; Romagnoli, M.; Parodi, A. Ciprofloxacin as a Trigger for Bullous Pemphigoid: The Second Case in the Literature. *Am. J. Ther.* **2016**, *23*, e1202–e1204. [CrossRef] [PubMed]

International Journal of *Molecular Sciences*

MDPI

Article

Anti-Fibrotic Effects of RF Electric Currents

María Luisa Hernández-Bule [1,*], Elena Toledano-Macías [1], Luis Alfonso Pérez-González [2], María Antonia Martínez-Pascual [1] and Montserrat Fernández-Guarino [2]

[1] Bioelectromagnetic Laboratory, Instituto Ramón y Cajal de Investigación Sanitaria (Irycis), Carretera de Colmenar Viejo, km. 9.100, 28034 Madrid, Spain; elena.toledano@hrc.es (E.T.-M.); m.antonia.martinez@hrc.es (M.A.M.-P.)

[2] Dermatology Service, Hospital Ramón y Cajal, Instituto Ramón y Cajal de Investigación Sanitaria (Irycis), Carretera de Colmenar Viejo, km. 9.100, 28034 Madrid, Spain; pg.l.alfonso@gmail.com (L.A.P.-G.); drafernandezguarino@gmail.com (M.F.-G.)

* Correspondence: mluisa.hernandez@hrc.es

Abstract: Hypertrophic scars and keloids are two different manifestations of excessive dermal fibrosis and are caused by an alteration in the normal wound-healing process. Treatment with radiofrequency (RF)-based therapies has proven to be useful in reducing hypertrophic scars. In this study, the effect of one of these radiofrequency therapies, Capacitive Resistive Electrical Transfer Therapy (CRET) on biomarkers of skin fibrosis was investigated. For this, in cultures of human myofibroblasts treated with CRET therapy or sham-treated, proliferation (XTT Assay), apoptosis (TUNEL Assay), and cell migration (Wound Closure Assay) were analyzed. Furthermore, in these cultures the expression and/or localization of extracellular matrix proteins such as α-SMA, Col I, Col III (immunofluorescence), metalloproteinases MMP1 and MMP9, MAP kinase ERK1/2, and the transcription factor NFκB were also investigated (immunoblot). The results have revealed that CRET decreases the expression of extracellular matrix proteins, modifies the expression of the metalloproteinase MMP9, and reduces the activation of NFκB with respect to controls, suggesting that this therapy could be useful for the treatment of fibrotic pathologies.

Keywords: fibrosis; hypertrophic scar; keloids; radiofrequency; myofibroblast; metalloproteinase; extracellular matrix proteins; MAP-Kinases; NFκB

Citation: Hernández-Bule, M.L.; Toledano-Macías, E.; Pérez-González, L.A.; Martínez-Pascual, M.A.; Fernández-Guarino, M. Anti-Fibrotic Effects of RF Electric Currents. *Int. J. Mol. Sci.* **2023**, *24*, 10986. https://doi.org/10.3390/ijms241310986

Academic Editors: Walter Wahli and Michal Zmijewski

Received: 10 May 2023
Revised: 21 June 2023
Accepted: 29 June 2023
Published: 1 July 2023

1. Introduction

The wound-healing process comprises a complex succession of events that is organized into three consecutive phases: inflammation phase, proliferation phase, and remodeling phase [1–3].

During the proliferation phase, fibroblasts are activated and acquire the capacity to express alpha smooth muscle actin (α-SMA), differentiating into myofibroblasts. These differentiated fibroblasts allow the wound to contract and close. Once the wound is closed, under normal physiological conditions, the myofibroblasts enter into apoptosis and are replaced by fibroblasts. In wound healing, various biochemical/cellular signals, such as Wnt and Notch signaling, AKT/mTOR, transforming growth factor beta (TGF-β), mitogen-activated protein kinase (MAPK), or binding protein to the nuclear factor kappa enhancer (NF-κB) intervene in a tightly coordinated cascade to repair the damage [4]. When this process is deregulated, abnormal or excessive scarring can occur, leading to the development of cutaneous fibrosis, which clinically manifests as hypertrophic and keloid scars.

Both types of fibrosis are differentiated by their etiology, symptoms, causes, and location, among others [3]. The main causes of hypertrophic scars are surgery, severe burns, trauma, or even insect bites, while keloids usually develop several months or even years after an injury or inflammation of the skin, and can be due to minor skin damage such as piercings, vaccinations, or acne [5]. Although the etiology of keloids is unknown, a strongly associated genetic, racial, and anatomical component has been observed, since they are more frequent in African Americans and Asians, and in the upper part of the thorax or earlobe [6]. Chronic infections and repeated injuries can also promote hypertrophic scar formation and tissue fibrosis [7].

At the tissue level, hypertrophic scars and keloids present hyperplasia, swelling, and redness, with aberrant growth being a specific characteristic of keloids, which usually invades beyond the margins of the original wound, unlike hypertrophic scars, which remain circumscribed to the original margins of the lesion [8]. In both pathologies, the myofibroblasts are not replaced by fibroblasts, but remain in the proliferating lesion with low rates of apoptosis [6]. These myofibroblasts generate persistent chronic inflammation, due to the continuous production of profibrotic cytokines and chemokines, such as TGF-β1, TGF-β2, VEGF, FGF, and CTGF [9], and synthesize a large amount of fibrotic extracellular matrix, composed by collagen types I and III, and α-SMA, which prevents the normal functioning of the affected tissues [10]. This dysfunction causes itching and pain in most patients for long periods of time [11]. In addition, from a psychological point of view, these pathologies generate a negative cosmetic and emotional impact on patients, which can even limit their social interaction and affect their self-esteem [12].

Currently, hypertrophic scars and keloids represent a great challenge for dermatologists and surgeons due to the lack of effective specific treatments. Corticosteroid administration, surgical excision, silicone gels, local radiotherapy, hormonal therapy, or laser have been the conventional treatments, but often do not achieve complete cure, especially in the case of keloids due to high rates of recurrence [13]. There is experimental evidence that hyperthermia induced by radiofrequency (RF) is effective in scar or keloid regeneration treatments. In this regard, clinical evidence indicates that the application of RF [14,15], alone or in combination with other physical therapies such as laser [16] or ultrasound [17], can be effective for the treatment of hypertrophic and keloid scars. Thus, physical therapies induce a remodeling of the collagen derived from the denaturation of the fibers due to hyperthermia. In particular, therapies using capacitive RF have been shown to be useful for reducing hypertrophic scars and increasing the flexibility of fibrotic skin tissue [18]. One of these capacitive therapies is Capacitive Resistive Electrical Transfer Therapy (CRET). This non-invasive therapy uses frequency currents around 0.5 MHz to induce deep heating in the treated tissues. Under thermal conditions, it has been shown to be effective in skin regeneration in animal models through increased skin thickening and an increase in collagen production and angiogenesis [19]. Additionally, previous research by our group has revealed that this therapy, under non-thermal conditions, can promote skin regeneration through fibroblast migration and keratinocytes, fibroblasts, and stem cell proliferation [2,20], as well as induce differentiation [21]. These effects would be mediated by changes in the expression and localization of intercellular adhesion proteins or cell–substrate adhesion proteins, and in kinases involved in cell proliferation and migration. In this way, electrical stimulation would promote the formation of granulation tissue before the closure of the external tissue layers, thus avoiding abnormal healing of the wound or its chronification.

However, in relation to fibrotic processes, besides cases of favorable effects of CRET observed in the clinic, the published experimental evidence is null and the biological bases of these effects are unknown. Given the absence of effective strategies for the treatment of these fibroses, it is of great interest to promote new therapeutic alternatives to the existing ones for their treatment. On this basis, the objective of this study was to investigate, in human cell models under normothermic conditions, the potential capacity of CRET to regenerate already formed hypertrophic or keloid scars and/or to prevent their formation in the initial phases of healing prior to their consolidation, in patients with a clinical predisposition to generate them.

2. Results

2.1. Extracellular Matrix Production

The immunoblot revealed a statistically significant reduction of 20 ± 6.3% ($p = 0.011$; Student's t-test) over the control in α-SMA expression, in cultures treated with CRET for 48 h (Figure 1A). This protein was also analyzed with immunofluorescence, and image analysis confirmed the decrease (38% over controls) in the amount of α-SMA in CRET-treated cultures versus controls (Figure 1B,C). Furthermore, collagen type I also decreased by 23% and collagen type III content by 16%, compared to the control. The results were statistically significant in all three analyses (Figure 1B,C).

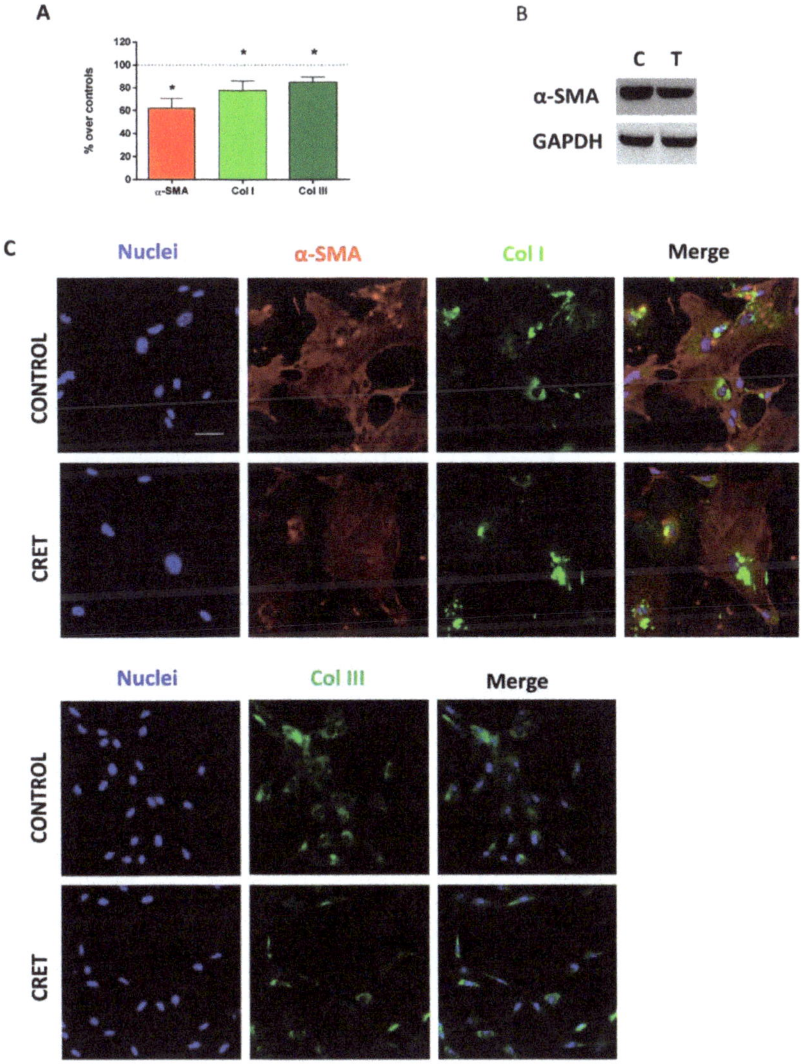

Figure 1. α-SMA, Col I and Col III expression. (**A**) α-SMA, Col I, and Col III protein expression of myofibroblasts at 48 h of CRET or sham treatment. Fluorescence intensity measurement per MHC channel. Data normalized over the corresponding sham-exposed controls (dashed line represents the

over the corresponding sham-exposed controls (dashed line represents the control group 100%). Means ± SD of the protein/GAPDH ratios of at least three experimental repeats per protein and time interval. **: $0.001 \leq p < 0.01$. *: $0.05 > p \geq 0.01$. Student's *t*-test. (**B**) Representative blots at 12 h or 24 h of CRET or sham treatment (100 μg protein/lane). GAPDH were used as loading control. C: Control. T: CRET treatment.

3. Discussion

Cutaneous fibrosis is a skin pathology that involves pain, itching, lack of functionality and psychological problems for patients who suffer from it. The main treatments for hypertrophic scars or keloids are not considered fully satisfactory since they are not very effective, can cause pain, or have adverse side effects. Laser is one of the first line treatments, however, it is expensive and requires repeated sessions. Other alternatives, such as intralesional treatments with corticosteroids, bleomycin, or 5-fluorouracil are painful and require multiple infiltrations. Local radiotherapy is a good treatment alternative but it needs to be applied in specialized centers and in several sessions that produce the patient's radiation. In any case, the approach needs to be multidirectional, which is why the combination of treatments is generally chosen. For this reason, these fibroses represent a challenge for medicine, and it is of great interest to find alternative therapies for their treatment.

Currently, progress is being made in understanding the molecular mechanism of these fibroses, which is generating new therapeutic strategies for the treatment of this pathology. Since the pathological characteristics of cutaneous fibrosis are characterized by an excess of extracellular matrix produced by fibroblasts at the tissue level, the action mechanisms of these new therapies aim to achieve one or more of the following objectives: reduction or inhibition of the proliferation of fibroblasts and myofibroblasts, reduction or inhibition of the production of extracellular matrix (collagen, α -SMA and fibronectin), increased apoptosis or necrosis of fibroblasts, decreased expression of TGF-β1 (a key regulator of collagen synthesis), decreased expression of the GFR β1/Smad2/3 signaling pathway, changes in the activity of metalloproteinases, decreased or modulated inflammation, and/or increased production of IFN-α (due to its antifibrogenic capacity or increased normal angiogenic activity) [22]. In this study we have investigated whether CRET therapy can act on one or several of these key action mechanisms in skin fibrosis.

Due to the relevance of extracellular matrix (ECM) production in the generation of the fibrotic process, we first investigated whether CRET could reduce the synthesis of matrix components or degrade the existing one. In fact, numerous investigations aimed at finding new pharmacological strategies focus on the reduction of collagen and extracellular matrix deposits such as hypertensives including the angiotensin-converting enzyme ACE-inhibitor [23], calcineurin inhibitors [24], doxorubicin [25], shock wave therapy [25,26], stem cell therapy, interferons [5], tamoxifen [27], or RNA-based therapies [28]. Some electrical therapies have also shown the ability to reduce collagen deposits in fibrotic processes through its degradation. Thus, electrical therapies with degenerate waves have shown an improvement in pain and itching, as well as a reduction in the formation of excess collagen in keloids [29]. In RF-based therapies, treatment of hypertrophic scars with moderate thermal increases (below 40 °C) generated by monopolar radiofrequency induces remodeling of collagen fibers, whether applied as a single therapy [14] or in association with negative pressure [18]. Other RF therapies have also shown changes in the morphology or production of collagen fiber [15] or a reduction in the amount of collagen I, collagen III, and TGF-β1 in scars, when RF is combined with pulsed light versus laser [16]. In our study conducted under subthermal conditions, CRET treatment of myofibroblasts significantly decreased the amount of collagen type I, type III, and α-SMA in their ECM. It is known that the changes induced in the connective tissue by RF-based therapies are not explained solely by the increase in temperature [30]. Given that the CRET therapy in our experiments has been applied under normothermia conditions (37 °C), the changes observed in the collagen content would not be related to denaturation and rearrangement of the fibers but to other molecular mechanisms such as the modulation of the activity of metalloproteinases (MMPs) or the Smad2/3 pathway.

Indeed, MMPs also seem to play a critical role in wound healing and scar formation, and their inhibition could be a strategy to treat fibrosis. MMPs are endopeptidases with a catalytic domain of Zn^{2+} ions that interact with multiple components of the extracellular matrix [31]. It has been reported that the expression of MMPs is elevated in skin lesions compared to intact skin, while hypertrophic scar fibroblasts appear to have low MMP-1 [32] and MMP9 [33] activity, which would favor the accumulation of collagen. For this reason, some novel therapies have sought to modulate the expression of MMPs. Thus, for example, shock waves have been shown to be capable of reducing the collagen fibers of keloids due to increases in the expression of MMP13 [25], while stem cell therapies attenuated the expression of tissue inhibitor of metalloproteinases 1 (TIMP-1) in keloid fibroblasts [34], which would promote the activity of MMPs. Similarly, pressure therapies were able to increase the expression of MMP9 and MMP12 in tissue from hypertrophic scars [35]. In this study, it was analyzed whether the observed decrease in electrically induced collagen expression and content could be due to a modulation in the expression of two of these MMPs: MMP1 and MMP9. The results showed that MMP9 increases significantly after 24 h of CRET treatment, while no changes in MMP1 expression were detected compared to the control. Thus, this activation of MMP9 could be responsible for the degradation of collagen I and collagen III observed after electrical stimulation, which would promote the reduction of fibrosis in CRET treatments.

Another of the objectives pursued by numerous emerging therapies for the treatment of fibrosis is the reduction of the proliferation of fibroblasts, responsible for most of the collagen and ECM deposition that occurs in wound healing, both normal and pathological. These actions are promoted by fibrogenic growth factors, such as TGF-β1, PDGF, fibroblast growth factor β (FGF-β), and insulin-like growth factor I (IGF-I). Fibroblasts isolated from keloid tissue have elevated expressions of TGF-β1, periostin, PAI-2, and inhibin beta A compared to normal healthy tissues [6]. For this reason, numerous therapies have focused on reducing the proliferation of fibroblasts such as the ACE-inhibitor lisinopril [23], botulinum toxin [36], calcineurin inhibitors [24], doxorubicin [37], microneedles [38], stem cell therapy [34,39], imidazoquinolines [40], or interferons [5]. CRET therapy has been shown to slightly reduce myofibroblast proliferation and decrease ERK1/2 expression relative to control, which could lead to an anti-proliferative effect. However, since no changes in the activation of the protein were observed, but only in its expression, and the effect on proliferation was weak, it is possible that such changes play a secondary role in the potential anti-fibrotic effect of the CRET therapy. Furthermore, in wound regeneration, proliferating mesenchymal stem cells (MSCs) play a key role, and recent studies have shown that exosomal microRNA derived from adipose-derived mesenchymal stem cells (ADSC) suppresses proliferation and exerts a pro-angiogenic role in keloid fibroblasts [41]. Therefore, a therapy that promotes stem cell proliferation could improve tissue fibrosis. This is the case of CRET therapy, which is capable of promoting the proliferation of ADSC [20]. Thus, CRET could also reduce or prevent the generation of hypertrophic scars by promoting stem cell proliferation while reducing that of myofibroblasts.

On the other hand, fibroblasts derived from hypertrophic scars overexpress transglutaminase that could inhibit their apoptosis, thus enhancing the fibrotic phenotype by increasing the number of cells capable of generating extracellular matrix [42]. For this reason, this enzyme has been the target of physical therapies such as degenerate electrical waveform stimulation in combination with photodynamic therapy [43]. In our study, treatment with CRET induced a decrease in apoptosis in cultures compared to those not treated electrically, although the actual proportion of apoptosis detected was very low. The proliferative phase of wound healing also involves the active migration of fibroblasts [6]. In our CRET assays, the myofibroblast migratory rate did not change with respect to control. Therefore, CRET would not significantly alter the migration and apoptosis processes of myofibroblasts.

The skin is considered a neuroendocrine organ that has immunological, endocrine, and neurological functions to maintain the body's homeostasis. For this reason, its resident cells, and the circulating cells of the immune system express neuropeptides and neurotransmitters, and produce endocrine factors and cytokines in response to stress [44]. This organizational system has been called the cutaneous hypothalamus-pituitary-adrenal axis (cHPA) and its functions are regulated through two main signaling pathways: the corticotropin-releasing hormone (CRH) pathway, and the proopiomelancortin (POMC) pathway.

Skin cells activate the CRH signaling pathway under physiological, pathological conditions, or after stimulation with microbial antigens or UVB spectrum radiation. Through the CRH pathway, these cells regulate cell proliferation and differentiation, as well as activities of the immune or endocrine system [45]. CRH can act as a pro-inflammatory agent since it has been described that the activation of this CRH pathway stimulates the activity of NFkB [46], a key transcription factor that regulates a multitude of genes responsible for triggering the inflammatory response. NFkB has been shown to be activated in keratinocytes and fibroblasts from keloids [8]. Furthermore, in fibrosis, myofibroblasts generate persistent chronic inflammation, due to the continuous production of profibrotic cytokines and chemokines, such as TGF-β1, TGF-β2, VEGF, FGF, and CTGF [9].

NFkB is also modulated by the proopiomelanocortin POMC signaling pathway. In skin cells such as keratinocytes, NFkB is indirectly inhibited by α-melanocyte-stimulating hormones (α-MSH) [45], while in fibroblasts, α-MSH reduces NFkB activation [47]. On the other hand, POMC gene expression, and POMC peptides and proteins production, can be enhanced by electromagnetic radiation such as UVB, among others [45]. Recent studies show that therapies based on the POMC pathway could be a new therapeutic strategy for the treatment of diseases related to fibrotic conditions, since melanocortin drugs have been shown to be able to reduce collagen deposition, myofibroblast activation, and the production of pro-inflammatory mediators [47]. The results of our study show that CRET decreases the activation of NFkB in myofibroblasts, and reduces the expression of collagens through MMP9. Considering these results, and given that POMC and CRH are activated by electromagnetic radiation, it cannot be ruled out that CRET radiofrequency currents could also act through these POMC- or CRH-signaling pathways. If so, CRET physical treatment could reduce the pro-inflammatory response in myofibroblasts through this cutaneous neuroendocrine mechanism, without excluding other potential pathways yet to be studied.

4. Materials and Methods

4.1. Cell Culture

Human dermal fibroblasts (HF) isolated from neonatal foreskin (cat. no. C-004-5C, Thermo Fisher, Carlsbad, CA, USA) were seeded in medium composed of high-glucose D-MEM (Biowhittaker, Lonza, Verviers, Belgium) supplemented with 10% inactivated fetal bovine serum (Gibco, Waltham, MA, USA), 1% glutamine, and 1% penicillin-streptomycin (Gibco) and maintained in a 5% CO_2 atmosphere at a temperature of 37 °C inside CO_2 incubators (Thermo Fisher Scientific, Waltham, MA, USA). The cells were subcultured once a week.

HF were plated at 450 cells/cm^2 density on the bottom of 60 mm Petri dishes (Nunc, Roskilde, Denmark), except for immunofluorescence assays, in which the cells were seeded on glass coverslips placed on the bottom of the plates. One day after seeding, cells were incubated with complete DMEM supplemented with 2 ng/mL of TGF-β1 (Peprotech, Rocky Hill, NJ, USA) for an additional 12 or 13 days depending on the experiment, renewing this conditioned culture medium every 4 days (Figure S1). Depending on the aim of the corresponding experiment, a total of 5 or 10 Petri dishes were used for experimental replicate.

4.2. Electric Treatment

The procedure for RF exposure has been described in detail elsewhere [48,49]. Briefly, 11 days after seeding, pairs of sterile stainless-steel electrodes designed ad hoc for in vitro stimulation were inserted in all Petri dishes and connected in series. Only the electrodes of dishes for electrical stimulation were energized using a signal generator (Indiba Activ HCR 902, INDIBA®, Barcelona, Spain), while the remaining plates were sham-exposed simultaneously inside an identical, separate CO_2 incubator. The intermittent stimulation pattern consisted of 5-min pulses of 448 kHz, sine wave current delivered at subthermal densities of 100 $\mu A/mm^2$, separated by 4-h interpulse lapses, and administered for a total of 12, 24, or 48 h. Such exposure parameters have been shown to stimulate the proliferation and early differentiation of human, adipose-derived stem cells [20,21,50] and in human dermal fibroblasts and keratinocytes [2].

4.3. *XTT Proliferation Assay*

Cell proliferation was determined with XTT assay (Roche, Switzerland). After 48 h of CRET or sham treatment, the cells were incubated for 3 h with the tetrazolium salt XTT in a 37 °C and 6.5% CO_2 atmosphere, as recommended by the manufacturer. The cell culture confluence reached 60–70%. The metabolically active cells reduced XTT into colored formazan compounds that were quantified with a microplate reader (TECAN, Männedorf, Switzerland) at a 492 nm wavelength. At least 3 experimental replicates per cell type were conducted.

4.4. *TUNEL Assay*

Apoptosis in cultures was assessed with the TUNEL assay. For this, the DeadEnd™ Fluorometric TUNEL System (Promega, Madison, WI, USA) was used. Cells treated for 48 h with CRET or sham exposure were fixed with 4% paraformaldehyde (Merck, Darmstadt, Germany) and then proceeded according to the manufacturer's instructions. The fluorescence of apoptotic cells was detected with fluorescence microscopy. Nuclei were counterstained with ProLongTM Gold antifade reagent whit DAPI (Invitrogen, Eugene, OR, USA). TUNEL+ cells were assessed using an inverted fluorescence microscope (Nikon Eclipse Ts2R, Nikon, Tokyo, Japan) coupled to a digital camera (Nikon DS-Ri2). Photomicrographs were taken and the images were computer-analyzed with NIS-Elements Br image software (version 4.40, Nikon, Japan). TUNEL+ cell identification and quantification were based on fixed thresholds of fluorescence (MHC mode) determined and automated for all images at the beginning of the analysis. The values obtained were normalized with respect to the number of cells per field. Three experimental replicates were performed.

4.5. *Wound Assay*

In each experimental replicate of the wound closure assay, HF were seeded on 8 plates and incubated at 37 °C. After 10 days of incubation with TGF-β1, a wound was scratched on the confluent monolayer of each of the plates, using a glass pipette tip. Dishes were washed with PBS (Gibco) to eliminate debris, and the cultures were maintained in high-glucose D-MEM medium supplemented with 10% inactivated fetal bovine serum (Gibco), 1% glutamine, 1% penicillin-streptomycin (Gibco), and 2 ng/mL of TGF-β1. Next, 4 plates were exposed to CRET for 24 or 48 h, while the remaining plates were sham-exposed for the same intervals. At 0, 24 and 48 h after scratching, 6 micrographs were taken of 3 equidistant points in the wounds, using a digital camera (Nikon DS-Ri2) coupled to an inverted microscope (Nikon Eclipse Ts2R). The wound closure rate was determined with dual analyses of the obtained images, using standard Photoshop software (Adobe Photoshop CS3, Extended version 10.0). Five experimental replicates were performed.

4.6. *Immunofluorescence for α-SMA, Collagen Type I and Collagen Type III*

At the end of 48 h RF- or sham-exposure, the samples were fixed with 4% paraformaldehyde (Merck, Darmstadt, Germany) and incubated overnight at 4 °C with mouse monoclonal anti- α-smooth muscle actin antibody α-SMA (1:400; cat. no. A 2547; Sigma Aldrich, St. Louis, MO, USA), rabbit polyclonal anti-collagen type I antibody (1:400; cat. no. NB600-408-0.1 mg; Novus; Centennial, CO, USA) and rabbit polyclonal anti-collagen type III alpha 1 antibody (1:400, cat. no. NB600-594SS; Novus; CO, USA). Afterwards, the samples were fluorescence-stained with Alexa Fluor^{TM} 568 goat anti-mouse IgG (1:500; cat. no. A11031; Invitrogen; Eugene, OR, USA) or Alexa Fluor^{TM} 488 goat anti-rabbit IgG (1:500; cat. no. A11031; Invitrogen) for 1 h at room temperature, and the cell nuclei were counterstained with ProLong^{TM} Gold antifade reagent whit DAPI (Invitrogen). Photomicrographs were taken using an inverted fluorescence microscope (Nikon Eclipse Ts2R) coupled to a digital camera (Nikon DS-Ri2) and the images were computer-analyzed with NIS-Elements Br image software (Nikon). Fluorescence intensity measurement per MHC channel was used to assess the fluorescence of samples labeled with Alexa Green or Alexa Red. Prior to analysis, MHC mode fluorescence thresholds were set and applied to all images. The values obtained were normalized with respect to the number of cells per field. At least three replicates of each protein were performed.

4.7. Immunoblot for α-SMA, MMP1, MMP9, ERK, P-ERK, NF-κB and p-NF-κB

Cultures were RF- or sham-exposed for 12 or 24 h. At the end of electric treatment, the cells were lysed for protein extraction. The immunoblot procedure has been described in detail elsewhere [21,48]. Briefly, the protein samples (100 µg protein aliquots) were separated in 10% sodium dodecyl sulphate-polyacrylamide gel and electrophoretically transferred to nitrocellulose membrane (Amersham, Buckinghamshire, UK). Blots were incubated at 4 °C overnight in mouse monoclonal anti- α-smooth muscle actin antibody α-SMA (1:400; cat. no. A 2547; Sigma Aldrich), rabbit monoclonal anti-MMP-9 antibody (1:1000, cat. no. ab76003; Abcam, Cambridge, UK), rabbit monoclonal anti-MMP1 antibody (1:1000; cat. no. ab134184; Abcam), rabbit monoclonal anti-p44/42 MAPK (ERK1/2) (1:1000; cat.no. 4695; Cell Signaling, Danvers, MA, USA), rabbit polyclonal anti Phospho-ERK1/ERK2), mouse monoclonal anti-NF-KB p65 (f-6) (1:1000; cat.no.sc-800; Santa Cruz, CA, USA), and rabbit monoclonal anti-phospho-NF-κB p65 (Ser536) (93H1) (1:1000; cat.no. 3033; Cell Signaling). Rabbit polyclonal anti-GAPDH antibody (1:500, cat. No. sc-25778; Santa Cruz Biotechnology) was used as loading controls. The membranes were incubated for one hour at room temperature with anti-mouse IgG horseradish peroxidase conjugated antibody (1:10,000 NA931; GE Heathcare, Hatfield, UK) and with anti-rabbit IgG horseradish peroxidase conjugated antibody (1:5000 NA934; GE Heathcare). Then, the membranes were scanned with a Bio-Rad imaging system (Hercules, CA, USA). The obtained bands were densitometry evaluated (PDI Quantity One 4.5.2 software, BioRad). At least three experimental replicates were conducted per protein. All values were normalized over the loading control.

4.8. Statistical Analysis

All procedures and analyses were conducted in blind conditions for treatment. At least three independent replicates were conducted per experiment or exposure interval. Results were expressed as means ± standard deviation (SD) or standard error of the mean (SEM). Unpaired Student's *t*-test was applied using GraphPad Prism 6.01 software (GraphPad Software, San Diego, CA, USA). Differences $p < 0.05$ were considered significant statistically.

5. Conclusions

This study reveals that CRET therapy could act on cutaneous fibrosis, reducing the fibrotic extracellular matrix, intervening in the control of the expression of the proteins involved in its degradation, and reducing the activation of pro-inflammatory transcription factors such as NFkB. Thus, this study provides some of the biological bases of the effects of CRET. However, although the results would suggest the utility of this therapy for the treatment of cutaneous fibrosis, a deeper understanding of the cellular and molecular mechanisms of response to CRET is necessary. On the other hand, this study was carried out in vitro, which is a limitation for direct extrapolation to patients. Thus, it is essential to carry out studies at the organism level and preferably in humans through clinical trials, to determine the real usefulness of CRET therapy in this pathology.

Supplementary Materials: The following supporting information can be downloaded at: https://www.mdpi.com/article/10.3390/ijms241310986/s1.

Author Contributions: Conceptualization, M.L.H.-B.; methodology, M.L.H.-B. and M.A.M.-P.; software, E.T.-M. and M.L.H.-B.; validation, M.L.H.-B.; formal analysis, M.L.H.-B.; investigation, M.L.H.-B., E.T.-M., M.F.-G., M.A.M.-P. and L.A.P.-G.; resources, M.L.H.-B. and M.A.M.-P.; data curation, M.L.H.-B. and E.T.-M.; writing—original draft preparation, M.L.H.-B.; writing—review and editing, M.L.H.-B., E.T.-M., M.F.-G., M.A.M.-P. and L.A.P.-G.; visualization, M.L.H.-B., E.T.-M., M.F.-G., M.A.M.-P. and L.A.P.-G.; supervision, M.L.H.-B.; project administration, M.L.H.-B.; funding acquisition, M.L.H.-B. All authors have read and agreed to the published version of the manuscript.

Funding: This work was financially supported by Fundación para la Investigación Biomédica del Hospital Ramón y Cajal, through Project FiBio-HRC No. 2015/0050.

Institutional Review Board Statement: Not applicable.

Informed Consent Statement: Not applicable.

Data Availability Statement: The data presented in this study are available on request from the corresponding author. The data are not publicly available due to privacy restrictions.

Conflicts of Interest: The authors declare no conflict of interest.

References

1. Martin, P.; Nunan, R. Cellular and Molecular Mechanisms of Repair in Acute and Chronic Wound Healing. *Br. J. Dermatol.* **2015**, *173*, 370–378. [CrossRef] [PubMed]
2. Hernández-Bule, M.L.; Toledano-Macías, E.; Naranjo, A.; de Andrés-Zamora, M.; Úbeda, A. In Vitro Stimulation with Radiofrequency Currents Promotes Proliferation and Migration in Human Keratinocytes and Fibroblasts. *Electromagn. Biol. Med.* **2021**, *40*, 338–352. [CrossRef] [PubMed]
3. Fernández-Guarino, M.; Bacci, S.; Pérez González, L.A.; Bermejo-Martínez, M.; Cecilia-Matilla, A.; Hernández-Bule, M.L. The Role of Physical Therapies in Wound Healing and Assisted Scarring. *Int. J. Mol. Sci.* **2023**, *24*, 7487. [CrossRef]
4. Park, Y.R.; Sultan, M.T.; Park, H.J.; Lee, J.M.; Ju, H.W.; Lee, O.J.; Lee, D.J.; Kaplan, D.L.; Park, C.H. NF-KB Signaling Is Key in the Wound Healing Processes of Silk Fibroin. *Acta Biomater.* **2018**, *67*, 183–195. [CrossRef] [PubMed]
5. Lee, H.J.; Jang, Y.J. Recent Understandings of Biology, Prophylaxis and Treatment Strategies for Hypertrophic Scars and Keloids. *Int. J. Mol. Sci.* **2018**, *19*, 711. [CrossRef] [PubMed]
6. Andrews, J.P.; Marttala, J.; Macarak, E.; Rosenbloom, J.; Uitto, J. Keloids: The Paradigm of Skin Fibrosis—Pathomechanisms and Treatment. *Matrix Biol.* **2016**, *51*, 37–46. [CrossRef]
7. Vinaik, R.; Barayan, D.; Auger, C.; Abdullahi, A.; Jeschke, M.G. Regulation of Glycolysis and the Warburg Effect in Wound Healing. *JCI Insight* **2020**, *5*, e138949. [CrossRef]
8. Wang, Z.-C.; Zhao, W.-Y.; Cao, Y.; Liu, Y.-Q.; Sun, Q.; Shi, P.; Cai, J.-Q.; Shen, X.Z.; Tan, W.-Q. The Roles of Inflammation in Keloid and Hypertrophic Scars. *Front. Immunol.* **2020**, *11*, 603187. [CrossRef]
9. Lingzhi, Z.; Meirong, L.; Xiaobing, F. Biological Approaches for Hypertrophic Scars. *Int. Wound J.* **2020**, *17*, 405–418. [CrossRef]
10. Jiang, D.; Rinkevich, Y. Scars or Regeneration?—Dermal Fibroblasts as Drivers of Diverse Skin Wound Responses. *Int. J. Mol. Sci.* **2020**, *21*, 617. [CrossRef]
11. Lee, S.-S.; Yosipovitch, G.; Chan, Y.-H.; Goh, C.-L. Pruritus, Pain, and Small Nerve Fiber Function in Keloids: A Controlled Study. *J. Am. Acad. Dermatol.* **2004**, *51*, 1002–1006. [CrossRef] [PubMed]
12. González, N.; Goldberg, D.J. Update on the Treatment of Scars. *J. Drugs Dermatol.* **2019**, *18*, 550–555. [PubMed]
13. Arno, A.I.; Gauglitz, G.G.; Barret, J.P.; Jeschke, M.G. Up-to-Date Approach to Manage Keloids and Hypertrophic Scars: A Useful Guide. *Burns* **2014**, *40*, 1255–1266. [CrossRef] [PubMed]
14. Pinheiro, N.M.; Melo, P.R.; Crema, V.O.; Mendonça, A.C. Effects of Radiofrequency Procedure on Hypertrophic Scar Due to Burns. *J. Eur. Acad. Dermatol. Venereol.* **2015**, *29*, 187–189. [CrossRef] [PubMed]
15. Meshkinpour, A.; Ghasri, P.; Pope, K.; Lyubovitsky, J.G.; Risteli, J.; Krasieva, T.B.; Kelly, K.M. Treatment of Hypertrophic Scars and Keloids with a Radiofrequency Device: A Study of Collagen Effects. *Lasers Surg. Med.* **2005**, *37*, 343–349. [CrossRef] [PubMed]
16. Khedr, M.M.; Mahmoud, W.H.; Sallam, F.A.; Elmelegy, N. Comparison of Nd:YAG Laser and Combined Intense Pulsed Light and Radiofrequency in the Treatment of Hypertrophic Scars: A Prospective Clinico-Histopathological Study. *Ann. Plast. Surg.* **2020**, *84*, 518–524. [CrossRef]
17. Trelles, M.A.; Martínez-Carpio, P.A. Clinical and Histological Results in the Treatment of Atrophic and Hypertrophic Scars Using a Combined Method of Radiofrequency, Ultrasound, and Transepidermal Drug Delivery. *Int. J. Dermatol.* **2016**, *55*, 926–933. [CrossRef]
18. Nicoletti, G.; Perugini, P.; Bellino, S.; Capra, P.; Malovini, A.; Jaber, O.; Tresoldi, M.; Faga, A. Scar Remodeling with the Association of Monopolar Capacitive Radiofrequency, Electric Stimulation, and Negative Pressure. *Photomed. Laser Surg.* **2017**, *35*, 246–258. [CrossRef]

19. Meyer, P.F.; de Oliveira, P.; Silva, F.K.B.A.; da Costa, A.C.S.; Pereira, C.R.A.; Casenave, S.; Valentim Silva, R.M.; Araújo-Neto, L.G.; Santos-Filho, S.D.; Aizamaque, E.; et al. Radiofrequency Treatment Induces Fibroblast Growth Factor 2 Expression and Subsequently Promotes Neocollagenesis and Neoangiogenesis in the Skin Tissue. *Lasers Med. Sci.* **2017**, *32*, 1727–1736. [CrossRef]
20. Hernández-Bule, M.L.; Paíno, C.L.; Trillo, M.Á.; Úbeda, A. Electric Stimulation at 448 KHz Promotes Proliferation of Human Mesenchymal Stem Cells. *Cell. Physiol. Biochem.* **2014**, *34*, 1741–1755. [CrossRef]
21. Hernandez Bule, M.L.; Angeles Trillo, M.; Martinez Garcia, M.A.; Abilahoud, C.; Ubeda, A. Chondrogenic Differentiation of Adipose-Derived Stem Cells by Radiofrequency Electric Stimulation. *J. Stem Cell Res. Ther.* **2017**, *7*, 12. [CrossRef]
22. Memariani, H.; Memariani, M.; Moravvej, H.; Shahidi-Dadras, M. Emerging and Novel Therapies for Keloids: A Compendious Review. *Sultan Qaboos Univ. Med. J.* **2021**, *21*, e22–e33. [CrossRef] [PubMed]
23. Fang, Q.-Q.; Wang, X.-F.; Zhao, W.-Y.; Ding, S.-L.; Shi, B.-H.; Xia, Y.; Yang, H.; Wu, L.-H.; Li, C.-Y.; Tan, W.-Q. Angiotensin-Converting Enzyme Inhibitor Reduces Scar Formation by Inhibiting Both Canonical and Noncanonical TGF-B1 Pathways. *Sci. Rep.* **2018**, *8*, 3332. [CrossRef] [PubMed]
24. Wu, C.-S.; Wu, P.-H.; Fang, A.-H.; Lan, C.-C.E. FK506 Inhibits the Enhancing Effects of Transforming Growth Factor (TGF)-B1 on Collagen Expression and TGF-β/Smad Signalling in Keloid Fibroblasts: Implication for New Therapeutic Approach. *Br. J. Dermatol.* **2012**, *167*, 532–541. [CrossRef]
25. Wang, C.-J.; Ko, J.-Y.; Chou, W.-Y.; Cheng, J.-H.; Kuo, Y.-R. Extracorporeal Shockwave Therapy for Treatment of Keloid Scars. *Wound Repair Regen.* **2018**, *26*, 69–76. [CrossRef]
26. Cui, H.S.; Hong, A.R.; Kim, J.-B.; Yu, J.H.; Cho, Y.S.; Joo, S.Y.; Seo, C.H. Extracorporeal Shock Wave Therapy Alters the Expression of Fibrosis-Related Molecules in Fibroblast Derived from Human Hypertrophic Scar. *Int. J. Mol. Sci.* **2018**, *19*, 124. [CrossRef]
27. Soares-Lopes, L.R.; Soares-Lopes, I.M.; Filho, L.L.; Alencar, A.P.; da Silva, B.B. Morphological and Morphometric Analysis of the Effects of Intralesional Tamoxifen on Keloids. *Exp. Biol. Med.* **2017**, *242*, 926–929. [CrossRef]
28. Aoki, M.; Miyake, K.; Ogawa, R.; Dohi, T.; Akaishi, S.; Hyakusoku, H.; Shimada, T. SiRNA Knockdown of Tissue Inhibitor of Metalloproteinase-1 in Keloid Fibroblasts Leads to Degradation of Collagen Type I. *J. Investig. Dermatol.* **2014**, *134*, 818–826. [CrossRef]
29. Perry, D.; Colthurst, J.; Giddings, P.; McGrouther, D.A.; Morris, J.; Bayat, A. Treatment of Symptomatic Abnormal Skin Scars with Electrical Stimulation. *J. Wound Care* **2010**, *19*, 447–453. [CrossRef]
30. Nicoletti, G.; Cornaglia, A.I.; Faga, A.; Scevola, S. The Biological Effects of Quadripolar Radiofrequency Sequential Application: A Human Experimental Study. *Photomed. Laser Surg.* **2014**, *32*, 561–573. [CrossRef]
31. Chuang, H.-M.; Chen, Y.-S.; Harn, H.-J. The Versatile Role of Matrix Metalloproteinase for the Diverse Results of Fibrosis Treatment. *Molecules* **2019**, *24*, 4188. [CrossRef]
32. Eto, H.; Suga, H.; Aoi, N.; Kato, H.; Doi, K.; Kuno, S.; Tabata, Y.; Yoshimura, K. Therapeutic Potential of Fibroblast Growth Factor-2 for Hypertrophic Scars: Upregulation of MMP-1 and HGF Expression. *Lab. Investig.* **2012**, *92*, 214–223. [CrossRef]
33. Xue, M.; Jackson, C.J. Extracellular Matrix Reorganization During Wound Healing and Its Impact on Abnormal Scarring. *Adv. Wound Care* **2015**, *4*, 119–136. [CrossRef] [PubMed]
34. Wang, X.; Ma, Y.; Gao, Z.; Yang, J. Human Adipose-Derived Stem Cells Inhibit Bioactivity of Keloid Fibroblasts. *Stem Cell Res. Ther.* **2018**, *9*, 40. [CrossRef] [PubMed]
35. Dong, H.; Kuan-hong, S.; Hong-gang, W. Pressure Therapy Upregulates Matrix Metalloproteinase Expression and Downregulates Collagen Expression in Hypertrophic Scar Tissue. *Chin. Med. J.* **2013**, *126*, 3321–3324.
36. Austin, E.; Koo, E.; Jagdeo, J. The Cellular Response of Keloids and Hypertrophic Scars to Botulinum Toxin A: A Comprehensive Literature Review. *Dermatol. Surg.* **2018**, *44*, 149–157. [CrossRef]
37. Sasaki, T.; Holeyfield, K.C.; Uitto, J. Doxorubicin-Induced Inhibition of Prolyl Hydroxylation during Collagen Biosynthesis in Human Skin Fibroblast Cultures. Relevance to Imparied Wound Healing. *J. Clin. Investig.* **1987**, *80*, 1735–1741. [CrossRef]
38. Yeo, D.C.; Balmayor, E.R.; Schantz, J.-T.; Xu, C. Microneedle Physical Contact as a Therapeutic for Abnormal Scars. *Eur. J. Med. Res.* **2017**, *22*, 28. [CrossRef]
39. Fang, F.; Huang, R.-L.; Zheng, Y.; Liu, M.; Huo, R. Bone Marrow Derived Mesenchymal Stem Cells Inhibit the Proliferative and Profibrotic Phenotype of Hypertrophic Scar Fibroblasts and Keloid Fibroblasts through Paracrine Signaling. *J. Dermatol. Sci.* **2016**, *83*, 95–105. [CrossRef]
40. Lin, W.-C.; Liou, S.-H.; Kotsuchibashi, Y. Development and Characterisation of the Imiquimod Poly(2-(2-Methoxyethoxy)Ethyl Methacrylate) Hydrogel Dressing for Keloid Therapy. *Polymers* **2017**, *9*, 579. [CrossRef]
41. Wu, D.; Liu, X.; Jin, Z. Adipose-derived Mesenchymal Stem Cells-sourced Exosomal microRNA-7846-3p Suppresses Proliferation and Pro-angiogenic Role of Keloid Fibroblasts by Suppressing Neuropilin 2. *J. Cosmet. Dermatol.* 2023, ahead of print. [CrossRef]
42. Linge, C.; Richardson, J.; Vigor, C.; Clayton, E.; Hardas, B.; Rolfe, K.J. Hypertrophic Scar Cells Fail to Undergo a Form of Apoptosis Specific to Contractile Collagen—The Role of Tissue Transglutaminase. *J. Investig. Dermatol.* **2005**, *125*, 72–82. [CrossRef] [PubMed]
43. Sebastian, A.; Syed, F.; McGrouther, D.A.; Colthurst, J.; Paus, R.; Bayat, A. A Novel in Vitro Assay for Electrophysiological Research on Human Skin Fibroblasts: Degenerate Electrical Waves Downregulate Collagen I Expression in Keloid Fibroblasts. *Exp. Dermatol.* **2011**, *20*, 64–68. [CrossRef] [PubMed]
44. Slominski, A.; Wortsman, J. Neuroendocrinology of the Skin1. *Endocr. Rev.* **2000**, *21*, 457–487. [CrossRef] [PubMed]
45. Slominski, A.T.; Slominski, R.M.; Raman, C.; Chen, J.Y.; Athar, M.; Elmets, C. Neuroendocrine Signaling in the Skin with a Special Focus on the Epidermal Neuropeptides. *Am. J. Physiol.-Cell Physiol.* **2022**, *323*, C1757–C1776. [CrossRef] [PubMed]

46. Zbytek, B.; Pfeffer, L.; Slominski, A. Corticotropin-Releasing Hormone Stimulates NF-KappaB in Human Epidermal Keratinocytes. *J. Endocrinol.* **2004**, *181*, R1–R7. [CrossRef]
47. Khodeneva, N.; Sugimoto, M.A.; Davan-Wetton, C.S.A.; Montero-Melendez, T. Melanocortin Therapies to Resolve Fibroblast-Mediated Diseases. *Front. Immunol.* **2023**, *13*, 1084394. [CrossRef]
48. Hernández-Bule, M.L.; Trillo, M.A.; Cid, M.A.; Leal, J.; Ubeda, A. In Vitro Exposure to 0.57-MHz Electric Currents Exerts Cytostatic Effects in HepG2 Human Hepatocarcinoma Cells. *Int. J. Oncol.* **2007**, *30*, 583–592. [CrossRef]
49. Hernández-Bule, M.L.; Trillo, M.Á.; Úbeda, A. Molecular Mechanisms Underlying Antiproliferative and Differentiating Responses of Hepatocarcinoma Cells to Subthermal Electric Stimulation. *PLoS ONE* **2014**, *9*, e84636. [CrossRef]
50. Hernández-Bule, M.L.; Martínez-Botas, J.; Trillo, M.Á.; Paíno, C.L.; Úbeda, A. Antiadipogenic Effects of Subthermal Electric Stimulation at 448 KHz on Differentiating Human Mesenchymal Stem Cells. *Mol. Med. Rep.* **2016**, *13*, 3895–3903. [CrossRef]

International Journal of
Molecular Sciences

MDPI

Review

Vitiligo: Pathogenesis and New and Emerging Treatments

Javier Perez-Bootello, Ruth Cova-Martin, Jorge Naharro-Rodriguez and Gonzalo Segurado-Miravalles *

Ramon y Cajal University Hospital, Road M-607, 9, 100, 28034 Madrid, Spain; jpbootello@gmail.com (J.P.-B.); ruth.cova.97@gmail.com (R.C.-M.); jorgenrmed@gmail.com (J.N.-R.)
* Correspondence: gonzalo.segurado@salud.madrid.org

Abstract: Vitiligo is a complex disease with a multifactorial nature and a high impact on the quality of life of patients. Although there are multiple therapeutic alternatives, there is currently no fully effective treatment for this disease. In the current era, multiple drugs are being developed for the treatment of autoimmune diseases. This review assesses the available evidence on the pathogenesis of vitiligo, and a comprehensive review of treatments available for vitiligo now and in the near future is provided. This qualitative analysis spans 116 articles. We reviewed the mechanism of action, efficacy and safety data of phototherapy, afamelanotide, cyclosporine, phosphodiesterase 4 inhibitors, trichloroacetic acid, basic fibroblast growth factor, tumor necrosis factor (TNF) inhibitors, secukinumab, pseudocatalase and janus kinase (JAK) inhibitors. At the moment, there is no clearly outstanding option or fully satisfactory treatment for vitiligo, so it is necessary to keep up the development of new drugs as well as the publication of long-term effectiveness and safety data for existing treatments.

Keywords: vitiligo; JAK inhibitor; pathogenesis; therapeutics

Citation: Perez-Bootello, J.; Cova-Martin, R.; Naharro-Rodriguez, J.; Segurado-Miravalles, G. Vitiligo: Pathogenesis and New and Emerging Treatments. *Int. J. Mol. Sci.* **2023**, *24*, 17306. https://doi.org/10.3390/ijms242417306

Academic Editors: Montserrat Fernández-Guarino, Asunción Ballester-Martinez and Andrés González-García

Received: 31 October 2023
Revised: 2 December 2023
Accepted: 8 December 2023
Published: 9 December 2023

1. Introduction

Vitiligo is a disease characterized by the appearance of white depigmented patches on the skin due to a selective loss of melanocytes [1]. It affects 0.1–2% of the world's population, with no significant differences in gender, ethnicity or geographic region [2,3]. Although it is not a disease that shortens life expectancy, it causes a significant negative psychological impact, comparable to other skin diseases such as eczema or psoriasis [4,5].

Vitiligo is a disease that is currently classified as an autoimmune disease [6]. It is a complex disease, in which genetics plays an important, but yet not fully elucidated role [7]. Heritability—the fraction of disease risk attributable to genetic variation—is high, estimated to be in European population between 0.75 and 0.83 [8]. More than 50 susceptibility loci for vitiligo have been discovered [7]. However, the occurrence of vitiligo is not solely explained by genetic factors: instead, the convergence theory proposes that vitiligo occurs as a result of the interaction between immunological, biochemical and environmental factors in genetically predisposed patients [9].

There are several reviews of the literature on medical treatments for vitiligo. These include reviews of specific emerging drug groups such as anti-JAK drugs [10], the emergence of new drugs in animal research [11] or global considerations in vitiligo [12].

Herein, we provide an updated review of the molecular pathogenesis of vitiligo, as well as a review of new treatments currently being studied from a clinical perspective without losing the molecular approach.

2. Pathogenesis of Vitiligo

2.1. Autoimmunity

Cell-mediated immunity drives vitiligo.

It is postulated that the main mechanism by which vitiligo is initiated and perpetuated is cell-mediated immunity [13]. There is ample evidence to support this theory, such as the existence of CD8+ T-cell infiltrates in skin biopsies taken at the margin of vitiligo lesions [14]. In addition, patients with vitiligo have a higher number of CD8+ T cells that are autoreactive to melanocyte-specific antigens such as tyrosinase, Melan-A/MART-1, gp100, TRP-1 and TRP-2 [15]. These autoreactive cells have been shown to induce vitiligo-like lesions in autologous skin tissue ex vivo [16]. Finally, another finding that supports the involvement of cell-mediated immunity is the high prevalence—up to 4%—of vitiligo-like lesions in patients treated with immunotherapy for melanoma [17]. This immunotherapy blocks T-cell checkpoint inhibitors, thus allowing these T cells to act uncontrollably on melanocytes [18].

Vitiligo pathogenesis acts through the activation of the JAK-STAT pathway.

The action of these T cells is highly dependent on the interferon gamma chemokine (IFN-γ) axis [19]. T cells secrete IFN-γ, which induces the production of chemokines CXCL9 and CXCL10 by keratinocytes [20]. These chemokines bind to the T-cell receptor CXCR3, increasing T-cell recruitment, thereby leading to the initiation, progression and maintenance of vitiligo lesions [21].

The IFNγ pathway is related to the JAK-STAT pathway through IFNγ binding to a specific cell surface receptor (IFNγR), which forms a heterodimeric protein that activates JAK proteins via phosphorylation. JAK proteins phosphorylate STAT, thereby activating it. Phosphorylated STAT proteins translocate to the nucleus and act as a transcription factor, thereby binding to DNA, regulating transcription of a variety of genes and affecting cell growth and apoptosis [22]. This is the physiological basis of JAK inhibitors' utility in the treatment of vitiligo [23].

Resident memory T cells play an important role in the persistence and relapse of vitiligo.

In addition, the importance of resident memory T cells (T_{RM} cells) has been identified in multiple studies. These are a type of CD8+ T cells expressing CD69, CD103 and CD49a that have the ability to remain in tissues and induce early immune responses [24]. It has been shown that there is a large population of T_{RM} cells in vitiligo skin, which appear to be involved in relapse induction by recruiting circulating T cells through the release of IFN-γ pathway cytokines [25].

IL-15 has a central role in the maintenance and function of T_{RM} cells.

IL-15 and IL-7 are key cytokines in the generation and maintenance of memory T cells [26]. IL-15-deficient mice show reduced production of T_{RM} cells, and IL-15 promotes TRM cell function ex vivo.

Therefore, blockade of one of the IL-15 receptor subunits (CD122) [27] has been tested in murine models of vitiligo with a specific monoclonal antibody, leading to a decrease in short-term effector function of T_{RM} cells through a reduction in IFNγ production, resulting in significant repigmentation in the group of mice treated. In addition, long-term depletion of T_{RM} cells, as well as other memory T-cell pools, was observed [21]. This is a mechanism that has been explored in the search for new therapeutic targets.

Humoral immunity does not play a central role in the pathophysiology of vitiligo.

On the other hand, humoral immunity does not appear to be fundamental for the pathogenesis of vitiligo, as serum titers of melanocyte-reactive antibodies do not correlate with disease activity [28] and the uniform distribution of circulating antibodies cannot explain the patchy appearance of vitiligo lesions [29].

2.2. Oxidative Stress

Another key element in the pathogenesis of vitiligo is the impact of oxidative stress. Available evidence suggests that oxidative stress may be the initial event that triggers the appearance of lesions [30]. Vitiligo patients' melanocytes are more sensitive to oxidative stress, and they are more difficult to culture than melanocytes from healthy controls [31].

The skin of patients with vitiligo shows alterations in the antioxidant system.

Melanocytes release reactive oxygen species (ROS) in response to cellular stress. In addition, melanogenesis itself is an active process that generates a pro-oxidant state in the skin [32]. All this leads to an imbalance between pro-oxidants and anti-oxidants. Pro-oxidant molecules and enzymes are favored, such as superoxide dismutase (responsible for the degradation of the O_2^- radical into H_2O_2 and O_2) and xanthine oxidase, whereas there is a total or functional deficit of antioxidants, such as catalase (which transforms H_2O_2 into H_2O and O_2) [33].

This increases cells' susceptibility to external and internal oxidants, leading to structural damage to DNA, proteins and lipids, as well as cell organelles such as mitochondria [34], with a functional impairment of the melanocyte.

ROS production triggers the activation of protective molecular pathways.

Oxidative stress to which melanocytes are exposed alters the protein folding machinery of the endoplasmic reticulum, leading to the accumulation of defective peptides and activating a cellular stress phenomenon known as the "unfolded protein response" (UPR). ROS also trigger the overexpression of calcium-channel-related proteins such as CGRP (calcitonin gene-related peptide) and TRPM2 (transient receptor potential cation channel subfamily M member 2), which are involved in mitochondria-dependent melanocyte apoptosis [33].

Melanocytes in vitiligo have also been shown to be deficient in protective pathways against oxidative stress such as the nuclear factor E2-related factor (Nrf2)-p62 pathway, which makes them more vulnerable to the presence of ROS [1].

Oxidative stress leads to T-cell activation.

In connection with the other fundamental pathogenic mechanism already mentioned, oxidative stress in patients with vitiligo leads to an increase in local levels of the cytokine CXCL16 due to the activation of the UPR in stressed keratinocytes. This increased expression of CXCL16 leads to the recruitment of CD8+ CXCR6+ T cells, whose expression is accompanied by loss of melanocytes in vitiligo patients [35]. A similar T-cell recruitment phenomenon occurs upon release of CXCL12 and CCL5 from melanocytes under oxidative stress, as demonstrated in animal models [36].

Finally, the presence of oxidative stress leads to a decrease in WNT expression, which negatively affects melanocyte differentiation, especially in skin affected by vitiligo in ex vivo skin models [37].

Oxidative stress may be responsible for the presence of the Koebner phenomenon in vitiligo.

Oxidative damage may be the mechanism that explains the Koebner phenomenon in vitiligo. According to this model, chronic mechanical stimulation of susceptible skin leads to increased release of oxidative particles. This oxidative damage alters the expression of cadherins that bind keratinocytes and melanocytes, thereby decreasing melanocyte adhesion and inducing the appearance of depigmented lesions [38].

3. Literature Search

For the first part of the narrative review (introduction and pathogenesis of vitiligo), a PubMed search was performed using the terms "Vitiligo", "Vitiligo AND pathogenesis" and "Vitiligo AND genetics". A collaborative selection was carried out among all authors of the most relevant articles related to this topic. Original articles, systematic and narrative reviews, guidelines and protocols were included. All sources with a similar level of evidence were analyzed, compiled and structured, and they are summarized in Section 1 of this review.

An expert consensus on vitiligo has recently been published, which provides a brief review of the therapeutic tools available for the treatment of vitiligo and makes specific recommendations for its use [39]. This document provides recommendations for the use of several well-established therapeutic modalities in the treatment of vitiligo: topical corticosteroids, topical immunomodulators, phototherapy, home light therapy, oral steroid minipulses, surgery and depigmenting therapies. These therapies are already established in routine clinical practice, so for the design of this review, their individual discussion was not considered. Despite this, the terms related to these therapies were included in the literature search so as not to rule out articles discussing the combination of these traditional modalities with other newer therapies. These conventional treatments will be briefly discussed at the end of this review.

For the literature search, the drugs mentioned in this expert consensus as drugs with little available evidence (methotrexate, cyclosporine, JAK inhibitors, anti-TNF α, IL-17 inhibitors and catalase) were included, as well as drugs mentioned in other reviews on the treatment of vitiligo [11] and other treatments known to us from our own clinical experience or from having been presented at medical congresses related to the subject.

Therefore, for the second part of the narrative review (new and emerging treatments), a PubMed search was conducted using the terms: (vitiligo) AND (afamelanotide OR JAK inhibitor OR ritlecitinib OR baricitinib OR ruxolitinib OR fluorouracil OR methotrexate OR FGF OR fibroblast growth factor OR laser OR apremilast OR crisaborole OR phosphodiesterase-4 inhibitor OR home light therapy OR home light phototherapy OR trichloroacetic acid OR THF inhibitor OR secukinumab) on 12 June 2023.

Firstly, the titles and abstracts of the articles obtained in the first search were reviewed to assess relevant studies. The inclusion criteria were (1) studies written in English or Spanish; (2) studies addressing effectiveness, tolerability and adverse effects of approved, off-label and under-research treatments for vitiligo. Systematic and narrative reviews, guidelines, protocols and conference abstracts were excluded. Articles prior to the year 2003 were excluded. Articles reporting surgical and non-surgical procedures except phototherapy were also excluded.

Secondly, the full text of articles that met the inclusion criteria was reviewed. Previous systematic and narrative reviews were examined to ensure the accuracy of our search and to manually check their reference lists. Figure 1 shows the article selection process used for this narrative review.

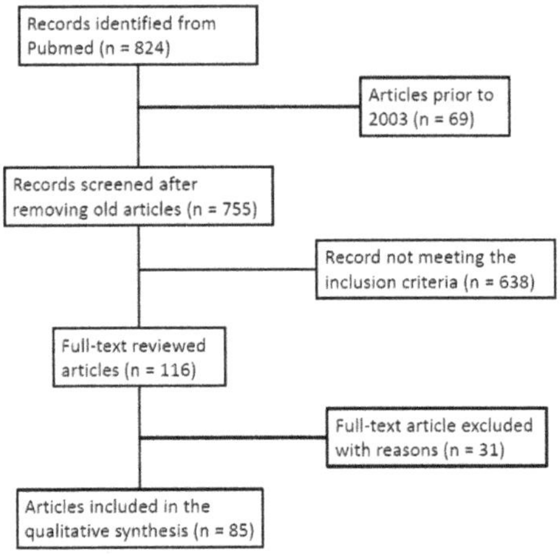

Figure 1. Flow chart showing the article selection process used in this narrative review.

4. Conventional Treatments

4.1. Phototherapy

Phototherapy in its different modalities (narrow-band ultraviolet B (NB-UVB), photochemotherapy, home-based and excimer or laser devices) has been a mainstay in the treatment of vitiligo for decades [40]. Its effect seems to be justified by the induction of T-lymphocyte apoptosis, the down-regulation of inflammatory cytokines (decreasing CXLCL9 and CXCL10 expression at keratinocytes) and the up-regulation of interleukin-10, which induces T-regulatory lymphocyte differentiation. Phototherapy also decreases the number of intraepithelial Langerhans cells and induces tyrosinase activity, thereby increasing melanin production as well as melanocyte proliferation and migration from epidermal hair follicles, favoring repigmentation of the affected area [41].

Throughout the last century, the efficacy of phototherapy in vitiligo, especially psolaren-UVA (PUVA) and NB-UVB, has been widely reported [39]. In recent years, scientific efforts have been especially oriented toward studying the efficacy of the emerging home-based phototherapy as well as targeted phototherapy.

Regarding the use of home-based NB-UVB phototherapy, a single-branched study conducted by Khandpur et al. [42] demonstrated its utility in vitiligo, while Eleftheriadou et al. [43] showed its efficacy compared to a placebo. When compared to hospital-based NB-UVB, similar efficacy has been demonstrated based on various endpoints (VASI, VitiQoL, BSA) in different clinical trials [44–46] and a retrospective study [47]. In one of the studies, patient-perceived satisfaction was significantly lower in home-based phototherapy [47]. Regarding intervention cost, all studies are consistent in reporting that home-based NB-UVB is cheaper in the long term despite the initial investment required, especially after 3 months of treatment [44]. Some studies showed an increase in intervention-related adverse effects (especially grade 3 erythema or burns) with home-based phototherapy [44,46].

Regarding targeted phototherapy, Raghuwanshi et al. [48] reported a 37% moderate response and a 4.5% excellent response in 134 patients with localized vitiligo treated weekly for 11 weeks with targeted NB-UVB. The use of an excimer lamp could be especially useful in localized vitiligo on the face, as recently reported by Juntongjin et al. [49]. A study involving 44 patients found no statistically significant difference in the efficacy of home-based NB-UVB when compared with a hospital excimer lamp [50].

In conclusion, phototherapy remains a cornerstone in the management of vitiligo, especially in generalized vitiligo, as confirmed by Sakhiya et al. [51] in a retrospective study including 3000 patients comparing its efficacy with that of topical treatment. Targeted phototherapy modalities appear to be a useful alternative in localized forms of vitiligo. Home-based phototherapy provides a cost-effective alternative for prolonged treatments.

4.2. *Afamelanotide*

Afamelanotide is a potent synthetic linear analogue of α-MSH in a controlled-release formulation. Subcutaneous injections result in increased skin pigmentation owing to increased expression of eumelanin. In recent years, pivotal pilot studies [52–54] have been undertaken to assess the effectiveness of afamelanotide in conjunction with NB–UV-B phototherapy for repigmenting non-segmental vitiligo. These studies included a comparison to NB–UV-B phototherapy as the control. During these investigations, patients underwent NB–UV-B phototherapy sessions 2–3 times weekly for 6–7 months. This regimen was either combined or not with a subcutaneously administered 16 mg implant of afamelanotide every 28 days for a duration of 4 to 6 months. The results demonstrated the superiority of the combination therapy group over the NB–UV-B monotherapy group in the experimental studies [53,54] A higher percentage of patients in the combination therapy group achieved repigmentation, and this occurred at earlier time points. In the observational study of Grimes et al. [52], a median of 66.25% repigmentation (ranging from 50% to 90%) was obtained, with 75% of cases exhibiting stability after 3 months. The most common secondary effects were hyperpigmentation along with limited cases of headaches, dizziness and nausea reported.

4.3. *Cyclosporine*

In addition to its classic role in arresting vitiligo progression, cyclosporine might be useful as an adjunctive treatment in an autologous noncultured melanocyte–keratinocyte cell transplantation (NCMKT) procedure. Although an in-depth description of NCMKT is beyond the remit of this review, the incorporation of cyclosporine has been proposed to ameliorate the depigmented halo surrounding the transplantation—an aesthetically significant sequelae frequently ascribed to the presence of CD8 T lymphocytes in perilesional skin. In accordance with this premise, Mutalik et al. [55] conducted a study involving 50 patients with stable localized vitiligo who underwent NCMKT. Of these, 25 received cyclosporine at a dosage of 3 mg/kg for 3 weeks, followed by 1.5 mg/kg for 6 weeks, in contrast to the control group, which received no adjuvant treatment. Consequently, all patients in the cyclosporine-treated group achieved a repigmentation percentage exceeding 75% (median 90.7%), whereas only seven individuals in the control group reached this threshold.

5. New and Emerging Therapies

5.1. Phosphodiesterase 4 (PDE-4) Inhibitors

PDE-4 physiologically degrades cyclic adenosine monophosphate (cAMP) to 5′-adenosine monophosphate. Inhibition of this enzyme increases intracellular cAMP and thus modifies the regulation of inflammatory mediators. These include a decrease in IL-17, 23, alfa-TNF and gamma-interferon while increasing IL-10, overall decreasing proinflammatory cytokines (which are increased in vitiligo-affected skin) and increasing suppressive cytokines [56,57]. The available evidence for PDE-4 inhibitors in vitiligo is limited to oral apremilast and a case report of topical crisaborole.

Regarding apremilast, all selected studies utilize a dose of 30 mg twice daily [57–62]. In 2019, a case series [58] and a case report [57] showed the utility of apremilast in monotherapy in vitiligo. Two clinical trials compared the improvement with the addition of apremilast to NB-UVB treatment with conflicting results [60,61]. Recently, Sharma et al. [62] have reported an improved response of vitiligo after adding apremilast to standard treatment. In most studies, headache and gastrointestinal discomfort have been reported as the main adverse effects of the treatment.

Apremilast seems to provide a comfortable option with an acceptable safety profile for vitiligo patients; however, its cost and conflicting evidence concerning its efficacy require further research in order to establish specific recommendations.

5.2. Trichloroacetic Acid (TCA)

The mechanism by which TCA induces repigmentation is presumably related to the ability to induce inflammation and subsequent post-inflammatory hyperpigmentation [63]. In addition, TCA-induced necrosis and subsequent trauma could theoretically stimulate melanocyte proliferation through the production of pro-opiomelanocortin and melanocortin and the release of growth factors and inflammatory mediators [64].

Regarding reported efficacy, Nofal et al. [63] published a 100-patient study reporting an 80% response rate in eyelid vitiligo, with a lower response rate in the face, torso and extremities with the application of variable concentrations of TCA every 2 weeks for 12 months. Two studies investigated the combination of microneedling and TCA, interestingly finding better response rates with the application of 70% TCA [65] than with 100% TCA [66]. The single application of 15% TCA in combination with NB-UVB achieved an excellent response in 70% of patients in a clinical trial [67]. Reported adverse effects included pain, erythema, post-inflammatory hyperpigmentation, infection and scarring.

Further research is needed on the role of TCA application in the treatment of vitiligo in monotherapy or as an adjuvant as well as to define optimal concentrations of TCA for vitiligo depending on location.

5.3. Basic Fibroblast Growth Factor (bFGF)

bFGF is a growth factor released by keratinocytes in response to certain stimuli. Its potential benefit in vitiligo seems to be related to its key role in melanocyte growth, migration and survival. In this regard, an increase in the release of growth factors, mainly bFGF, by keratinocytes after the application of NB-UVB has been observed [68].

Concerning its efficacy, an upgraded response has been found according to disease scales with the addition of bFGF-related decapeptide 0.1% solution treatment to tacrolimus 0.1% topical therapy in stable vitiligo [69] and to PUVA therapy [70]. Monotherapy application of bFGF-related decapeptide 0.1% solution in a retrospective study in 65 patients showed a 12% significant response at 5 months [71].

5.4. TNF Inhibitors

The existing data on the potential correlation between vitiligo and anti-TNF-α agents remain inconclusive due to limited evidence. Recent investigations into the utilization of anti-TNFs for vitiligo treatment have yielded controversial outcomes, characterized by a predominantly low level of evidential support in the current literature. Upon a thorough examination of the latest publications in this field, we have compiled data from case series therapeutic trials involving two patients treated with subcutaneous adalimumab [72], three patients with intravenous infliximab [72,73] and seven patients administered subcutaneous etanercept [72,74,75]. All subjects exhibited generalized vitiligo vulgaris, with the body surface area (BSA) ranging between 10% and 30%. Among these cases, there are only two reported instances wherein infliximab and etanercept demonstrated potential efficacy in vitiligo therapy. In the remaining cases, although no exacerbation in depigmented areas was observed, repigmentation was not achieved in any patient. Consequently, it can be concluded that anti-TNF-α agents have not proven effective in the treatment of vitiligo, based on current evidence. Larger-scale and long-term studies are warranted to comprehensively assess the efficacy of anti-TNF-α agents in vitiligo treatment.

5.5. Secukinumab

A vitiligo paradoxical adverse reaction following TNF-α agents has been documented during psoriasis treatment. The management of such cases poses a notable challenge. A recent case report describes the onset of vitiligo after the administration of adalimumab for psoriasis treatment [76], leading to its suspension and the initiation of secukinumab, an anti-interleukin-17A monoclonal antibody approved for psoriasis treatment. Complete repigmentation of vitiligo lesions and resolution of psoriasis were achieved. Despite empirical evidence affirming elevated circulating interleukin-17 (IL-17) levels and increased Th17 lymphocyte counts in vitiligo patients, along with heightened expression levels of IL-17A messenger RNA in vitiligo lesions [77], the precise role of IL-17 remains elusive. Further research is needed to elucidate IL-17's role and ascertain its viability as a therapeutic target.

5.6. Pseudocatalase

The oxidative stress observed in vitiligo, related to hydrogen peroxide (H_2O_2)-mediated lipid peroxidation, constitutes an additional proposed mechanism contributing to the pathogenesis of vitiligo. This phenomenon has been observed in vivo through direct measurements of H_2O_2 levels within the depigmented epidermis. Notably, synthetic catalysts capable of oxidizing H_2O_2 to O_2 and H_2O can eliminate epidermal H_2O_2 [78]. One such active catalyst is a NB-UV-B-activated bis-MnII(EDTA)2(HCO_3^-)2 complex (EDTA, ethylenediaminetetraacetate), denoted as "pseudocatalase PC-KUS". This topically applied pseudocatalase has been proposed as a potential agent to arrest disease progression. The most extensive patient cohort treated with this approach was documented by Schallreuter et al. Their study enrolled 71 patients presenting generalized vitiligo, categorized in two groups: control group of 10 patients subject to NB-UVB radiation and 61 individuals also receiving daily topical application of pseudocatalase. Cessation of progression was achieved in 99% of patients with low-dose PC-KUS, compared with 30% in the control group. Also, repigmentation rates above 75% were achieved in most body areas except acral areas, with results showing statistically significant differences compared with the control group.

In the most extensive patient cohort, documented by Schallreuter et al. [79], 61 individuals received daily topical application of pseudocatalase with NB-UVB radiation versus a control group of 10 patients treated with NB-UVB radiation alone. Cessation of progression was achieved in 99% of patients with low-dose PC-KUS, compared with 30% in the control group. Also, repigmentation rates above 75% were achieved in most body areas except acral areas, with results showing statistically significant differences.

These were promising results; however, subsequent clinical trials conducted by Patel et al. [80], Bakis-Petsoglou et al. [81] and Alshiyab et al. [82], among others, proved that the use of pseudocatalase was not superior to the use of placebo cream or was not associated with a therapeutic effect when combined with other treatments. In conclusion, despite initial promise, pseudocatalase has not demonstrated efficacy in the management of vitiligo, as evidenced by several clinical trials.

5.7. *JAK Inhibitors*

JAK-STAT pathway inhibition is a promising target for the treatment of vitiligo [83]. Elevated levels of interferon gamma (IFN-γ) have been observed in human skin with vitiligo, which activates via JAK 1/2 the transcription of the cytokines CXCL9 and CXCL10. These cytokines are necessary for the recruitment of cytotoxic T-lymphocytes, which are responsible for melanocyte destruction [84]. This is the reason why inhibition of JAK proteins is postulated as an effective therapeutic strategy for the treatment of vitiligo.

5.7.1. Case Reports and Case Series

Clinical experience with JAK inhibitors (iJAKs) dates back to 2015 and 2016 with isolated case reports. Craiglow et al. [85] published a case report in 2015 in which an off-label therapeutic trial with oral tofacitinib (JAK 1 and JAK 3 inhibitor) was performed in a patient with generalized vitiligo, presenting almost complete repigmentation in the forehead and hands after 5 months of treatment. In 2016, Harris et al. [86] published another report in which oral ruxolitinib was initiated in a patient with coexisting vitiligo and alopecia areata. A great improvement in facial vitiligo was achieved after 20 weeks of treatment, although there was loss of pigment after withdrawal of the drug. There are other case reports in which oral tofacitinib is initiated for other pathologies and improvement of concomitant vitiligo is achieved, such as in the reports of Komnitski et al. [87] in a patient with rheumatoid arthritis and Vu et al. [88]'s report in which a marginal improvement of vitiligo was observed in a patient in whom tofacitinib was initiated for atopic dermatitis and alopecia areata. Other case reports have been published reporting improvement of vitiligo with oral iJAKs, both with tofacitinib [89] and with other drugs such as oral baricitinib, as shown in the article by Li et al. [90] in which two patients treated with baricitinib, phototherapy and topical corticosteroids and calcineurin inhibitors showed great improvement, or even upadacitinib, as in a patient with concomitant atopic dermatitis described in Pan et al.'s [91] article as having great facial repigmentation after starting this drug.

A number of case series have also been published in which oral tofacitinib was tested off-label for the treatment of vitiligo. These case series have shown heterogeneous results: Liu et al. [92] present a case series of 10 patients in which only 5 showed improvement with oral tofacitinib in sun-exposed areas or in concomitance with phototherapy. These results are consistent with those of Gianfaldoni et al. [93], who combined treatment with oral tofacitinib with phototherapy and achieved a better repigmentation rate (reaching 92% repigmentation) than with phototherapy alone. However, not all reports have yielded the same results. For instance, Fang et al. [94], in a first study, observed a poor response to treatment with oral tofacitinib and phototherapy with narrow-band UVB in four patients, although in a second study, they did find an improvement after treatment with oral tofacitinib and phototherapy with a 308 nm excimer light [95].

Finally, a series of 12 patients treated with oral upadacitinib in monotherapy has recently been published, which, in line with the results of studies with other oral iJAKs, showed moderate improvement, especially in the facial area [96].

No serious adverse effects were reported after treatment with oral iJAK, with the only adverse events reported being upper respiratory infection [92] and worsening of acne [91], with most patients being asymptomatic.

Multiple case reports and real-life case series have also been published reporting the effectiveness and safety data of topical iJAK.

In 2018, Joshipura et al. [97] reported on two patients treated with 1.5% ruxolitinib cream, who showed an improvement of vitiligo in sun-exposed areas.

Most reports, however, refer to topical iJAK tofacitinib cream in its 2% formulation. The studies by McKesey et al. [98], Mobasher et al. [99], Olamiju et al. [100] and Berbert-Ferreira et al. [101] reported the results of treatment of vitiligo with tofacitinib 2% cream in a total of 29 patients, allowing treatment with concomitant phototherapy. In all of these publications, a high degree of facial repigmentation was observed, with mixed results in extrafacial locations.

Local and systemic adverse effects have been reported with topical iJAK. Two patients treated with 1.5% ruxolitinib cream presented myalgias, which caused self-discontinuation on both of them. One of the patients even presented mild elevation of the phosphokinase level (CPK) [102]. Adverse effects with 2% tofacitinib cream were minor, such as transient erythema [101], skin contour changes on the chin [99] and acneiform lesions [99,101].

A synthesis of case reports and case series reported to date on the use of iJAK for vitiligo is shown in Table 1.

Table 1. Case reports and case series reported to date on the use of iJAK for vitiligo.

Drug	Publication Data (Author/Year/Country)	Report Data (Drug and Route of Administration/Patients (n)/Treatment Duration/Area Affected/Follow-Up)	Outcome	Side Effects
Tofacitinib	Craiglow et al. [85]/2015/USA	5 mg tofacitinib citrate orally, initially 5 mg every other day; after 2 weeks, the dosage was increased to 5 mg/d 1 patient with forehead, torso and extremities vitiligo (10% BSA) treated and followed for 22 weeks (5 months)	Nearly complete repigmentation of the forehead and hands, partial repigmentation of extremities (5% BSA remained depigmented)	No adverse effects, no laboratory abnormalities
Ruxolitinib	Harris et al. [86]/2016/USA	20 mg ruxolitinib orally, twice daily. 1 patient with face, torso and extremities vitiligo treated for 20 weeks and followed for 16 more weeks	Improvement in facial pigmentation from 0.8% to 51%. 12 weeks after discontinuation of ruxolitinib, much of the regained pigment had regressed, from 51% to 16%	No side effects
Tofacitinib	Liu et al. [92]/2017/USA	5–10 mg tofacitinib orally QD-BID 10 patients treated for at least 3 months, an average of 9.9 months. 8 patients had generalized vitiligo and 2 patients had primarily acral involvement, with 1–100% BSA	A mean decrease of 5.4% BSA involvement with vitiligo was observed in 5/10 patients, while the other 5 patients did not achieve any repigmentation In the 5 patients who achieved some reversal of disease, repigmentation occurred only in sun-exposed areas of skin in 3 of them, diffusely in another patient undergoing concomitant full-body nbUVB phototherapy and to the dorsal hands in another patient after starting concomitant hand nbUVB phototherapy	Upper respiratory infection in 2 patients. 1 patient reported weight gain of 5 pounds and 1 patient reported arthralgias. Mild elevations of lipids were noted in 4 patients. There were no serious adverse events

Table 1. *Cont.*

Drug	Publication Data (Author/Year/Country)	Report Data (Drug and Route of Administration/Patients (n)/Treatment Duration/Area Affected/Follow-Up)	Outcome	Side Effects
Tofacitinib	Vu et al. [88]/2017/Australia	5 mg tofacitinib orally twice daily. 1 patient with multifocal vitiligo treated and followed for 6 months	Patient with concomitant atopic dermatitis and alopecia areata, both with great improvement. Marginal improvement in the vitiligo (decline in VASI score from 4.68 at baseline to 3.95 at 5 months)	Two episodes of self-resolving upper respiratory tract infections and diarrhea, no treatment interruption required
Ruxolitinib	Joshipura et al. [97]/2018/USA	Topical 1.5% ruxolitinib cream, twice daily. 2 patients with face, torso and extremities vitiligo treated for 38 and 12 weeks, respectively	Improvement in sun-exposed areas only (face and forearms)	No side effects
Tofacitinib	Gianfaldoni et al. [93]/2018/Italy	Tofacitinib citrate (10 mg orally every day) + cold light generator micro-focused phototherapy. 9 patients treated for at least 36 weeks	Repigmentation rate of 92% in the phototherapy + tofacitinib group, better than the phototherapy-alone group, in which only 72% obtained a repigmentation rate higher than 75%	No side effects
Tofacitinib	Kim et al. [89]/2018/USA	5 mg tofacitinib twice daily orally and narrow-band UV-B (360–500 mJ) 2 patients Patient 1: face (75% area affected), neck, torso and extremities vitiligo, results reported after 3 months Patient 2: face (90% area affected), torso and arms vitiligo, results reported after 6 months	Patient 1: complete repigmentation of her face, 75% or greater repigmentation of her neck, chest, forearms and shins, and only minimal freckling of the dorsal hands after full body phototherapy Patient 2: about 75% facial repigmentation. No repigmentation occurred at the other body sites (only facial phototherapy) Both had previously depigmented their faces using monobenzyl ether of hydroquinone (MBEH)	No side effects
Tofacitinib	McKesey et al. [98]/2019/USA	2% tofacitinib cream twice daily in conjunction with narrow-band ultraviolet B (NB-UVB) therapy thrice weekly 11 patients with face vitiligo treated for 12 ± 4 weeks and followed for a mean time of 112 days (range 84–154)	The mean facial VASI was 0.80 (range 0.1–2.25) at baseline and 0.23 (range 0.03–0.75) at follow-up, which is a mean improvement of 70% (range 50–87%)	No side effects

Table 1. *Cont.*

Drug	Publication Data (Author/Year/Country)	Report Data (Drug and Route of Administration/Patients (n)/Treatment Duration/Area Affected/Follow-Up)	Outcome	Side Effects
Tofacitinib	Mobasher et al. [99]/2020/USA	2% tofacitinib cream twice daily Concomitant treatment with topical steroids, topical calcineurin inhibitors, supplements (e.g., Polypodium leucotomos and Ginkgo biloba) or phototherapy was allowed 16 patients with "facial" or "non-facial" vitiligo followed for a mean time of 153 days (63–367)	13 experienced repigmentation with 4 patients experiencing > 90% repigmentation, 5 patients experiencing 25–75% repigmentation and 4 patients experiencing 5–15% repigmentation. 2 patients experienced no change and 1 patient experienced slow progression of depigmentation in the target lesion. Facial lesions improved more than non-facial lesions ($p = 0.0216$)	Acne-like papules on the face were reported by 1 patient. These lesions resolved with cessation of the medication. 1 patient reported subtle skin contour changes on his chin, which led to cessation of treatment after 2 weeks
Tofacitinib	Komnitski et al. [87]/2020/Brazil	5 mg tofacitinib orally twice daily. 1 patient with face, neck, elbows, hands and feet vitiligo, treated and followed for 104 weeks (2 years)	Complete repigmentation of the forehead and perilabial macules could be noted, as well as partial repigmentation in the posterior region of the neck and upper chest. No exposition to any source of ultraviolet radiation	No side effects
Tofacitinib	Olamiju et al. [100]/2020/USA	2% tofacitinib cream twice daily + narrow-band ultraviolet B phototherapy using a handheld unit 1 patient with face (segmental vitiligo) treated for 6 months and followed for 1 year	Freckling was observed within 4 weeks, almost complete repigmentation after 3 months and complete repigmentation at 6 months. The patient discontinued treatment after another month, and the area remained fully repigmented for approximately 6 months before a few depigmented macules began to reappear	No side effects
Ruxolitinib	Narla et al. [102]/2020/USA	1.5% ruxolitinib cream twice daily, for 2 patients presenting non-segmental vitiligo	Unspecified	Myalgias, which caused self-discontinuation in both patients. One of the patients presented mild elevation of the phosphokinase level (CPK)

Table 1. *Cont.*

Drug	Publication Data (Author/Year/Country)	Report Data (Drug and Route of Administration/Patients (n)/Treatment Duration/Area Affected/Follow-Up)	Outcome	Side Effects
Tofacitinib	Berbert-Ferreira et al. [101]/2021/Brazil	2% tofacitinib ointment twice daily only on facial lesions, combined with NB-UVB phototherapy, 3 times a week. The total dose for the face vitiligo was 1000 mJ/cm^2 1 patient presenting stable non-segmental vitiligo with acrofacial involvement treated for 9 months	Significant repigmentation of the forehead, nose, eyes and lips was observed	Minor adverse events such as erythema and transient acne
Tofacitinib	Fang et al. [94]/2021/Taiwan	5 mg tofacitinib orally once daily concomitant with nbUVB phototherapy. 4 patients with torso, arms, hands and leg vitiligo treated for 16 weeks	3 out of the 4 patients presented minimal or no change on vitiligo lesions. Only 1 of the patients had a partial response, with 14/42 (33%) of lesions showing signs of repigmentation. The results indicate that 5 mg daily tofacitinib concomitant with nbUVB phototherapy for 16 weeks is not sufficient for treating patients who showed an inadequate response to previous treatments	No side effects
Tofacitinib	Fang et al. [95]/2021/Taiwan	5 mg tofacitinib orally daily and 308 nm excimer light three times weekly 3 patients with torso, arms, hands, legs and feet vitiligo treated for 12 weeks	All patients had repigmentation and the mean reduction in VES was 32.7% (decreases of 38%, 44% and 16% in patients 1, 2 and 3, respectively). Of the 44 lesions, 14 (32%) showed follicular-patterned repigmentation, and of these, 6 repigmented lesions (43%) were in areas that were not sun-exposed regions. Acral lesions showed poor response	No side effects
Baricitinib	Li et al. [90]/2022/China	2 mg baricitinib orally twice daily + phototherapy + topical tacrolimus + topical steroids 2 patients with face, torso and extremities vitiligo treated for 6 months and 8 months, respectively	In patient 1, significant repigmentation after 8 months; in patient 2, over 75% repigmentation after 6 months	No side effects
Upadacitinib	Pan et al. [91]/2023/China	15 mg upadacitinib orally daily, combined with crisaborole. 1 patient with face, torso and extremities vitiligo treated for 4 months and followed for 7 months	After 4 months, there was nearly 90% repigmentation of his face and neck, 60% repigmentation of the chest and only a little repigmentation of the extremities	Worsening of acne

5.7.2. Clinical Trials

Topical ruxolitinib, in its 1.5% cream form, is the most studied iJAK. In 2017, Rothstein et al. [103] conducted a single-group, open-label, proof-of-concept trial (NCT02809976) in which 11 patients were treated with 1.5% ruxolitinib cream. After 20 weeks, patients showed generalized improvement in vitiligo, especially the four patients with facial involvement, who showed an improvement in fVASI of 76%. In addition, an open-label extension study was performed in eight of these patients, in which the application was continued for 52 weeks and UVB phototherapy was added in three patients, improving repigmentation on the face (reaching 92%), nonacral extremities and torso, especially those treated with phototherapy [104].

In 2020, Rosmarin et al. [84] published the results of a phase 2, randomized, double-blind and dose-ranging clinical trial (NCT03099304). In this study, 157 patients were treated with ruxolitinib cream at various concentrations (from 1.5% twice daily to 0.15% once daily, plus a placebo group) for 52 weeks. Patients who achieved significance for the primary endpoint (50% improvement in facial involvement) were the patients treated with the highest concentration of ruxolitinib (1.5%). Other publications on the same clinical trial report that a 1.5% ruxolitinib cream twice daily application produces the greatest improvement in extrafacial locations (around 50% in upper and lower limbs, 15.0% in hands and 29.4% in feet) [105], and that the addition of concomitant therapy with NB-UVB phototherapy produces an additional improvement of 50.2% for F-VASI and 29.5% for T-VASI over that achieved with ruxolitinib cream monotherapy [106].

The strongest evidence for the use of ruxolitinib cream is from the TRuE-V1 (NCT04052425) and TRuE-V2 (NCT04057573) clinical trials, two multinational, phase 3, double-blind, vehicle-controlled trials of identical design involving 661 patients. The primary endpoint was to achieve F-VASI75 at week 24. In both studies, the response was clearly better in patients treated with 1.5% ruxolitinib cream twice daily. In TRuE-V1, the percentage of patients with a F-VASI75 response at week 24 was 29.8% in the ruxolitinib-cream group and 7.4% in the vehicle group (relative risk, 4.0; 95% confidence interval (CI), 1.9 to 8.4; $p < 0.001$). In TRuE-V2, the percentages were 30.9% and 11.4%, respectively (relative risk, 2.7; 95% CI, 1.5 to 4.9; $p < 0.001$). Results of key secondary endpoints showed the superiority of ruxolitinib cream over the vehicle control (F-VASI50, F-VASI90, T-VASI50 and F-VASI75 in the 52-week extension study) [107]. Evidence from the latter two clinical trials led to FDA approval of 1.5% ruxolitinib cream in 2022, applied twice daily to affected areas of up to 10% of the body surface area in adult and pediatric patients aged 12 years and older.

In all of these studies, adverse effects were mild and consisted mainly of local itching, nasopharyngitis and acne at the application site.

A clinical trial (NCT04530344) has yet to publish its final results from a 52-week extension period in 458 patients who participated in the TRuE-V1 (NCT04052425) and TRuE-V2 (NCT04057573) clinical trials to assess the long-term efficacy and safety of ruxolitinib cream in participants with vitiligo [108].

Another ongoing clinical trial (NCT05247489) is investigating the effect of the addition of phototherapy to ruxolitinib cream compared to ruxolitinib cream monotherapy [109].

In 2023, the largest clinical trial of an oral iJAK was published (NCT03715829). Treatment with ritlecitinib, a JAK 3/TEC inhibitor, was tested in a phase 2b, randomized, double-blind, placebo-controlled, parallel-group, multicenter, dose-ranging, double-blind, phase 2b study. In this study, 364 patients were randomized to once-daily oral ritlecitinib ± a 4-week loading dose (200/50 mg, 100/50 mg, 30 mg or 10 mg) or a placebo for 24 weeks (dose adjustment period). Subsequently, 187 patients received ritlecitinib at 200/50 mg daily in a 24-week extension period. Significant differences from the placebo were observed in the percentage change from baseline in the facial vitiligo area score index in the 50 mg ritlecitinib groups with (−21.2 vs. 2.1; $p < 0.001$) or without (−18.5 vs. 2.1; $p < 0.001$) a loading dose and in the 30 mg ritlecitinib group (−14.6 vs. 2.1; $p = 0.01$). Accelerated improvement was observed after treatment with 200/50 mg ritlecitinib in the extension period (n = 187). The most common adverse events were nasopharyngitis (15.9%), upper respiratory tract infection (11.5%) and headache (8.8%). Four patients had confirmed cases of herpes zoster (all non-serious), two patients had malignancies (non-melanoma skin cancers) and no thromboembolic events occurred [110]. To date, oral ritlecitinib has not yet been approved in the USA nor Europe.

In addition, a real-world clinical practice out-of-label oral tofacitinib clinical trial was conducted on 15 patients and 19 controls, in conjunction with a topical corticosteroid, topical calcineurin inhibitors and phototherapy. Both groups showed great improvement, to the extent that the differences were not statistically significant in facial lesions. No other clinical trials specific to the use of tofacitinib for vitiligo have been reported [111].

Finally, it is worth mentioning that there is an ongoing placebo-controlled dose-ranging clinical trial to evaluate the safety and efficacy of upadacitinib in subjects with non-segmental vitiligo (NCT04927975) [112].

Other trials with topical iJAK (ARQ-252 [113], cerdulatinib [114] and ATI-50002 [115]) have been initiated but no publications are available due to termination of the trial by the sponsor or lack of clear effectiveness in the preliminary results published on Clinicaltrials.gov.

A summary of the clinical trials reviewed for this section is shown in Table 2.

Table 2. A summary of the clinical trials reviewed for this section.

Drug	Study Data (Authors/Year/Country/NCT)	Study Design	Results	Side Effects
Ruxolitinib (topical)	Rothstein et al. [103]/2017/USA/NCT02809976	1.5% topical ruxolitinib cream, twice daily Single group, open-label, phase 2 11 patients followed for 20 weeks, presenting facial, upper limbs, torso or acral vitiligo	23% improvement in overall VASI in all patients. The 4 patients with facial involvement presented 76% improvement in fVASI. 3/8 patients responded on body surfaces. 1/8 responded on acral surfaces	Minor (erythema, hyperpigmentation and transient acne)
Ruxolitinib (topical)	Josahipura et al. [104] (open-label extension study of Rothstein's)/2018/USA/ No registration	1.5% topical ruxolitinib cream, twice daily (all 8 patients) + optional UVB phototherapy (3/8 patients chose it) Open-label extension study Phase 2 8 patients followed for 32 weeks, presenting facial, upper limbs, torso or acral vitiligo	Mean improvement in overall VASI of 37.6% ± 31.2% ($p < 0.011$). 5/8 had treatment response. 4 patients with facial vitiligo had mean 92% improvement. 3/6 had a response on their nonacral upper extremities (2 of these 3 had been treated with combination phototherapy). 2/3 patients (both of whom had opted for combination phototherapy) responded on the torso with a mean VASI improvement of 16.7% ± 16.7%	Minor (erythema and transient acne)
Ruxolitinib (topical)	Rosmarin et al. [84]/2020/USA/NCT03099304	Ruxolitinib cream (1.5% twice daily, 1.5% once daily, 0.5% once daily or 0.15% once daily) or vehicle (control group) twice daily A randomized, double-blind, dose-ranging study. Phase 2. 157 patients with vitiligo affecting at least 0.5% of the total body surface area (BSA) on the face and at least 3% of the total BSA on nonfacial areas; followed for 52 weeks	The primary endpoint at week 24, F-VASI50, was reached by significantly more patients given the two highest doses of ruxolitinib cream (1.5% twice daily, 15 (45%) of 33 patients, odds ratio (OR) 24·7, 95% CI 3.3–1121.4; $p = 0.0001$; 1.5% once daily, 15 (50%) of 30 patients, OR 28.5, 95% CI 3.7–1305.2; $p < 0.0001$) and also by more patients who received the two lowest doses of ruxolitinib cream (0.5% once daily, eight (26%) of 31; 0.15% once daily, ten (32%) of 31) compared with the vehicle (one (3%) of 32 patients). T-VASI50 at week 52, a key secondary endpoint, was reached by patients in the total population in a dose-dependent manner (1.5% twice daily, 12 (36%) of 33; 1.5% once daily, 9 (30%) of 30; 0.5% once daily, 8 (26%) of 31)	Application site pruritus was the most common treatment-related adverse event among patients given ruxolitinib cream (1 (3%) of 33 in the 1.5% twice daily group; 3 (10%) of 30 in the 1.5% once daily group; 3 (10%) of 31 in the 0.5% once daily group; and 6 (19%) of 31 in the 0.15% once daily group), with 3 (9%) of 32 patients showing application site pruritis in the control group. Acne was noted as a treatment-related adverse event in 13 (10%) of 125 patients who received ruxolitinib cream and 1 (3%) of 32 patients who received vehicle cream. All treatment-related adverse events were mild or moderate in severity and similar across treatment groups. No serious adverse events were related to study treatment

Table 2. *Cont.*

Drug	Study Data (Authors/Year/Country/NCT)	Study Design	Results	Side Effects
Ruxolitinib (topical)	Hamzavi et al. [105]/2022/USA/NCT03099304	Ruxolitinib cream (1.5% twice daily, 1.5% once daily, 0.5% once daily or 0.15% once daily) or vehicle (control group) twice daily A randomized, double-blind, dose-ranging study. Phase 2. 157 patients with vitiligo affecting at least 0.5% of the total body surface area (BSA) on the face and at least 3% of the total BSA on nonfacial areas; followed for 52 weeks	Among patients with vitiligo affecting ≤ 20% of T-BSA at baseline, both doses of ruxolitinib cream (1.5% once daily and twice daily) produced notable T-VASI50 and T-VASI75 responses at week 52. The 1.5% ruxolitinib cream twice-daily dose produced the highest proportion of T-VASI50 responders in the head/neck region (60.0%), followed by the upper and lower extremities (52.9% and 52.6%, respectively). T-VASI50 of the hands and feet was noted for 15.0% and 29.4% of patients, respectively, who received 1.5% ruxolitinib cream twice daily	Unspecified
Ruxolitinib	Pandya et al. [106]/2022/USA/NCT03099304	Ruxolitinib cream with concomitant narrow-band UVB (NB-UVB) phototherapy during the open-label phase after week 52 A randomized, double-blind, dose-ranging study. Phase 2. 19 patients with vitiligo affecting at least 0.5% of the total body surface area (BSA) on the face and at least 3% of the total BSA on nonfacial areas; followed for 52 weeks	After the addition of NB-UVB phototherapy, F-VASI and T-VASI scores improved in 15 of 19 patients (78.9%) and 18 of 19 patients (94.7%), respectively. In these 19 patients, the mean percentage improvement at week 104 was 50.2% for F-VASI and 29.5% for T-VASI versus the improvement at the last visit before the addition of NB-UVB phototherapy. Postcombination therapy response parameters were similar to data at week 104 from 70 patients who remained on ruxolitinib cream alone from day 1; responses were higher at week 104 versus week 52 among patients who received ruxolitinib cream alone	No adverse events considered to be related to the treatment
Ruxolitinib	Rosmarin et al. [107]/2022/USA/TRuE-V1 (NCT04052425) and TRuE-V2 (NCT04057573)	1.5% ruxolitinib cream or matching vehicle cream twice daily to all depigmented vitiligo lesions, on a 2:1 ratio Two multinational, phase 3, double-blind, vehicle-controlled trials of identical design conducted across 101 centers 661 patients (330 TRuE-V1 and 331 TRuE-V2) with face and body vitiligo followed for 24 weeks	In TRuE-V1, the percentage of patients with an F-VASI75 response at week 24 was 29.8% in the ruxolitinib cream group and 7.4% in the vehicle group (relative risk, 4.0; 95% confidence interval (CI), 1.9 to 8.4; $p < 0.001$). In TRuE-V2, the percentages were 30.9% and 11.4%, respectively (relative risk, 2.7; 95% CI, 1.5 to 4.9; $p < 0.001$). The results for key secondary end points showed superiority of ruxolitinib cream over vehicle control (F-VASI50, F-VASI90, T-VASI50 and F-VASI75 in the 52-week extension study)	Among patients who applied ruxolitinib cream for 52 weeks, adverse events occurred in 54.8% in TRuE-V1 and 62.3% in TRuE-V2; the most common adverse events were application site acne (6.3% and 6.6%, respectively), nasopharyngitis (5.4% and 6.1%) and application site pruritus (5.4% and 5.3%)

Table 2. *Cont.*

Drug	Study Data (Authors/Year/Country/NCT)	Study Design	Results	Side Effects
Tofacitinib (oral)	Song et al. [111]/2022/China/ No registration	Oral tofacitinib at 5 mg twice daily. Both control and treatment group were treated with halometasone cream applied externally to the lesions on the torso and limbs twice a day, and 0.1% tacrolimus ointment or pimecrolimus cream applied externally on the face and neck twice a day. In addition, NB-UVB therapy was administered three times weekly for a period of 16 weeks Real-world clinical practice out-of-label tofacitinib clinical trial 15 patients in treatment group and 19 controls with face and body vitiligo followed for 16 weeks	From eighth week, the repigmentation level was significantly higher in the combination than the control group ($p < 0.05$). The repigmentation improved in the tofacitinib group on acral lesions, torso and extremities No significant differences in lesions on the face and neck were observed between the combination and control groups during 16 weeks of treatment ($p > 0.05$), probably because both groups had great improvement	One patient treated with tofacitinib developed mild pain in his right thumb and right hallux after 3 weeks of treatment, but the pain resolved with cessation of tofacitinib 1 week later. Mild effects related to phototherapy
Ritlecitinib (oral)	Ezzedine et al. [110]/2023/USA/NCT03715829	Patients were randomized to once-daily oral ritlecitinib ± 4-week loading dose (200/50 mg, 100/50 mg, 30 mg or 10 mg) or placebo for 24 weeks (dose-ranging period). 187 patients subsequently received ritlecitinib at 200/50 mg daily in a 24-week extension period Phase 2b, randomized, double-blind, placebo-controlled, parallel-group, multicenter and dose-ranging study 364 patients with face and body vitiligo treated for a 24-week dose-ranging period and 24-week extension period	Significant differences from placebo in percent change from baseline in Facial-Vitiligo Area Scoring Index were observed for the 50 mg ritlecitinib groups with (−21.2 vs. 2.1; $p < 0.001$) or without (−18.5 vs. 2.1; $p < 0.001$) a loading dose and 30 mg ritlecitinib group (−14.6 vs. 2.1; $p = 0.01$). Accelerated improvement was observed after treatment with 200/50 mg ritlecitinib in the extension period (n = 187)	The 3 most common TEAEs were nasopharyngitis (15.9%), upper respiratory tract infection (11.5%) and headache (8.8%). 4 patients had confirmed cases of herpes zoster (all non-serious), 2 patients had malignancies (nonmelanoma skin cancers) and there were no thromboembolic events. No serious adverse events
Upadacitinib (oral)	No results published/2023/USA/NCT04927975 [112]	Oral upadacitinib (dose ranging) vs. placebo A multicenter, randomized, double-blind, placebo-controlled, dose-ranging study to evaluate the safety and efficacy of upadacitinib in subjects with non-segmental vitiligo. Phase 2 185 patients with face and body vitiligo followed for at least 24 weeks, up to 52 weeks	Ongoing. No results published	Ongoing. No results published
Ruxolitinib (topical)	No results published/2023/USA/NCT05247489 [109]	Group A: 1.5% ruxolitinib cream + narrow-band ultraviolet B phototherapy (NB-UVB). Group B: 1.5% ruxolitinib cream monotherapy A randomized, phase 2, open-label interventional study. 55 patients with face and body vitiligo follows for 48 weeks	Ongoing. No results published	Ongoing. No results published

Table 2. *Cont.*

Drug	Study Data (Authors/Year/Country/NCT)	Study Design	Results	Side Effects
Ruxolitinib (topical)	No publications available/2023/USA/NCT04530344 [108]	1.5% ruxolitinib cream or matching vehicle cream twice daily A double-blind, vehicle-controlled, randomized withdrawal and treatment extension study to assess the long-term efficacy and safety of ruxolitinib cream in participants with vitiligo Phase 3 458 patients with face and body vitiligo followed for 52 weeks	Completed. No publications available	Completed. No publications available
ARQ-252 (topical)	No results published/2022/USA/NCT04811131 [113]	0.3% ARQ-252 cream BID or vehicle cream BID, and active phototherapy or sham phototherapy for 24 weeks Phase 2a, parallel-group, double-blind, vehicle-controlled study of the safety and efficacy of 0.3% ARQ-252 cream in combination with NB-UVB phototherapy treatment in subjects with non-segmental facial vitiligo 114 patients with face and body vitiligo followed for 24 weeks	Terminated. No publications available	Terminated. No publications available
Cerdulatinib (topical)	No publications available/2022/USA/NCT04103060 [114]	0.37% cerdulatinib gel applied topically twice daily vs. vehicle cream A phase 2a, randomized, double-blind, vehicle-controlled study to assess the safety, tolerability and systemic exposure of 0.37% cerdulatinib gel in adults with vitiligo 33 patients with face and body vitiligo followed for 6 weeks	No publications available	No publications available
ATI-50002 (topical)	No publications available/2020/USA/NCT03468855 [115]	ATI-50002 topical solution, high dose active, twice daily, 24 weeks An open-label pilot study of the safety, tolerability and efficacy of ATI-50002 topical solution administered twice daily in adult subjects with non-segmental facial vitiligo. Phase 2 34 patients with face vitiligo followed for 24 weeks	Mean change in facial depigmentation in quantified area of interest (AOI) from baseline (Visit 2) to week 24 worsened after treatment: mean change + 2 (standard deviation 8.41)	Alcoholic pancreatitis and acute myocardial infarction (in 1 patient, not related to the drug), application site acne, other minor local adverse events

5.8. 5-Fluorouracil

5-Fluorouracil (5-FU) is a therapeutic agent that has been subject to growing interest in recent years for vitiligo treatment, thanks to the convenience of its topical formulation with very good results and almost no side effects. 5-FU stands as a crucial systemic chemotherapy agent in the treatment of cancer patients. In the context of vitiligo, its topical and intradermal formulation has been employed with diverse outcomes, often coupled with manual and electric dermabrasion, needling and fractional CO_2 laser.

Among these approaches, microneedling has emerged as a promising technique, demonstrating favorable outcomes. This method, also known as collagen induction therapy, is a minimally invasive procedure that uses fine miniature needles to create superficial holes in the skin that are hypothesized to trigger the repair and release of growth factors, stimulate the migration of keratinocytes and facilitate the penetration of other drugs. While different therapeutic modalities have been explored, the procedural aspect remains consistent across most studies. This involves microneedling, followed by the application of a uniformly thin layer of 5% 5-FU cream or solution. This protocol is typically administered once or twice monthly for a duration ranging from 3 to 6 months. Subsequently, patients are advised to apply 5-fluorouracil cream over the same patch daily for one week following each session. Both observational [116–118] and experimental studies have been undertaken to compare the efficacy of combination therapy versus only microneedling [119–121], only 5-FU [122], and microneedling coupled with tacrolimus application [123,124] or 308 nm excimer light [125]. The overall qualitative response was better in the patches treated with the combinational therapy, 5-fluorouracil and microneedling, with statistically significant better repigmentation rates compared to those treated with tacrolimus or microneedling alone. All studies showed significantly higher and excellent responses, considered as repigmentation above 75%, and also lower (considered poor) response rates (<25%). In the study conducted by Saad et al. [125], the treatment with the combination of microneedling then application of 5-FU and excimer showed a significant and earlier response versus the excimer alone. Also, the percentage of repigmentation was higher in the patches treated with the combination, especially in the face and torso.

To facilitate the penetration of 5-FU, other techniques have also been tried, such as dermabrasion [126,127] with a similar procedure to microneedling. The most superficial layers of the skin are removed with a dermabrader until the papillary dermis is reached and then a layer of 5-FU is applied. Participants were then advised to apply topical 5% 5-FU over the abraded area once or twice daily for 2–4 weeks, with excellent repigmentation responses after the treatment. In both techniques, the most reported side effects were erythema and itching.

Recent studies have also tested intradermal infiltrations of 5-FU (50 mg/mL) every 2 weeks, comparing its effect with infiltrations of triamcinolone acetonide (3 mg/mL) with the same frequency [128]. Intradermal fluorouracil showed the best overall improvement when compared with triamcinolone. During follow-up, the vitiliginous patches continued to repigment for 6 months in fluorouracil. Finally, the combination of 5-FU with phototherapy [129] has shown better results than phototherapy alone. The main disadvantage of intradermal infiltration is the higher rate of side effects, with most patients reporting pain and a burning sensation during injections, blistering and ulcer formation.

5.9. Platelet-Rich Plasma

Alternative therapeutic interventions, such as platelet-rich plasma (PRP), present a regenerative treatment modality by cultivating a fertile environment rich in growth factors and cytokines. It has been proposed to stimulate the restoration of normal cellular function and holds the potential to encourage the differentiation, proliferation and maturation of melanocytes and keratinocytes, thereby contributing to epidermal repigmentation [130].

Its role has been predominantly examined in conjunction with laser [131,132], phototherapy [133] and surgical treatments [134], where it appears to exert a synergistic effect, that significantly amplifies repigmentation rates across different studies. Nevertheless, the available evidence supporting its efficacy in monotherapy remains limited. Given the current knowledge gaps, further studies are imperative to validate the effectiveness of PRP and establish comprehensive guidelines for its application in the management of vitiligo and related cases.

5.10. Other Regenerative Therapies

Microneedling consists of a roller with fine miniature needles used to produce micro-injuries that activate factors promoting collagen secretion by fibroblasts and stimulate melanocytes' migration to non-pigmented areas. This technique has proven effective in monotherapy [135]. However, the combination of microneedling with topical therapies or NB-UVB was more effective compared to microneedling monotherapy [135]. As stated before, it can also be beneficial when combined with 5-fluorouracil [121]. On the other hand, microneedling has not shown an additional benefit when added to other therapies [136,137].

Other surgical therapies, oriented to grafting functional melanocytes in affected regions, constitute an emerging and promising alternative for cases of stable vitiligo. Numerous modalities have been described with different efficacy and tolerability outcomes that exceed the scope of this review and should be discussed separately [39].

5.11. Conventional Therapies versus Emerging Therapies

As noted in Section 3, conventional therapies for vitiligo have not been considered individually in the development of this review as they are beyond its scope. A summary of the conventional therapies considered in the expert consensus [39] and the emerging therapies reviewed is shown in Table 3.

Table 3. Conventional [39] versus emerging therapies.

Treatment Modality	Conventional versus Emerging	Advantages/Data That Favor Its Use	Main Disadvantages
Topical corticosteroids (TCSs)	Conventional	Recommended for vitiligo, particularly for extrafacial locations and more limited treatment areas Wide experience on its use	More effective for stabilization of vitiligo than for repigmentation Local side effects if applied continuously (skin atrophy, telangiectasia, hypertrichosis, acneiform eruptions and striae)
Topical calcineurin inhibitors	Conventional	As affective as TCS on face and neck, with better safety profile in these locations No serious adverse events detected in patients with vitiligo treated with topical calcineurin inhibitors	Less effective than TCS on extrafacial lesions Off-label use
Narrow-band ultraviolet B phototherapy (NB-UVB)	Conventional	Preferred first-line therapy for widespread or rapidly progressing disease No significant association with greater incidence of basal cell carcinoma, squamous cell carcinoma or melanoma	Bad response of acral lesions and areas lacking melanocyte reservoir Erythema and xerosis are common Multiple sessions are required, so patients have to attend their healthcare center two or three times a week for several months
Excimer devices	Conventional	Equally effective or even superior compared to NB-UVB Safety and tolerability of excimer laser therapy is comparable to NB-UVB	The cost of therapy is higher than NB-UVB Long-term adverse events not well-established
Home phototherapy	Conventional	Better compliance, similar repigmentation outcomes, similar frequency of adverse effects and less time investment	Shortage of home phototherapy units, high initial cost, low energy output of the device over time, lack of mechanical servicing and unfamiliarity of patients with the modality

Table 3. *Cont.*

Treatment Modality	Conventional versus Emerging	Advantages/Data That Favor Its Use	Main Disadvantages
Oral steroid minipulse therapy (dexamethasone, metilprednisolone or prednisone)	Conventional	Useful to stop disease progression	Not suitable for repigmentation on monotherapy Relapse after discontinuation Systemic corticosteroid-class side effects: weight gain, insomnia, agitation, acne, menstrual disturbances, hypertrichosis, growth retardation in children and immunosuppression
Surgical interventions	Conventional/emerging	Many different techniques A treatment option for segmental vitiligo and other localized and stabilized forms of vitiligo (non-segmental) after the documented failure of medical interventions	Koebner phenomenon is possible High cost Pros and cons depend on the technique, but this topic exceeds the subject of this review and should be discussed separately
Afamelanotide	Conventional	Potential benefit for use in combination with phototherapy	Subcutaneous administration More data need to be collected
Cyclosporine	Conventional	Useful for arresting vitiligo progression Might be useful as adjunctive treatment in autologous noncultured melanocyte–keratinocyte cell transplantation procedure	Not suitable for long-term treatment
Phosphodiesterase 4 (PDE-4) inhibitors	Emerging	Case reports of improvement with apremilast or crisaborole in monotherapy	Conflicting data on its use in combination with phototherapy
Trichloroacetic acid	Emerging	Good response on face vitiligo in combination with microneedling or phototherapy	More data need to be collected
Basic fibroblast growth factor (bFGF)	Emerging	Could improve repigmentation when combined with phototherapy or tacrolimus ointment	More data need to be collected
TNF inhibitors	Emerging	Isolated case reports showing efficacy in repigmentation	Most studies show no response or even TNFα inhibitor-induced vitiligo
Secukinumab	Emerging	A suitable option to replace a TNFα inhibitor after new-onset vitiligo related to TNFα inhibitors	Not recommended for the treatment of isolated vitiligo
Pseudocatalase	Emerging	Oxidative stress plays a role in vitiligo pathogenesis Initial data supported its efficacy	All recent data show no improvement in repigmentation
JAK inhibitors	Emerging	Multiple case reports and clinical trials support its efficacy Ruxolitinib cream already approved for vitiligo Several ongoing clinical trials with promising results	Long-term efficacy and long-term safety data need to be assessed More expensive than conventional treatments Results when used in combination with other treatment modalities need to be studied

Table 3. *Cont.*

Treatment Modality	Conventional versus Emerging	Advantages/Data That Favor Its Use	Main Disadvantages
5-fluorouracil	Emerging	Useful to achieve repigmentation when used alongside phototherapy, microneedling and dermabrasion Intradermal infiltrations of 5-FU have also been tested	Local side effects (burning, pruritus, blistering)
Platelet-rich plasma	Emerging	Synergistic effect in conjunction with laser, phototherapy and surgical treatments	Limited data on monotherapy More data need to be collected
Microneedling	Emerging	Could improve repigmentation in monotherapy or when combined with phototherapy or 5-fluorouracil	More data need to be collected

6. Conclusions

Vitiligo is a disease with a complex and multifactorial pathogenesis, which has a great impact on the quality of life of patients.

New horizons are opening up in the treatment of this disease, both with long-known molecules such as 5-fluorouracil and with new molecules such as JAK inhibitors. The latter are postulated as a first-rate therapeutic tool for the treatment of vitiligo at present and in the near future, probably in conjunction with other traditional treatments such as UVB phototherapy.

At the moment, there is no clearly outstanding option or fully satisfactory treatment, so it is necessary to keep up the development of new drugs as well as the publication of long-term effectiveness and safety data for existing treatments.

Author Contributions: Conceptualization, J.P.-B. and G.S.-M.; methodology, J.P.-B.; software, J.P.-B.; validation, G.S.-M., R.C.-M. and J.N.-R.; formal analysis, J.P.-B., J.N.-R. and R.C.-M.; investigation, J.P.-B., J.N.-R. and R.C.-M.; resources, G.S.-M.; data curation, J.P.-B.; writing—original draft preparation, J.P.-B., J.N.-R. and R.C.-M.; writing—review and editing, J.P.-B., J.N.-R. and G.S.-M.; visualization, J.P.-B.; supervision, G.S.-M. All authors have read and agreed to the published version of the manuscript.

Funding: This research received no external funding.

Data Availability Statement: The data that support the findings of this study are available from the corresponding author upon reasonable request. The data are not publicly available due to privacy or ethical restrictions.

Conflicts of Interest: The authors declare no conflict of interest.

References

1. Bergqvist, C.; Ezzedine, K. Vitiligo: A Focus on Pathogenesis and Its Therapeutic Implications. *J. Dermatol.* **2021**, *48*, 252–270. [CrossRef]
2. Krüger, C.; Schallreuter, K.U. A Review of the Worldwide Prevalence of Vitiligo in Children/Adolescents and Adults. *Int. J. Dermatol.* **2012**, *51*, 1206–1212. [CrossRef] [PubMed]
3. Zhang, Y.; Cai, Y.; Shi, M.; Jiang, S.; Cui, S.; Wu, Y.; Gao, X.-H.; Chen, H.-D. The Prevalence of Vitiligo: A Meta-Analysis. *PLoS ONE* **2016**, *11*, e0163806. [CrossRef] [PubMed]
4. Bibeau, K.; Pandya, A.G.; Ezzedine, K.; Jones, H.; Gao, J.; Lindley, A.; Harris, J.E. Vitiligo Prevalence and Quality of Life among Adults in Europe, Japan and the USA. *J. Eur. Acad. Dermatol. Venereol.* **2022**, *36*, 1831–1844. [CrossRef] [PubMed]
5. Linthorst Homan, M.W.; Spuls, P.I.; de Korte, J.; Bos, J.D.; Sprangers, M.A.; van der Veen, J.P.W. The Burden of Vitiligo: Patient Characteristics Associated with Quality of Life. *J. Am. Acad. Dermatol.* **2009**, *61*, 411–420. [CrossRef] [PubMed]
6. Rodrigues, M.; Ezzedine, K.; Hamzavi, I.; Pandya, A.G.; Harris, J.E.; Vitiligo Working Group. New Discoveries in the Pathogenesis and Classification of Vitiligo. *J. Am. Acad. Dermatol.* **2017**, *77*, 1–13. [CrossRef]

7. Spritz, R.A.; Santorico, S.A. The Genetic Basis of Vitiligo. *J. Investig. Dermatol.* **2021**, *141*, 265–273. [CrossRef] [PubMed]
8. Roberts, G.H.L.; Santorico, S.A.; Spritz, R.A. Deep Genotype Imputation Captures Virtually All Heritability of Autoimmune Vitiligo. *Hum. Mol. Genet.* **2020**, *29*, 859–863. [CrossRef]
9. Kundu, R.V.; Mhlaba, J.M.; Rangel, S.M.; Le Poole, I.C. The Convergence Theory for Vitiligo: A Reappraisal. *Exp. Dermatol.* **2019**, *28*, 647–655. [CrossRef]
10. Qi, F.; Liu, F.; Gao, L. Janus Kinase Inhibitors in the Treatment of Vitiligo: A Review. *Front. Immunol.* **2021**, *12*, 790125. [CrossRef]
11. Feng, Y.; Lu, Y. Advances in Vitiligo: Update on Therapeutic Targets. *Front. Immunol.* **2022**, *13*, 986918. [CrossRef]
12. Bergqvist, C.; Ezzedine, K. Vitiligo: A Review. *Dermatology* **2020**, *236*, 571–592. [CrossRef] [PubMed]
13. Chang, W.-L.; Lee, W.-R.; Kuo, Y.-C.; Huang, Y.-H. Vitiligo: An Autoimmune Skin Disease and Its Immunomodulatory Therapeutic Intervention. *Front. Cell Dev. Biol.* **2021**, *9*, 797026. [CrossRef] [PubMed]
14. Le Poole, I.C.; van den Wijngaard, R.M.; Westerhof, W.; Das, P.K. Presence of T Cells and Macrophages in Inflammatory Vitiligo Skin Parallels Melanocyte Disappearance. *Am. J. Pathol.* **1996**, *148*, 1219–1228. [PubMed]
15. Palermo, B.; Campanelli, R.; Garbelli, S.; Mantovani, S.; Lantelme, E.; Brazzelli, V.; Ardigó, M.; Borroni, G.; Martinetti, M.; Badulli, C.; et al. Specific Cytotoxic T Lymphocyte Responses against Melan-A/MART1, Tyrosinase and Gp100 in Vitiligo by the Use of Major Histocompatibility Complex/Peptide Tetramers: The Role of Cellular Immunity in the Etiopathogenesis of Vitiligo. *J. Investig. Dermatol.* **2001**, *117*, 326–332. [CrossRef] [PubMed]
16. van den Boorn, J.G.; Konijnenberg, D.; Dellemijn, T.A.M.; van der Veen, J.P.W.; Bos, J.D.; Melief, C.J.M.; Vyth-Dreese, F.A.; Luiten, R.M. Autoimmune Destruction of Skin Melanocytes by Perilesional T Cells from Vitiligo Patients. *J. Investig. Dermatol.* **2009**, *129*, 2220–2232. [CrossRef] [PubMed]
17. Sibaud, V. Dermatologic Reactions to Immune Checkpoint Inhibitors: Skin Toxicities and Immunotherapy. *Am. J. Clin. Dermatol.* **2018**, *19*, 345–361. [CrossRef] [PubMed]
18. He, X.; Xu, C. Immune Checkpoint Signaling and Cancer Immunotherapy. *Cell Res.* **2020**, *30*, 660–669. [CrossRef]
19. Frisoli, M.L.; Essien, K.; Harris, J.E. Vitiligo: Mechanisms of Pathogenesis and Treatment. *Annu. Rev. Immunol.* **2020**, *38*, 621–648. [CrossRef]
20. Wang, X.X.; Wang, Q.Q.; Wu, J.Q.; Jiang, M.; Chen, L.; Zhang, C.F.; Xiang, L.H. Increased Expression of CXCR3 and Its Ligands in Patients with Vitiligo and CXCL10 as a Potential Clinical Marker for Vitiligo. *Br. J. Dermatol.* **2016**, *174*, 1318–1326. [CrossRef]
21. Richmond, J.M.; Bangari, D.S.; Essien, K.I.; Currimbhoy, S.D.; Groom, J.R.; Pandya, A.G.; Youd, M.E.; Luster, A.D.; Harris, J.E. Keratinocyte-Derived Chemokines Orchestrate T-Cell Positioning in the Epidermis during Vitiligo and May Serve as Biomarkers of Disease. *J. Investig. Dermatol.* **2017**, *137*, 350–358. [CrossRef] [PubMed]
22. Garcia-Melendo, C.; Cubiró, X.; Puig, L. Inhibidores de JAK: Usos en dermatología. Parte 1: Generalidades, aplicaciones en vitíligo y en alopecia areata. *Actas Dermo-Sifiliográficas* **2021**, *112*, 503–515. [CrossRef]
23. Solimani, F.; Meier, K.; Ghoreschi, K. Emerging Topical and Systemic JAK Inhibitors in Dermatology. *Front. Immunol.* **2019**, *10*, 2847. [CrossRef] [PubMed]
24. Tokura, Y.; Phadungsaksawasdi, P.; Kurihara, K.; Fujiyama, T.; Honda, T. Pathophysiology of Skin Resident Memory T Cells. *Front. Immunol.* **2020**, *11*, 618897. [CrossRef]
25. Richmond, J.M.; Strassner, J.P.; Rashighi, M.; Agarwal, P.; Garg, M.; Essien, K.I.; Pell, L.S.; Harris, J.E. Resident Memory and Recirculating Memory T Cells Cooperate to Maintain Disease in a Mouse Model of Vitiligo. *J. Investig. Dermatol.* **2019**, *139*, 769–778. [CrossRef] [PubMed]
26. Adachi, T.; Kobayashi, T.; Sugihara, E.; Yamada, T.; Ikuta, K.; Pittaluga, S.; Saya, H.; Amagai, M.; Nagao, K. Hair Follicle-Derived IL-7 and IL-15 Mediate Skin-Resident Memory T Cell Homeostasis and Lymphoma. *Nat. Med.* **2015**, *21*, 1272–1279. [CrossRef]
27. Yuan, X.; Dong, Y.; Tsurushita, N.; Tso, J.Y.; Fu, W. CD122 Blockade Restores Immunological Tolerance in Autoimmune Type 1 Diabetes via Multiple Mechanisms. *JCI Insight* **2018**, *3*, e96600. [CrossRef]
28. Kroon, M.W.; Kemp, E.H.; Wind, B.S.; Krebbers, G.; Bos, J.D.; Gawkrodger, D.J.; Wolkerstorfer, A.; van der Veen, J.P.W.; Luiten, R.M. Melanocyte Antigen-Specific Antibodies Cannot Be Used as Markers for Recent Disease Activity in Patients with Vitiligo. *J. Eur. Acad. Dermatol. Venereol.* **2013**, *27*, 1172–1175. [CrossRef]
29. Katz, E.L.; Harris, J.E. Translational Research in Vitiligo. *Front. Immunol.* **2021**, *12*, 624517. [CrossRef]
30. Speeckaert, R.; Dugardin, J.; Lambert, J.; Lapeere, H.; Verhaeghe, E.; Speeckaert, M.M.; van Geel, N. Critical Appraisal of the Oxidative Stress Pathway in Vitiligo: A Systematic Review and Meta-Analysis. *J. Eur. Acad. Dermatol. Venereol.* **2018**, *32*, 1089–1098. [CrossRef]
31. Puri, N.; Mojamdar, M.; Ramaiah, A. In Vitro Growth Characteristics of Melanocytes Obtained from Adult Normal and Vitiligo Subjects. *J. Investig. Dermatol.* **1987**, *88*, 434–438. [CrossRef]
32. Denat, L.; Kadekaro, A.L.; Marrot, L.; Leachman, S.A.; Abdel-Malek, Z.A. Melanocytes as Instigators and Victims of Oxidative Stress. *J. Investig. Dermatol.* **2014**, *134*, 1512–1518. [CrossRef]
33. Marchioro, H.Z.; Silva de Castro, C.C.; Fava, V.M.; Sakiyama, P.H.; Dellatorre, G.; Miot, H.A. Update on the Pathogenesis of Vitiligo. *An. Bras. Dermatol.* **2022**, *97*, 478–490. [CrossRef] [PubMed]
34. Kang, P.; Zhang, W.; Chen, X.; Yi, X.; Song, P.; Chang, Y.; Zhang, S.; Gao, T.; Li, C.; Li, S. TRPM2 Mediates Mitochondria-Dependent Apoptosis of Melanocytes under Oxidative Stress. *Free Radic. Biol. Med.* **2018**, *126*, 259–268. [CrossRef] [PubMed]

35. Li, S.; Zhu, G.; Yang, Y.; Jian, Z.; Guo, S.; Dai, W.; Shi, Q.; Ge, R.; Ma, J.; Liu, L.; et al. Oxidative Stress Drives CD8+ T-Cell Skin Trafficking in Patients with Vitiligo through CXCL16 Upregulation by Activating the Unfolded Protein Response in Keratinocytes. *J. Allergy Clin. Immunol.* **2017**, *140*, 177–189.e9. [CrossRef] [PubMed]
36. Rezk, A.F.; Kemp, D.M.; El-Domyati, M.; El-Din, W.H.; Lee, J.B.; Uitto, J.; Igoucheva, O.; Alexeev, V. Misbalanced CXCL12 and CCL5 Chemotactic Signals in Vitiligo Onset and Progression. *J. Investig. Dermatol.* **2017**, *137*, 1126–1134. [CrossRef]
37. Regazzetti, C.; Joly, F.; Marty, C.; Rivier, M.; Mehul, B.; Reiniche, P.; Mounier, C.; Rival, Y.; Piwnica, D.; Cavalié, M.; et al. Transcriptional Analysis of Vitiligo Skin Reveals the Alteration of WNT Pathway: A Promising Target for Repigmenting Vitiligo Patients. *J. Investig. Dermatol.* **2015**, *135*, 3105–3114. [CrossRef]
38. Wagner, R.Y.; Luciani, F.; Cario-André, M.; Rubod, A.; Petit, V.; Benzekri, L.; Ezzedine, K.; Lepreux, S.; Steingrimsson, E.; Taieb, A.; et al. Altered E-Cadherin Levels and Distribution in Melanocytes Precede Clinical Manifestations of Vitiligo. *J. Investig. Dermatol.* **2015**, *135*, 1810–1819. [CrossRef]
39. Seneschal, J.; Speeckaert, R.; Taïeb, A.; Wolkerstorfer, A.; Passeron, T.; Pandya, A.G.; Lim, H.W.; Ezzedine, K.; Zhou, Y.; Xiang, F.; et al. Worldwide Expert Recommendations for the Diagnosis and Management of Vitiligo: Position Statement from the International Vitiligo Task Force—Part 2: Specific Treatment Recommendations. *J. Eur. Acad. Dermatol. Venereol.* **2023**, *37*, 2185–2195. [CrossRef]
40. Bae, J.M.; Jung, H.M.; Hong, B.Y.; Lee, J.H.; Choi, W.J.; Lee, J.H.; Kim, G.M. Phototherapy for Vitiligo. *JAMA Dermatol.* **2017**, *153*, 666–674. [CrossRef]
41. Zubair, R.; Hamzavi, I.H. Phototherapy for Vitiligo. *Dermatol. Clin.* **2020**, *38*, 55–62. [CrossRef]
42. Khandpur, S.; Bhatia, R.; Bhadoria, A.S. Narrow-Band Ultraviolet B Comb as an Effective Home-Based Phototherapy Device for Limited or Localized Non-Segmental Vitiligo: A Pilot, Open-Label, Single-Arm Clinical Study. *Indian J. Dermatol. Venereol. Leprol.* **2020**, *86*, 298–301. [CrossRef] [PubMed]
43. Eleftheriadou, V.; Thomas, K.; Ravenscroft, J.; Whitton, M.; Batchelor, J.; Williams, H. Feasibility, Double-Blind, Randomised, Placebo-Controlled, Multi-Centre Trial of Hand-Held NB-UVB Phototherapy for the Treatment of Vitiligo at Home (HI-Light Trial: Home Intervention of Light Therapy). *Trials* **2014**, *15*, 51. [CrossRef] [PubMed]
44. Dillon, J.-C.P.; Ford, C.; Hynan, L.S.; Pandya, A.G. A Cross-Sectional, Comparative Study of Home vs in-Office NB-UVB Phototherapy for Vitiligo. *Photodermatol. Photoimmunol. Photomed.* **2017**, *33*, 282–283. [CrossRef] [PubMed]
45. Zhang, L.; Wang, X.; Chen, S.; Zhao, J.; Wu, J.; Jiang, M.; Zhang, C.; Xiang, L. Comparison of Efficacy and Safety Profile for Home NB-UVB vs. Outpatient NB-UVB in the Treatment of Non-Segmental Vitiligo: A Prospective Cohort Study. *Photodermatol. Photoimmunol. Photomed.* **2019**, *35*, 261–267. [CrossRef] [PubMed]
46. Liu, B.; Sun, Y.; Song, J.; Wu, Z. Home vs Hospital Narrowband UVB Treatment by a Hand-Held Unit for New-Onset Vitiligo: A Pilot Randomized Controlled Study. *Photodermatol. Photoimmunol. Photomed.* **2020**, *36*, 14–20. [CrossRef]
47. Wind, B.S.; Kroon, M.W.; Beek, J.F.; Van Der Veen, J.P.W.; Nieuweboer-Krobotová, L.; Meesters, A.A.; Bos, J.D.; Wolkerstorfer, A. Home vs. Outpatient Narrowband Ultraviolet B Therapy for the Treatment of Nonsegmental Vitiligo: A Retrospective Questionnaire Study: Correspondence. *Br. J. Dermatol.* **2010**, *162*, 1142–1144. [CrossRef]
48. Raghuwanshi, A.D.; Jambhore, M.W.; Viswanath, V.; Gopalani, V. A Retrospective Study of the Utility of Targeted Phototherapy in Vitiligo. *Indian J. Dermatol. Venereol. Leprol.* **2018**, *84*, 49–53. [CrossRef]
49. Juntongjin, P.; Toncharoenphong, N. Effectiveness of a Combined 308-Nm Excimer Lamp and Topical Mid-Potent Steroid Treatment for Facial Vitiligo: A Preliminary, Randomized Double-Blinded Controlled Study. *Lasers Med. Sci.* **2020**, *35*, 2023–2029. [CrossRef]
50. Tien Guan, S.T.; Theng, C.; Chang, A. Randomized, Parallel Group Trial Comparing Home-Based Phototherapy with Institution-Based 308 Excimer Lamp for the Treatment of Focal Vitiligo Vulgaris. *J. Am. Acad. Dermatol.* **2015**, *72*, 733–735. [CrossRef]
51. Sakhiya, J.; Sakhiya, D.; Virmani, N.; Gajjar, T.; Kaklotar, J.; Khambhati, R.; Daruwala, F.; Dudhatra, N. A Retrospective Study of 3,000 Indian Patients with Vitiligo Treated with Phototherapy or Topical Monotherapy. *J. Clin. Aesthet. Dermatol.* **2021**, *14*, 46–49. [PubMed]
52. Grimes, P.E.; Hamzavi, I.; Lebwohl, M.; Ortonne, J.P.; Lim, H.W. The Efficacy of Afamelanotide and Narrowband UV-B Phototherapy for Repigmentation of Vitiligo. *JAMA Dermatol.* **2013**, *149*, 68. [CrossRef] [PubMed]
53. Lim, H.W.; Grimes, P.E.; Agbai, O.; Hamzavi, I.; Henderson, M.; Haddican, M.; Linkner, R.V.; Lebwohl, M. Afamelanotide and Narrowband UV-B Phototherapy for the Treatment of Vitiligo: A Randomized Multicenter Trial. *JAMA Dermatol.* **2015**, *151*, 42. [CrossRef] [PubMed]
54. Toh, J.J.H.; Chuah, S.Y.; Jhingan, A.; Chong, W.-S.; Thng, S.T.G. Afamelanotide Implants and Narrow-Band Ultraviolet B Phototherapy for the Treatment of Nonsegmental Vitiligo in Asians. *J. Am. Acad. Dermatol.* **2020**, *82*, 1517–1519. [CrossRef] [PubMed]
55. Mutalik, S.; Shah, S.; Sidwadkar, V.; Khoja, M. Efficacy of Cyclosporine After Autologous Noncultured Melanocyte Transplantation in Localized Stable Vitiligo—A Pilot, Open Label, Comparative Study. *Dermatol. Surg.* **2017**, *43*, 1339–1347. [CrossRef]
56. Schafer, P. Apremilast Mechanism of Action and Application to Psoriasis and Psoriatic Arthritis. *Biochem. Pharmacol.* **2012**, *83*, 1583–1590. [CrossRef]
57. Huff, S.B.; Gottwald, L.D. Repigmentation of Tenacious Vitiligo on Apremilast. *Case Rep. Dermatol. Med.* **2017**, *2017*, 2386234. [CrossRef]

58. Majid, I.; Imran, S.; Batool, S. Apremilast Is Effective in Controlling the Progression of Adult Vitiligo: A Case Series. *Dermatologic. Therapy* **2019**, *32*, e12923. [CrossRef]
59. Plachouri, K.-M.; Kyriakou, G.; Chourdakis, V.; Georgiou, S.; Grafanaki, K. One Stone, Two Birds: Improvement of Early-Onset Vitiligo under Apremilast in a Patient with Plaque Psoriasis. *Dermatol. Ther.* **2019**, *32*, e13064. [CrossRef]
60. Khemis, A.; Fontas, E.; Moulin, S.; Montaudié, H.; Lacour, J.-P.; Passeron, T. Apremilast in Combination with Narrowband UVB in the Treatment of Vitiligo: A 52-Week Monocentric Prospective Randomized Placebo-Controlled Study. *J. Investig. Dermatol.* **2020**, *140*, 1533–1537.e2. [CrossRef]
61. Kim, H.J.; Singer, G.K.; Del Duca, E.; Abittan, B.J.; Chima, M.A.; Kimmel, G.; Bares, J.; Gagliotti, M.; Genece, J.; Chu, J.; et al. Combination of Apremilast and Narrowband Ultraviolet B Light in the Treatment of Generalized Vitiligo in Skin Phototypes IV to VI: A Randomized Split-Body Pilot Study. *J. Am. Acad. Dermatol.* **2021**, *85*, 1657–1660. [CrossRef]
62. Sharma, S.; Bhardwaj, A.; Dwivedi, P.; Yadav, S.S.; Shamim, M.A.; Singh, S.; Sharma, P.P.; Ambwani, S.; SIngh, K. Apremilast Add-On Benefits Over Conventional Drugs (ABCD) in Unstable Non-Segmental Vitiligo: A 12-Week Single-Center Randomized Controlled Trial. *Cureus* **2023**, *15*, e37180. [CrossRef]
63. Nofal, A.; Fawzy, M.M.; Alakad, R. Trichloroacetic Acid in Different Concentrations: A Promising Treatment Modality for Vitiligo. *Dermatol. Surg.* **2021**, *47*, e53–e57. [CrossRef]
64. Kimura, A.; Kanazawa, N.; Li, H.-J.; Yonei, N.; Yamamoto, Y.; Furukawa, F. Influence of Trichloroacetic Acid Peeling on the Skin Stress Response System. *J. Dermatol.* **2011**, *38*, 740–747. [CrossRef]
65. Khater, M.; Nasr, M.; Salah, S.; Khattab, F.M. Clinical Evaluation of the Efficacy of Trichloroacetic Acid 70% after Microneedling vs Intradermal Injection of 5-Fluorouracil in the Treatment of Nonsegmental Vitiligo; A Prospective Comparative Study. *Dermatol. Ther.* **2020**, *33*, e13532. [CrossRef]
66. Nofal, A.; Eldeeb, F.; Shalaby, M.; Al-Balat, W. Microneedling Combined with Pimecrolimus, 5-Fluorouracil, and Trichloroacetic Acid in the Treatment of Vitiligo: A Comparative Study. *Dermatol. Ther.* **2022**, *35*, e15294. [CrossRef] [PubMed]
67. Ibrahim, S.; Hunter, N.; Mashaly, H.; Dorgham, D.; Shaker, O. Trichloroacetic Acid Peel 15% + NB-UVB Versus Trichloroacetic Acid Peel 25% + NB-UVB for Stable Non-Segmental Vitiligo. *Med. J. Cairo Univ.* **2016**, *84*, 959–963.
68. Wu, C.S.; Lan, C.C.; Chiou, M.H.; Yu, H. Basic Fibroblast Growth Factor Promotes Melanocyte Migration via Increased Expression of P125(FAK) on Melanocytes. *Acta Derm. -Venereol.* **2006**, *86*, 498–502. [CrossRef] [PubMed]
69. Shah, B.; Godse, K.; Mahajan, S.; Grandhi, S.; Shendkar, S.; Sharma, A.; Teli, C.; Pathak, R.; Parsad, D. Efficacy and Safety of Basic Fibroblast Growth Factor (bFGF) Related Decapeptide Solution plus Tacrolimus 0.1% Ointment versus Tacrolimus 0.1% Ointment in the Treatment of Stable Vitiligo. *Dermatol. Ther.* **2019**, *32*, e13109. [CrossRef]
70. Nayak, C.S.; Kura, M.M.; Banerjee, G.; Patil, S.P.; Deshpande, A.; Sekar, S.; Sharma, A.; Pathak, R.; Sarma, P. Efficacy and Safety Comparison of Basic Fibroblast Growth Factor-Related Decapeptide 0.1% Solution (bFGFrP) Plus Oral PUVA Combination Therapy with Oral PUVA Monotherapy in the Treatment of Vitiligo. *J. Cutan. Aesthet. Surg.* **2023**, *16*, 28–33. [CrossRef]
71. Sharma, A.; Majid, I.; Kumar, H.K.; Banodkar, P.; Mhatre, M.; Mohod, B.; Jaiswal, A. The Safety and Effectiveness of Decapeptide in Patients With Vitiligo: A Real-World Study. *Cureus* **2023**, *15*, e41418. [CrossRef] [PubMed]
72. Alghamdi, K.M.; Khurrum, H.; Taieb, A.; Ezzedine, K. Treatment of Generalized Vitiligo with Anti-TNF-α Agents. *J. Drugs Dermatol.* **2012**, *11*, 534–539.
73. Simón, J.-A.; Burgos-Vargas, R. Vitiligo Improvement in a Patient with Ankylosing Spondylitis Treated with Infliximab. *Dermatology* **2008**, *216*, 234–235. [CrossRef] [PubMed]
74. Campanati, A.; Giuliodori, K.; Ganzetti, G.; Liberati, G.; Offidani, A.M. A Patient with Psoriasis and Vitiligo Treated with Etanercept. *Am. J. Clin. Dermatol.* **2010**, *11*, 46–48. [CrossRef]
75. Rigopoulos, D.; Gregoriou, S.; Larios, G.; Moustou, E.; Belayeva-Karatza, E.; Kalogeromitros, D. Etanercept in the Treatment of Vitiligo. *Dermatology* **2007**, *215*, 84–85. [CrossRef]
76. Palazzo, G. Resolution of Post-Adalimumab Vitiligo with Secukinumab in a Patient with Psoriasis Vulgaris. *Oxf. Med. Case Rep.* **2020**, *2020*, omz134. [CrossRef] [PubMed]
77. Bassiouny, D.A.; Shaker, O. Role of Interleukin-17 in the Pathogenesis of Vitiligo: Role of IL-17 in the Pathogenesis of Vitiligo. *Clin. Exp. Dermatol.* **2011**, *36*, 292–297. [CrossRef]
78. Schallreuter, K.U.; Moore, J.; Wood, J.M.; Beazley, W.D.; Gaze, D.C.; Tobin, D.J.; Marshall, H.S.; Panske, A.; Panzig, E.; Hibberts, N.A. In Vivo and In Vitro Evidence for Hydrogen Peroxide (H_2O_2) Accumulation in the Epidermis of Patients with Vitiligo and Its Successful Removal by a UVB-Activated Pseudocatalase. *J. Investig. Dermatol. Symp. Proc.* **1999**, *4*, 91–96. [CrossRef]
79. Schallreuter, K.U.; Krüger, C.; Würfel, B.A.; Panske, A.; Wood, J.M. From Basic Research to the Bedside: Efficacy of Topical Treatment with Pseudocatalase PC-KUS in 71 Children with Vitiligo. *Int. J. Dermatol.* **2008**, *47*, 743–753. [CrossRef]
80. Patel, D.C.; Evans, A.V.; Hawk, J.L.M. Topical Pseudocatalase Mousse and Narrowband UVB Phototherapy Is Not Effective for Vitiligo: An Open, Single-Centre Study. *Clin. Exp. Dermatol.* **2002**, *27*, 641–644. [CrossRef]
81. Bakis-Petsoglou, S.; Le Guay, J.L.; Wittal, R. A Randomized, Double-Blinded, Placebo-Controlled Trial of Pseudocatalase Cream and Narrowband Ultraviolet B in the Treatment of Vitiligo. *Br. J. Dermatol.* **2009**, *161*, 910–917. [CrossRef]
82. Alshiyab, D.M.; Al-Qarqaz, F.A.; Muhaidat, J.M.; Alkhader, Y.S.; Al-Sheyab, R.F.; Jafaar, S.I. Comparison of the Efficacy of Tacrolimus 0.1% Ointment and Tacrolimus 0.1% plus Topical Pseudocatalase/Superoxide Dismutase Gel in Children with Limited Vitiligo: A Randomized Controlled Trial. *J. Dermatol. Treat.* **2022**, *33*, 146–149. [CrossRef] [PubMed]

83. Garcia-Melendo, C.; Cubiró, X.; Puig, L. Janus Kinase Inhibitors in Dermatology: Part 2: Applications in Psoriasis, Atopic Dermatitis, and Other Dermatoses. *Actas Dermo-Sifiliográficas (Engl. Ed.)* **2021**, *112*, 586–600. [CrossRef] [PubMed]
84. Rosmarin, D.; Pandya, A.G.; Lebwohl, M.; Grimes, P.; Hamzavi, I.; Gottlieb, A.B.; Butler, K.; Kuo, F.; Sun, K.; Ji, T.; et al. Ruxolitinib Cream for Treatment of Vitiligo: A Randomised, Controlled, Phase 2 Trial. *Lancet* **2020**, *396*, 110–120. [CrossRef] [PubMed]
85. Craiglow, B.G.; King, B.A. Tofacitinib Citrate for the Treatment of Vitiligo: A Pathogenesis-Directed Therapy. *JAMA Dermatol.* **2015**, *151*, 1110–1112. [CrossRef]
86. Harris, J.E.; Rashighi, M.; Nguyen, N.; Jabbari, A.; Ulerio, G.; Clynes, R.; Christiano, A.M.; Mackay-Wiggan, J. Rapid Skin Repigmentation on Oral Ruxolitinib in a Patient with Coexistent Vitiligo and Alopecia Areata (AA). *J. Am. Acad. Dermatol.* **2016**, *74*, 370–371. [CrossRef]
87. Komnitski, M.; Komnitski, A.; Komnitski Junior, A.; Silva de Castro, C.C. Partial Repigmentation of Vitiligo with Tofacitinib, without Exposure to Ultraviolet Radiation. *An. Bras. Dermatol.* **2020**, *95*, 473–476. [CrossRef]
88. Vu, M.; Heyes, C.; Robertson, S.J.; Varigos, G.A.; Ross, G. Oral Tofacitinib: A Promising Treatment in Atopic Dermatitis, Alopecia Areata and Vitiligo. *Clin. Exp. Dermatol.* **2017**, *42*, 942–944. [CrossRef]
89. Kim, S.R.; Heaton, H.; Liu, L.Y.; King, B.A. Rapid Repigmentation of Vitiligo Using Tofacitinib Plus Low-Dose, Narrowband UV-B Phototherapy. *JAMA Dermatol.* **2018**, *154*, 370–371. [CrossRef]
90. Li, X.; Sun, Y.; Du, J.; Wang, F.; Ding, X. Excellent Repigmentation of Generalized Vitiligo with Oral Baricitinib Combined with NB-UVB Phototherapy. *Clin. Cosmet. Investig. Dermatol.* **2023**, *16*, 635–638. [CrossRef]
91. Pan, T.; Mu, Y.; Shi, X.; Chen, L. Concurrent Vitiligo and Atopic Dermatitis Successfully Treated with Upadacitinib: A Case Report. *J. Dermatol. Treat.* **2023**, *34*, 2200873. [CrossRef]
92. Liu, L.Y.; Strassner, J.P.; Refat, M.A.; Harris, J.E.; King, B.A. Repigmentation in Vitiligo Using the Janus Kinase Inhibitor Tofacitinib May Require Concomitant Light Exposure. *J. Am. Acad. Dermatol.* **2017**, *77*, 675–682.e1. [CrossRef]
93. Gianfaldoni, S.; Tchernev, G.; Wollina, U.; Roccia, M.G.; Fioranelli, M.; Lotti, J.; Rovesti, M.; Satolli, F.; Valle, Y.; Goren, A.; et al. Micro—Focused Phototherapy Associated To Janus Kinase Inhibitor: A Promising Valid Therapeutic Option for Patients with Localized Vitiligo. *Open Access Maced. J. Med. Sci.* **2018**, *6*, 46–48. [CrossRef] [PubMed]
94. Fang, W.-C.; Chiu, S.-H.; Lin, S.-Y.; Huang, S.-M.; Lan, C.-C.E. Evaluation of Low-Dose Tofacitinib Combining Narrowband UVB Therapy for Treating Vitiligo Patients Who Had Failed Previous Therapy: A Pilot Study. *Photodermatol. Photoimmunol. Photomed.* **2021**, *37*, 345–347. [CrossRef] [PubMed]
95. Fang, W.-C.; Lin, S.-Y.; Huang, S.-M.; Lan, C.-C.E. Low-Dose Tofacitinib with 308-Nm Excimer Therapy Successfully Induced Repigmentation in Patients with Refractory Vitiligo. *Clin. Exp. Dermatol.* **2022**, *47*, 782–783. [CrossRef] [PubMed]
96. Su, X.; Luo, R.; Ruan, S.; Zhong, Q.; Zhuang, Z.; Xiao, Z.; Zhang, P.; Cheng, B.; Gong, T.; Ji, C. Efficacy and Tolerability of Oral Upadacitinib Monotherapy in Patients with Recalcitrant Vitiligo. *J. Am. Acad. Dermatol.* **2023**, *89*, 1257–1259. [CrossRef] [PubMed]
97. Joshipura, D.; Plotnikova, N.; Goldminz, A.; Deverapalli, S.; Turkowski, Y.; Gottlieb, A.; Rosmarin, D. Importance of Light in the Treatment of Vitiligo with JAK-Inhibitors. *J. Dermatol. Treat.* **2018**, *29*, 98–99. [CrossRef]
98. McKesey, J.; Pandya, A.G. A Pilot Study of 2% Tofacitinib Cream with Narrowband Ultraviolet B for the Treatment of Facial Vitiligo. *J. Am. Acad. Dermatol.* **2019**, *81*, 646–648. [CrossRef] [PubMed]
99. Mobasher, P.; Guerra, R.; Li, S.J.; Frangos, J.; Ganesan, A.K.; Huang, V. Open-Label Pilot Study of Tofacitinib 2% for the Treatment of Refractory Vitiligo. *Br. J. Dermatol.* **2020**, *182*, 1047–1049. [CrossRef]
100. Olamiju, B.; Craiglow, B.G. Tofacitinib Cream plus Narrowband Ultraviolet B Phototherapy for Segmental Vitiligo in a Child. *Pediatr. Dermatol.* **2020**, *37*, 754–755. [CrossRef]
101. Berbert Ferreira, S.; Berbert Ferreira, R.; Neves Neto, A.C.; Assef, S.M.C.; Scheinberg, M. Topical Tofacitinib: A Janus Kinase Inhibitor for the Treatment of Vitiligo in an Adolescent Patient. *Case Rep. Dermatol.* **2021**, *13*, 190–194. [CrossRef]
102. Narla, S.; Oska, S.; Lyons, A.B.; Lim, H.W.; Hamzavi, I.H. Association of Myalgias with Compounded Topical Janus Kinase Inhibitor Use in Vitiligo. *JAAD Case Rep.* **2020**, *6*, 637–639. [CrossRef]
103. Rothstein, B.; Joshipura, D.; Saraiya, A.; Abdat, R.; Ashkar, H.; Turkowski, Y.; Sheth, V.; Huang, V.; Au, S.C.; Kachuk, C.; et al. Treatment of Vitiligo with the Topical Janus Kinase Inhibitor Ruxolitinib. *J. Am. Acad. Dermatol.* **2017**, *76*, 1054–1060.e1. [CrossRef]
104. Joshipura, D.; Alomran, A.; Zancanaro, P.; Rosmarin, D. Treatment of Vitiligo with the Topical Janus Kinase Inhibitor Ruxolitinib: A 32-Week Open-Label Extension Study with Optional Narrow-Band Ultraviolet B. *J. Am. Acad. Dermatol.* **2018**, *78*, 1205–1207.e1. [CrossRef]
105. Hamzavi, I.; Rosmarin, D.; Harris, J.E.; Pandya, A.G.; Lebwohl, M.; Gottlieb, A.B.; Butler, K.; Kuo, F.I.; Sun, K.; Grimes, P. Efficacy of Ruxolitinib Cream in Vitiligo by Patient Characteristics and Affected Body Areas: Descriptive Subgroup Analyses from a Phase 2, Randomized, Double-Blind Trial. *J. Am. Acad. Dermatol.* **2022**, *86*, 1398–1401. [CrossRef]
106. Pandya, A.G.; Harris, J.E.; Lebwohl, M.; Hamzavi, I.H.; Butler, K.; Kuo, F.I.; Wei, S.; Rosmarin, D. Addition of Narrow-Band UVB Phototherapy to Ruxolitinib Cream in Patients with Vitiligo. *J. Investig. Dermatol.* **2022**, *142*, 3352–3355.e4. [CrossRef] [PubMed]
107. Rosmarin, D.; Passeron, T.; Pandya, A.G.; Grimes, P.; Harris, J.E.; Desai, S.R.; Lebwohl, M.; Ruer-Mulard, M.; Seneschal, J.; Wolkerstorfer, A.; et al. Two Phase 3, Randomized, Controlled Trials of Ruxolitinib Cream for Vitiligo. *N. Engl. J. Med.* **2022**, *387*, 1445–1455. [CrossRef] [PubMed]
108. Incyte Corporation. *A Double-Blind, Vehicle-Controlled, Randomized Withdrawal and Treatment Extension Study to Assess the Long-Term Efficacy and Safety of Ruxolitinib Cream in Participants with Vitiligo*; ClinicalTrials: Bethesda, MD, USA, 2023.

109. Incyte Corporation. *A Safety and Efficacy Study of Ruxolitinib Cream Combined with Narrow-Band Ultraviolet B Phototherapy in Participants with Vitiligo*; ClinicalTrials: Bethesda, MD, USA, 2023.
110. Ezzedine, K.; Peeva, E.; Yamaguchi, Y.; Cox, L.A.; Banerjee, A.; Han, G.; Hamzavi, I.; Ganesan, A.K.; Picardo, M.; Thaçi, D.; et al. Efficacy and Safety of Oral Ritlecitinib for the Treatment of Active Nonsegmental Vitiligo: A Randomized Phase 2b Clinical Trial. *J. Am. Acad. Dermatol.* **2023**, *88*, 395–403. [CrossRef] [PubMed]
111. Song, H.; Hu, Z.; Zhang, S.; Yang, L.; Liu, Y.; Wang, T. Effectiveness and Safety of Tofacitinib Combined with Narrowband Ultraviolet B Phototherapy for Patients with Refractory Vitiligo in Real-World Clinical Practice. *Dermatol. Ther.* **2022**, *35*, e15821. [CrossRef]
112. AbbVie. *A Multicenter, Randomized, Double-Blind, Placebo-Controlled Dose-Ranging Study to Evaluate the Safety and Efficacy of Upadacitinib in Subjects with Non-Segmental Vitiligo*; ClinicalTrials: Bethesda, MD, USA, 2023.
113. Arcutis Biotherapeutics, Inc. *A Phase 2a, Proof of Concept, 24-Week, Parallel Group, Double Blind, Vehicle-Controlled Study of the Safety and Efficacy of ARQ-252 Cream 0.3% in Subjects with Non-Segmental Facial Vitiligo*; ClinicalTrials: Bethesda, MD, USA, 2022.
114. Dermavant Sciences GmbH. *A Phase 2a, Randomized, Double-Blind, Vehicle-Controlled Study to Assess the Safety, Tolerability, and Systemic Exposure of Cerdulatinib Gel, 0.37% in Adults with Vitiligo*; ClinicalTrials: Bethesda, MD, USA, 2020.
115. Aclaris Therapeutics, Inc. *An Open-Label Pilot Study of the Safety, Tolerability and Efficacy of ATI-50002 Topical Solution Administered Twice-Daily in Adult Subjects with Non-Segmental Facial Vitiligo*; ClinicalTrials: Bethesda, MD, USA, 2020.
116. Marasca, C.; Fabbrocini, G.; D'Andrea, M.; Luciano, M.A.; De Maio, G.; Ruggiero, A. Low Dose Oral Corticosteroids, Microneedling, and Topical 5-fluorouracil: A Novel Treatment for Recalcitrant Pediatric Vitiligo. *Pediatr. Dermatol.* **2021**, *38*, 322–323. [CrossRef]
117. Kumar, A.; Bharti, R.; Agarwal, S. Microneedling with Dermaroller 192 Needles along with 5-Fluorouracil Solution in the Treatment of Stable Vitiligo. *J. Am. Acad. Dermatol.* **2019**, *81*, e67–e69. [CrossRef] [PubMed]
118. Shashikiran, A.; Gandhi, S.; Murugesh, S.; Kusagur, M. Sugareddy Efficacy of Topical 5% Fluorouracil Needling in Vitiligo. *Indian J. Dermatol. Venereol. Leprol.* **2018**, *84*, 203. [CrossRef] [PubMed]
119. Jartarkar, S.; Manjunath, K.; Harini, S.; Sampath, S. A single blind active controlled study to compare the efficacy of microneedling and microneedling with 5-flurouracil in treatment of stable vitiligo. *Przegląd Dermatol.* **2021**, *108*, 275–284. [CrossRef]
120. Attwa, E.M.; Khashaba, S.A.; Ezzat, N.A. Evaluation of the Additional Effect of Topical 5-fluorouracil to Needling in the Treatment of Localized Vitiligo. *J. Cosmet. Dermatol.* **2020**, *19*, 1473–1478. [CrossRef]
121. Abdou, A.G.; Farag, A.G.A.; Rashwan, M.; Shehata, W.A. The Clinical and Pathological Effectiveness of Microneedling and Topical 5-fluorouracil in Vitiligo Treatment: An Association with Matrix Metalloproteinase 2 Immunohistochemical Expression. *J. Cosmet. Dermatol.* **2022**, *21*, 2153–2161. [CrossRef]
122. Zahra, F.; Adil, M.; Amin, S.; Mohtashim, M.; Bansal, R.; Khan, H. Efficacy of Topical 5% 5-Fluorouracil with Needling versus 5% 5-Fluorouracil Alone in Stable Vitiligo: A Randomized Controlled Study. *J. Cutan. Aesthet. Surg.* **2020**, *13*, 197. [CrossRef]
123. Mina, M.; Elgarhy, L.; Al-saeid, H.; Ibrahim, Z. Comparison between the Efficacy of Microneedling Combined with 5-fluorouracil vs Microneedling with Tacrolimus in the Treatment of Vitiligo. *J. Cosmet. Dermatol.* **2018**, *17*, 744–751. [CrossRef]
124. Pazyar, N.; Hatami, M.; Yaghoobi, R.; Parvar, S.Y.; Radmanesh, M.; Hadibarhaghtalab, M. The Efficacy of Adding Topical 5-fluorouracil to Micro-needling in the Treatment of Vitiligo: A Randomized Controlled Trial. *J. Cosmet. Dermatol.* **2023**, *22*, 1513–1520. [CrossRef]
125. Saad, M.A.; Tawfik, K.M.; Abdelaleem, H.L. Efficacy and Safety of Micro-needling Combined with Topical 5-fluorouracil and Excimer Light vs. Excimer Light Alone in Treatment of Non-segmental Vitiligo: A Comparative Study. *J. Cosmet. Dermatol.* **2023**, *22*, 810–821. [CrossRef]
126. Sethi, S.; Mahajan, B.B.; Gupta, R.R.; Ohri, A. Comparative Evaluation of the Therapeutic Efficacy of Dermabrasion, Dermabrasion Combined with Topical 5% 5-fluorouracil Cream, and Dermabrasion Combined with Topical Placentrex Gel in Localized Stable Vitiligo. *Int. J. Dermatol.* **2007**, *46*, 875–879. [CrossRef]
127. Garg, T.; Chander, R.; Jain, A. Combination of Microdermabrasion and 5-Fluorouracil to Induce Repigmentation in Vitiligo: An Observational Study. *Dermatol. Surg.* **2011**, *37*, 1763–1766. [CrossRef]
128. Zohdy, H.A.; Hussein, M.S. Intradermal Injection of Fluorouracil versus Triamcinolone in Localized Vitiligo Treatment. *J. Cosmet. Dermatol.* **2019**, *18*, 1430–1434. [CrossRef]
129. Abd El-Samad, Z.; Shaaban, D. Treatment of Localized Non-Segmental Vitiligo with Intradermal 5-Flurouracil Injection Combined with Narrow-Band Ultraviolet B: A Preliminary Study. *J. Dermatol. Treat.* **2012**, *23*, 443–448. [CrossRef] [PubMed]
130. Hesseler, M.J.; Shyam, N. Platelet-Rich Plasma and Its Utility in Medical Dermatology: A Systematic Review. *J. Am. Acad. Dermatol.* **2019**, *81*, 834–846. [CrossRef] [PubMed]
131. Khattab, F.M.; Abdelbary, E.; Fawzi, M. Evaluation of Combined Excimer Laser and Platelet-Rich Plasma for the Treatment of Nonsegmental Vitiligo: A Prospective Comparative Study. *J. Cosmet. Dermatol.* **2020**, *19*, 869–877. [CrossRef] [PubMed]
132. Abdelghani, R.; Ahmed, N.A.; Darwish, H.M. Combined Treatment with Fractional Carbon Dioxide Laser, Autologous Platelet-Rich Plasma, and Narrow Band Ultraviolet B for Vitiligo in Different Body Sites: A Prospective, Randomized Comparative Trial. *J. Cosmet. Dermatol.* **2018**, *17*, 365–372. [CrossRef] [PubMed]
133. Ibrahim, Z.A.; El-Ashmawy, A.A.; El-Tatawy, R.A.; Sallam, F.A. The Effect of Platelet-Rich Plasma on the Outcome of Short-Term Narrowband-Ultraviolet B Phototherapy in the Treatment of Vitiligo: A Pilot Study. *J. Cosmet. Dermatol.* **2016**, *15*, 108–116. [CrossRef] [PubMed]

134. Parambath, N.; Sharma, V.K.; Parihar, A.S.; Sahni, K.; Gupta, S. Use of Platelet-Rich Plasma to Suspend Noncultured Epidermal Cell Suspension Improves Repigmentation after Autologous Transplantation in Stable Vitiligo: A Double-Blind Randomized Controlled Trial. *Int. J. Dermatol.* **2019**, *58*, 472–476. [CrossRef]
135. Salloum, A.; Bazzi, N.; Maalouf, D.; Habre, M. Microneedling in Vitiligo: A Systematic Review. *Dermatol. Ther.* **2020**, *33*, e14297. [CrossRef]
136. Kaur, A.; Barman, K.D.; Sahoo, B.; Choudhary, P. A Comparative Interventional Study of Narrowband Ultraviolet B Alone and Narrowband Ultraviolet B in Combination with Microneedling in Patients with Stable Vitiligo. *Photodermatol. Photoimmunol. Photomed.* **2023**, *39*, 357–363. [CrossRef]
137. Stanimirovic, A.; Kovacevic, M.; Korobko, I.; Šitum, M.; Lotti, T. Combined Therapy for Resistant Vitiligo Lesions: NB-UVB, Microneedling, and Topical Latanoprost, Showed No Enhanced Efficacy Compared to Topical Latanoprost and NB-UVB. *Dermatol. Ther.* **2016**, *29*, 312–316. [CrossRef] [PubMed]

International Journal of
Molecular Sciences

MDPI

Article

Predictive Performances of Blood-Count-Derived Inflammatory Markers for Liver Fibrosis Severity in Psoriasis Vulgaris

Oana Mirela Tiucă [1,2,3], Silviu Horia Morariu [2,3,*], Claudia Raluca Mariean [1,4], Robert Aurelian Tiucă [1,5,6], Alin Codrut Nicolescu [7] and Ovidiu Simion Cotoi [4,8]

1 Doctoral School of Medicine and Pharmacy, George Emil Palade University of Medicine, Pharmacy, Science, and Technology of Targu Mures, 540142 Targu Mures, Romania
2 Dermatology Department, George Emil Palade University of Medicine, Pharmacy, Science, and Technology of Targu Mures, 540142 Targu Mures, Romania
3 Dermatology Clinic, Mures Clinical County Hospital, 540342 Targu Mures, Romania
4 Pathophysiology Department, George Emil Palade University of Medicine, Pharmacy, Science, and Technology of Targu Mures, 540142 Targu Mures, Romania
5 Endocrinology Department, George Emil Palade University of Medicine, Pharmacy, Science, and Technology of Targu Mures, 540142 Targu Mures, Romania
6 Endocrinology Department, Mures Clinical County Hospital, 540139 Targu Mures, Romania
7 Agrippa Ionescu Emergency Clinical Hospital, 011773 Bucharest, Romania
8 Pathology Department, Mures Clinical County Hospital, 540011 Targu Mures, Romania
* Correspondence: silviu.morariu23@gmail.com

Abstract: Psoriasis is an immune-mediated, chronic disorder that significantly alters patients' quality of life and predisposes them to a higher risk of comorbidities, including liver fibrosis. Various non-invasive tests (NITs) have been validated to assess liver fibrosis severity, while blood-count-derived inflammatory markers have been proven to be reliable in reflecting inflammatory status in psoriatic disease. The fibrosis-4 (FIB-4) index became part of the newest guideline for monitoring psoriasis patients undergoing systemic treatment. Patients with psoriasis vulgaris and fulfilling inclusion criteria were enrolled in this study, aiming to assess for the first time in the literature whether such inflammatory markers are useful in predicting liver fibrosis. Based on internationally validated FIB-4 index values, patients were divided into two study groups: a low risk of significant fibrosis (LR-SF) and a high risk of significant fibrosis (HR-SF). Patients from HR-SF were significantly older and had higher values of the monocyte-to-lymphocyte ratio (MLR) ($p < 0.001$), which further significantly correlated with fibrosis severity ($p < 0.001$). Platelet-to-lymphocyte ratio (PLR), systemic immune inflammation index (SII), platelet-to-white blood cell ratio (PWR), and aggregate index of systemic inflammations (AISI) significantly correlated negatively with liver fibrosis ($p < 0.001$). PWR proved to be the most reliable inflammatory predictor of fibrosis severity (AUC = 0.657). MLR, PWR, and AISI were independent inflammatory markers in multivariate analysis ($p < 0.001$), while the AST to platelet ratio index (APRI) and AST to ALT ratio (AAR) can be used as additional NITs for significant liver fibrosis ($p < 0.001$). In limited-resources settings, blood-count-derived inflammatory markers such as MLR, PWR, and AISI, respectively, and hepatic indexes APRI and AAR prove to be of particular help in predicting significant liver fibrosis.

Keywords: psoriasis; inflammation; fibrosis; non-invasive; risk-assessment

Citation: Tiucă, O.M.; Morariu, S.H.; Mariean, C.R.; Tiucă, R.A.; Nicolescu, A.C.; Cotoi, O.S. Predictive Performances of Blood-Count-Derived Inflammatory Markers for Liver Fibrosis Severity in Psoriasis Vulgaris. *Int. J. Mol. Sci.* **2023**, *24*, 16898. https://doi.org/10.3390/ijms242316898

Academic Editors: Montserrat Fernández-Guarino, Asunción Ballester-Martinez and Andrés González-García

Received: 31 October 2023
Revised: 24 November 2023
Accepted: 26 November 2023
Published: 29 November 2023

1. Introduction

Psoriasis is an immune-mediated, chronic disorder that significantly alters patients' quality of life (QoL), affecting between 1.5% and 5% of the population in developed countries [1] (recently estimated at 4.99% in Romania [2]).

Cutaneous lesions may vary depending on the psoriasis subtype, but the most common morphology refers to well-defined erythematous and scaly plaques, reflecting skin inflammation, epidermal hyperplasia, and angiogenesis due to altered immune pathways. A continuous interaction between dendritic cells, T cells, and keratinocytes leads to increased production of pro-inflammatory molecules, promoting an increased inflammatory state, that transcends skin level and has a systemic impact.

Patients with psoriasis have a higher risk of developing cardiovascular diseases, especially hypertension [3] and atherosclerosis, metabolic disorders, inflammatory bowel disease, psychiatric disorders, and kidney disease [4]. Additionally, psoriasis is linked to major cardiovascular events, such as myocardial infarction and stroke, especially in those with severe and prolonged courses of disease.

Psoriasis patients are more likely to have liver fibrosis [5], partly due to the interleukin-17 pathway [6]. Drug-induced fibrosis, especially methotrexate-related, should also be taken into account. Even though previous guidelines recommended monitoring possible liver disease with routine blood analysis and liver biopsy [7], more recent evidence considers routine liver enzymes to be non-reliable [8] and liver biopsy to be too invasive.

Recent advances in the field revealed that non-invasive tests (NITs) are of great help in clinical practice and can confidently rule out the presence of advanced fibrosis (AF) [9], with patients at a high risk of AF being offered further testing, and those at low risk of AF benefiting from annual re-evaluation. NITs have become an integral part of the most recent AAD guideline [10] for baseline evaluation of liver fibrosis. Patients should benefit first-hand from liver fibrosis evaluation by the means of NITs, such as Fibrosis-4 (FIB-4) index, Fibrosure, Fibrometer, or Hepascore, and if proven to be at low risk of AF, methotrexate treatment can safely be initiated. Additionally, NITs, such as AST to platelet ratio index (APRI), AST to ALT ratio (AAR), and GGT to platelet ratio index (GPR) have been described, but their usefulness has not been until now widely accepted.

Blood-count-derived inflammatory markers, such as neutrophil-to-lymphocyte ratio (NLR), platelet-to-lymphocyte ratio (PLR), or systemic immune inflammation index (SII) have gained increased interest in recent years. They were proven to be associated with and predicted outcomes in patients with cardiovascular disease [11–13], tumors [14–18], and kidney disease [19,20]. For skin disorders, the usefulness of these markers has been assessed in erythema nodosum [21], Behcet disease [22], and sarcoidosis [23]. In psoriasis, these markers have been proven to be reliable in assessing both the disease's presence and its severity [24–26]. The platelet-to-white blood cell ratio (PWR), a potential biomarker of vascular inflammation predicting acute ischemic stroke and cardiovascular risk [27,28], has never been assessed in relation to psoriasis. Moreover, the usefulness of PWR in hepatic diseases has been, until now, tested only in acute-to-chronic liver failure (ACLF) [29], HBV-positive patients [30], and pyogenic liver abscesses [31].

To the best of our knowledge, until now, no study has evaluated the reliability of blood-count-derived inflammatory markers in assessing liver fibrosis. This study aimed to establish the prognostic value of inflammatory markers in predicting liver fibrosis severity in patients with psoriasis based on an international consensus regarding NITs.

2. Results

2.1. Patients' Clinical Profile

A total of 359 patients diagnosed with psoriasis were included in this study. Most of them were males (n = 216), with a mean age at enrollment of 54.76 ± 16.36. Regarding psoriasis severity, 177 presented with mild disease, while 182 had moderate-to-severe psoriasis. As depicted in Table 1, 246 patients had mild fibrosis (LR-SF, median FIB-4 = 0.69; 95% CI: 0.65–0.75), while 113 presented moderate-to-severe liver fibrosis (HR-SF, median FIB-4 = 2.08; 95% CI: 1.78–2.66). Patients in the HR-SF group were significantly older ($p < 0.001$) than those in the non-AF group. Most patients in the LR-SF group had mild psoriasis (53.66%), while in the HR-SF group most patients presented with moderate-to-severe psoriasis (60.18%).

Table 1. Clinical and laboratory characteristics of the study population.

Variables	All Patients	LR-SF (n = 246)	HR-SF (n = 113)	*p*-Value
Age	54.76 ± 16.36	50.07 ± 16.10	64.98 ± 11.63	<0.001
Gender				
Male	216 (60.17%)	141 (57.32%)	75 (66.37%)	0.100
Female	143 (39.83%)	105 (42.68%)	38 (33.63%)	
Disease severity				
Mild	177 (49.30%)	132 (53.66%)	45 (39.82%)	0.015
Moderate-severe	182 (50.70%)	114 (46.34%)	68 (60.18%)	
AST	19 [18–20.56]	16 [15–17]	31 [26–37]	<0.001
ALT	22 [21–24]	21 [19–22.86]	28 [23.61–33]	0.001
GGT	30 [27–32]	24.5 [20.14–28]	48 [36–68.40]	<0.001
Platelets	238.02 [228.90–243.00]	270.44 [261.67–279.21]	188.67 [178.59–198.75]	<0.001
WBC	7.50 [7.17–7.85]	7.73 [7.37–8.09]	6.84 [6.43–7.67]	0.001
Neutrophils	4.44 [4.23–4.75]	4.53 [4.28–4.88]	4.12 [3.77–4.66]	0.02
Lymphocytes	2.08 [1.97–2.23]	2.22 [2.08–2.30]	1.85 [1.67–2.00]	<0.001
Monocytes	0.50 [0.48–0.53]	0.49 [0.46–0.52]	0.53 [0.48–0.56]	0.33
PLR	115.19 [110.12–120.96]	117.49 [112.46–153.81]	102.51 [89.95–117.91]	<0.001
NLR	2.05 [1.91–2.21]	2.04 [1.82–2.23]	2.08 [1.95–2.32]	0.58
d-NLR	1.56 [1.44–1.66]	1.55 [1.42–1.67]	1.60 [1.44–1.73]	0.96
MLR	0.24 [0.22–0.25]	0.22 [0.21–0.23]	0.28 [0.26–0.30]	<0.001
ESR	15 [12.74–17.26]	14.26 [12.47–16.53]	17 [13.63–20]	0.07
SII	480.22 [453.86–524.81]	526.07 [480.15–570.06]	431.53 [387.45–462.05]	<0.001
SIRI	1.04 [0.94–1.11]	0.99 [0.90–1.11]	1.07 [0.98–1.28]	0.42
AISI	258.40 [231.92–274]	273.26 [248.12–285.65]	214.55 [187.50–250.25]	0.001
APRI	0.22 [0.20–0.23]	0.18 [0.16–0.19]	0.49 [0.41–0.55]	<0.001
AAR	0.88 [0.82–0.93]	0.75 [0.70–0.81]	1.10 [1.02–1.25]	<0.001
PWR	32.86 [30.99–33.98]	34.49 [22.05–36.53]	27.40 [25.39–31.12]	<0.001
GPR	0.12 [0.11–0.13]	0.09 [0.08–0.10]	0.24 [0.20–0.33]	<0.001

AST, aspartate aminotransferase; ALT, alanine aminotransferase; GGT, gamma-glutamyl transferase; WBC, white blood cell count; PLR, platelet-to-lymphocyte ratio; NLR, neutrophil-to-lymphocyte ratio; d-NLR, derived neutrophil-to-lymphocyte ratio; MLR, monocyte-to-lymphocyte ratio; ESR, erythrocyte sedimentation rate; SII, systemic immune inflammation index; SIRI, systemic inflammation response index; AISI, aggregate index of systemic inflammation; APRI, AST to platelet ratio; AAR, AST to ALT ratio; PWR, platelet-to-white blood cell ratio; GPR, GGT to platelet ratio index.

Patients in the HR-SF group had significantly higher values of ALT, AST, GGT, MLR, APRI, AAR, and GPR, while those with LR-SF presented higher levels of WBC, platelets, neutrophils, lymphocytes, PLR, SII, AISI, and PWR. No statistically significant differences were identified regarding monocyte count, NLR, d-NLR, and SIRI between the two study groups. Nevertheless, patients with HR-SF had higher NLR and d-NLR than those with LR-SF. Moreover, thrombocytopenia was more frequently encountered in HR-SF (22/113; 19%), while only two patients from LR-SF presented this blood alteration (0.008%).

2.2. Serological Markers and Liver Fibrosis Scores

The association of serological markers with liver fibrosis was further analyzed. As fibrosis progressed, PLR decreased. Spearman's correlation analysis revealed (Table 2) that platelet count, WBC, neutrophil and lymphocyte count, PLR, SII, AISI, and PWR were significantly and negatively correlated with liver fibrosis. On the other hand, AST, ALT,

GGT, MLR, APRI, AAR, and GPR were strongly positively correlated with liver fibrosis. No correlation was identified between NLR, d-NLR, and SIRI values and liver fibrosis.

Table 2. Correlation between serological markers and liver fibrosis severity.

Marker	r	*p*-Value	Marker	r	*p*-Value
AST	0.49	<0.001	MLR	0.20	<0.001
ALT	0.21	<0.001	SII	−0.22	<0.001
GGT	0.39	<0.001	AISI	−0.17	<0.001
Platelets	−0.546	<0.001	PWR	−0.25	<0.001
WBC	−0.17	0.001	APRI	0.63	<0.001
Lymphocytes	−0.20	<0.001	AAR	0.44	<0.001
PLR	−0.19	<0.001	GPR	0.46	<0.001

AST, aspartate aminotransferase; ALT, alanine aminotransferase; GGT, gamma-glutamyl transferase; WBC, white blood cell count; PLR, platelet-to-lymphocyte ratio.

2.3. Performance of Inflammatory Biomarkers for the Evaluation of Liver Fibrosis

The diagnostic performances of different markers are demonstrated in Table 3. The AUC of PLR for evaluating significant fibrosis was 0.618 (95% CI = 0.565–0.668) with a cut-off value of 94.68, while the AUC of MLR for evaluating significant fibrosis was 0.624 (95% CI = 0.571–0.674) with a cut-off of 0.26. The AUC of SII for evaluating significant fibrosis was 0.640 (95% CI = 0.588–0.690) with a cut-off at 828.77, AISI predicted significant fibrosis with an AUC of 0.607 (95% CI = 0.555–0.658) and a cut-off value of 273.09, while PWR predicted significant fibrosis with an AUC of 0.657 (95% CI = 0.606–0.706) and a threshold value of 27.59.

Table 3. Predictive performance of hepatic NITs.

	AUC (95% CI)	*p*-Value	Cut-Off	Se (%)	Sp (%)	Youden Index J	*p*-Value *
PLR	0.618 (0.565–0.668)	<0.001	94.68	46.90	76.42	0.23	0.19
MLR	0.624 (0.571–0.674)	<0.001	0.26	58.41	65.85	0.24	0.44
SII	0.640 (0.588–0.690)	<0.001	828.77	93.81	26.42	0.20	0.71
AISI	0.607 (0.555–0.658)	<0.001	273.09	66.37	50.00	0.16	0.33
PWR	0.657 (0.606–0.706)	<0.001	27.59	52.21	74.80	0.27	-

Se: sensitivity; Sp: specificity; * Compared to PWR; PLR, platelet-to-lymphocyte ratio; MLR, monocyte-to-lymphocyte ratio; MLR, monocyte-to-lymphocyte ratio; AISI, aggregate index of systemic inflammation; PWR, platelet-to-white blood cell ratio.

SII had the highest sensitivity, while PLR had the highest specificity. Comparing AUCs of different serum models for predicting significant liver fibrosis, the AUC of PWR was the highest, but comparable with PLR ($p = 0.19$), MLR ($p = 0.44$), SII ($p = 0.71$), and AISI ($p = 0.33$) (Figure 1).

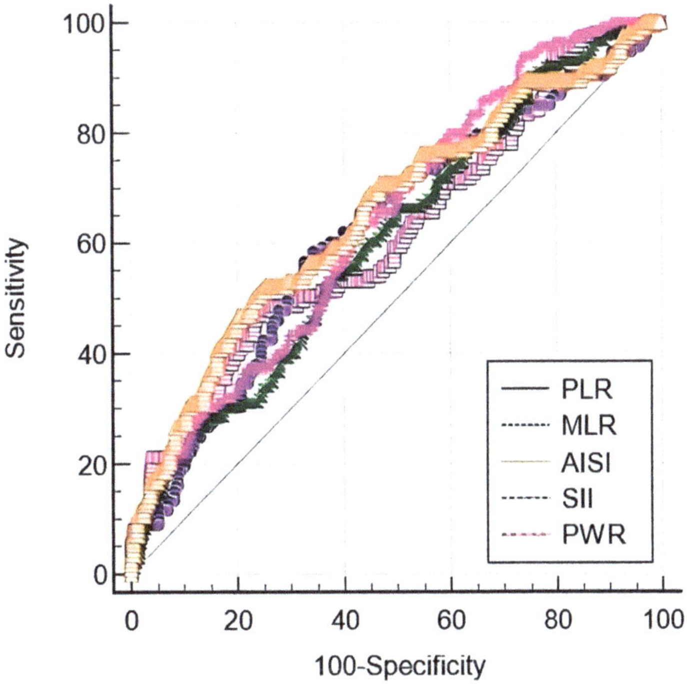

Figure 1. ROC comparison of PLR, MLR, AISI, SII, and PWR in predicting significant liver fibrosis.

2.4. Performance of Hepatic NITs for the Evaluation of Liver Fibrosis

APRI (r = 0.63; $p < 0.001$), AAR (r = 0.44; $p < 0.001$), and GPR (0.46; $p < 0.001$) were positively and statistically significantly correlated with liver fibrosis severity. The AUCs of APRI, AAR, and GPR for assessing liver fibrosis were 0.889 (95% CI = 0.852–0.920), 0.774 (95% CI = 0.727–0.816), and 0.786 (95% CI = 0.740–0.828), respectively, with cut-offs 0.22, 0.89, and 0.14, respectively (Table 4).

Table 4. Predictive performance of hepatic NITs.

	AUC (95% CI)	*p*-Value	Cut-Off	Se (%)	Sp (%)	Youden Index J	*p*-Value *
APRI	0.889 (0.852–0.920)	<0.001	0.22	91.15	69.11	0.60	-
AAR	0.774 (0.727–0.816)	<0.001	0.89	75.22	66.67	0.42	<0.001
GPR	0.786 (0.740–0.828)	<0.001	0.14	74.34	73.98	0.48	<0.001

Se: sensitivity; Sp: specificity; * Compared to APRI; APRI, AST to platelet ratio; AAR, AST to ALT ratio; GPR, GGT to platelet ratio index.

Out of these indexes, APRI had the highest sensitivity, while GPR had the highest specificity. The AUC of APRI was higher compared to AAR ($p < 0.001$) and GPR ($p < 0.001$), as depicted in Figure 2.

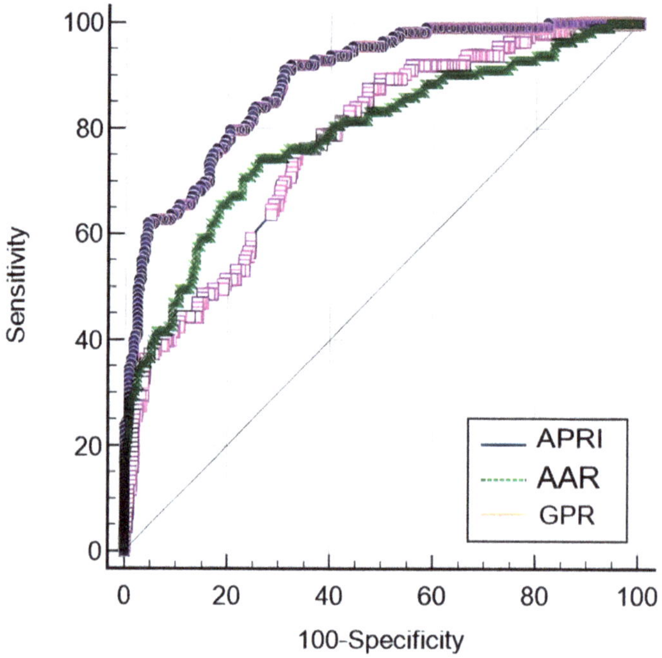

Figure 2. ROC comparison of APRI, AAR, and GPR for predicting significant liver fibrosis.

2.5. The Reliability of Blood-Count-Derived Markers for Predicting Liver Fibrosis Severity

In a multivariate logistic regression model (Table 5), patients aged more than 50 years old (OR: 4.63, $p < 0.001$) and presenting with moderate-to-severe psoriasis (OR: 1.70, $p = 0.028$) were identified to have a higher risk of significant liver fibrosis. Moreover, higher levels of MLR (OR:3.51, $p < 0.001$), APRI (OR = 11.68, $p < 0.001$), and AAR (OR = 13.26, $p < 0.001$), and lower levels of AISI (OR = 0.98, $p = 0.009$) and PWR (OR = 0.94, $p < 0.001$) were independent predictors of significant liver fibrosis.

Table 5. Predictors of significant liver fibrosis in psoriasis patients.

Parameter	OR	95% CI	*p*-Value
Demographic characteristics			
Age > 50 years old	4.63	2.57–8.36	<0.001
Male sex	0.78	0.48–1.27	0.127
Moderate-severe psoriasis	1.70	1.06–2.73	0.028
Inflammatory markers			
PLR	1.02	0.99–1.06	0.097
MLR	3.51	1.69–7.29	<0.001
PWR	0.94	0.99–1.02	<0.001
SII	0.99	0.99–1.01	0.150
AISI	0.98	0.98–0.99	0.009
Hepatic NITs			
APRI	11.68	7.44–18.32	<0.001
AAR	13.26	5.37–32.78	<0.001
GPR	4.54	0.70–29.43	0.110

PLR, platelet-to-lymphocyte ratio; MLR, monocyte-to-lymphocyte ratio; PWR, platelet-to-white blood cell ratio; SII, systemic immune inflammation index; AISI, aggregate index of systemic inflammation; APRI, AST to platelet ratio; AAR, AST to ALT ratio; GPR, GGT to platelet ratio index.

3. Discussion

Early detection and a proper assessment of liver inflammation and fibrosis are important not only for disease progression but also necessary when dealing with multifactorial and complex diseases such as psoriasis, which very often require systemic treatment. Additionally, psoriatic patients may require a personalized approach, taking into account associated comorbidities and data reported in the literature.

Keratinocytes play a key role in psoriasis etiopathogenesis. By providing antimicrobial peptides like S100A7 that bind to host DNA, they initiate the stimulation of dendritic cells. Activated dendritic cells lead to increased production of proinflammatory markers such as IL-12, IL-23, IL-8, IL-17, and TNF-α [32–36]. Moreover, the genetic bases of psoriasis, defined by more than 50 psoriasis susceptibility loci with PSOR1 being the most important, modulate immune pathways that further increase disease susceptibility, such as the IL-23/IL-17 axis and the type I IFN pathway [37]. Nevertheless, even though these cytokines are the hallmarks of psoriasis etiopathogenesis and are proven to be reliable markers of disease progression, they are not widely used in daily clinical practice, most likely due to highly specialized techniques used for their detections and high costs.

Blood-count-derived inflammatory markers have been reported to be reliable in cardiovascular diseases, tumors, and kidney disease. Studies referring to psoriasis tested the reliability of these markers both as diagnostic and prognostic factors and also their usefulness in assessing a patient's response to different therapeutical means, such as conventional immunosuppressants and innovative (both biological and non-biological) drugs [38–43]. Andersen et al. [43] identified that a higher pretreatment with PLR and SII were less likely to respond to conventional systemic agents, while Asahina et al. [39] proved that NLR and PLR decrease in the same manner as C-reactive protein (CRP) in patients undergoing biological therapy, no matter the biologic agent that was used. Anti-TNF agents, such as adalimumab, infliximab, and etanercept, seem to be more effective in decreasing NLR and CRP values compared to IL inhibitors ustekinumab and secukinumab [44]. Moreover, biologics seem to decrease the proinflammatory cytokines TNF-α [45], IL-6, and IL-22 [46]. Additionally, infliximab [47] and secukinumab [48] decrease oxidative stress levels and increase total antioxidant status [47], adalimumab and etanercept increase superoxide dismutase and glutathione levels and decrease nitric oxide [49], while efalizumab [47] and ustekinumab [50] decrease malondialdehyde levels. On the other hand, methotrexate elevates malondialdehyde, caspase-3, and oxidative stress levels [51]. As such, apart from decreasing inflammatory status, biologics may have protective effects against oxidative stress, a key pathogenic factor in psoriasis development.

An increased inflammatory status in psoriatic disease is further reflected in associated comorbidities. It should be noted that patients with psoriasis present an additional comorbid risk derived from the choice of treatment.

Psoriasis patients are prone to liver fibrosis, partly due to the interleukin-17 pathway. IL-17 signaling increases the expression of a fibrogenic cytokine, the transforming growth factor-1, and induces the production of type 1 collagen in hepatic stellate cells by activating the Stat3 pathway [6]. On the other hand, methotrexate leads to liver fibrosis by increasing extracellular adenosine in stellate cells [52], while acitretin promotes fibrogenesis by impacting the mitochondrial function of stellate cells and leading to apoptosis and necrosis of these cells. In addition, IL-22 and IL-23 seem to decrease liver fibrosis [6]. As such, screening for liver fibrosis is essential because it identifies patients at risk and guides treatment decisions.

Our study was based on FIB-4 and not other NITs due to the fact this marker was integrated into the latest guidelines [10] for assessing liver fibrosis. While in resource-limited settings, liver fibrosis scores calculated from simple laboratory values, such as the FIB-4 index, are useful for identifying patients who may need additional testing, allowing, therefore, better resource management and therapeutic decisions. Patients with an FIB-4 lower than 1.3 are considered to being of having a low risk of significant fibrosis (F0-F1) and should benefit from periodical monitoring, while those with values higher than this cut-off benefit from further testing. Additionally, a FIB-4 > 3.25 is considered to indicate significant liver fibrosis (>F2) [53,54].

Our study identified that patients with HR-SF presented with decreased values of peripheral neutrophils and lymphocytes, probably due to the migration of these cells from the blood to the liver. Patients with significant liver fibrosis lose more lymphocytes than neutrophils in their peripheral blood, as indicated by elevated NLR and d-NLR in HR-SF. On the other hand, high levels of monocytes in HR-SF can be attributed to ongoing bone marrow inflammation and monocyte mobilization to the periphery. The relationship between NLR and liver fibrosis was explored in other studies, with conflicting results [55,56]. In a study published by Kara et al. [56], NLR was not associated with the severity of liver fibrosis, while Ülger et al. [55] described that low NLR values are useful in predicting advanced liver fibrosis in HCV-positive patients. In our study, NLR and d-NLR did not exhibit differences between LR-SF and HR-SF. MLR significantly differed between study groups and correlated positively with fibrosis severity, while PLR, SII, AISI, and PWR negatively correlated with liver fibrosis. Other studies reported that PLR is useful in evaluating liver fibrosis and inflammation [57] and could perform comparably to FIB-F [58]. All markers were good indicators of liver fibrosis, with an AUC > 0.60. Our study reports for the first time in the literature, PWR as an inflammatory marker in psoriasis and its usefulness in predicting liver fibrosis severity. It had the highest performance to assess HR-SF with an AUC of 0.657. However, after running a multivariate regression model, only MLR, PWR, and AISI proved to be significant independent predictors of liver fibrosis. Thrombocytopenia was more frequently encountered in HR-SF, most likely due to decreased thrombopoietin levels in advanced liver disease and direct bone marrow suppression [59].

Significant differences were also noted between the two study groups regarding AST, ALT, and GGT. However, these markers should not be individually used to assess liver fibrosis since they can easily be influenced by various factors, such as diet, living habits, and metabolic status. We also evaluated combined parameters such as AAR, APRI, and GPR, which were proved to indicate the presence and severity of liver fibrosis in chronic hepatitis C [60–63]. AAR and GPR displayed good predictive value (AUC > 0.60), while APRI, which had the highest performance to stage HR-SF with an AUC of 0.889 and was superior to AAR and GPR, had a very good predictive value. Our analysis also identified that APRI and AAR can be used as prognostic factors of liver fibrosis. Additionally, APRI and AAR proved to be prognostic factors of HR-SF.

Disease severity, male sex, and age > 50 years old were also identified as predictors of HR-SF. This indicates the need for additional screening for these patients and exemplifies once more the direct link between psoriatic disease and systemic comorbidities.

The main limitation of this study lies in its single-center retrospective character. Alcohol intake was evaluated based on clinical records and patients with psoriasis vulgaris who reported a daily intake of alcohol were excluded; no systematically quantified level of alcohol intake was available due to the retrospective nature of data collection. Psoriasis severity was assessed using only the BSA score. Future ideas might include a prospective enrollment of psoriasis patients, disease severity assessment using combined scores, such as PGAxBSA, modified PASI (mPASI), and psoriasis log-based area and severity index (PLASI), and a calculation of the FIB-4 cut-off value in the study population for discriminating between LR-SF and HR-SF. In this study, we used FIB-4 threshold values as reported by international consensus. A cut-off value determined in the study population might eliminate possible populational intervariability.

Nevertheless, to our knowledge, this is the first study, to date, to assess the usefulness of blood-count-derived inflammatory markers in predicting liver fibrosis. Additionally, this is the first study reporting PWR as an inflammatory marker in liver fibrosis, and, as our results showed, it proves to be the most reliable one for discriminating liver fibrosis severity.

4. Materials and Methods

4.1. Study Population

We conducted a retrospective observational study that included patients diagnosed with psoriasis vulgaris in the Dermatology Department of Mures Clinical County Hospital, Romania, between January 2017 and December 2022. The inclusion criteria were patients older than 18 years of age, presenting for the first time in our department, diagnosed with psoriasis vulgaris in the aforementioned timeframe, and for whom data regarding disease severity and laboratory investigations were available. The following patients were excluded: patients diagnosed with other clinical forms of psoriasis, of pediatric age, for whom there were no available laboratory investigations or information regarding disease severity, patients with a known history of psoriatic arthritis, cardiovascular disease, liver diseases, malignant tumors, active infections, or diabetes, patients reporting daily alcohol use, and those who underwent 3 months of systemic treatment before enrollment with one of the following: steroids, classic immunosuppressive drugs (Methotrexate, Azathioprine, Cyclosporine), or innovative drugs (any type of biologics or PDE-4 inhibitors) were excluded.

4.2. Data Collection

The data was collected using the hospital's electronic databases. For each patient, information regarding demographics (age, sex), clinical presentation, and laboratory parameters were extracted. Psoriasis severity was assessed using the Body Surface Area (BSA) score and defined as follows: mild (BSA < 5%), and moderate-to-severe (BSA > 10%). The following laboratory parameters were analyzed: complete white blood cell count (WBC), leucocyte subsets (neutrophils, lymphocytes, and monocytes) count, platelet count, alanine-aminotransferase (ALT), aspartate aminotransferase (AST), and gamma-glutamyl transferase (GGT) levels. For patients presenting multiple times in our department in the aforementioned time interval, data referring to the first presentation was taken into account.

4.3. Biomarkers

The following blood count-derived inflammatory markers were calculated: NLR, derived neutrophil-to-lymphocyte ratio (d-NLR), PLR, monocyte-to-lymphocyte ratio (MLR), SII, systemic inflammation response index (SIRI), aggregate index of systemic inflammation (AISI), and PWR. Liver fibrosis assessment was established based on the FIB-4 index. Additional non-invasive fibrosis markers, such as APRI, AAR, and GPR were evaluated. The formulas for the aforementioned markers are depicted in Table 6.

Table 6. Formulas of blood-count-derived markers.

Marker	Formula
NLR	Neutrophil count/lymphocyte count [$\times 10^3/\mu L$]
d-NLR	Neutrophil count/(WBC-neutrophil count) [$\times 10^3/\mu L$]
PLR	Platelet count/lymphocyte count [$\times 10^3/\mu L$]
MLR	Monocyte count/lymphocyte count [$\times 10^3/\mu L$]
SII	(Neutrophil count × platelet count)/lymphocyte count [$\times 10^3/\mu L$]
SIRI	(Neutrophil count × monocyte count)/lymphocyte count [$\times 10^3/\mu L$]
AISI	(Neutrophil count × monocyte count × platelet count)/lymphocyte count [$\times 10^3/\mu L$]
PWR	Platelet count/WBC [$\times 10^3/\mu L$]
FIB-4	(Age [years] × AST [U/L])/(platelet count [$\times 10^3/\mu L$] × $\sqrt{}$ALT [U/L])
APRI	[(AST/upper limit of the normal AST range) × 100]/platelet count [$\times 10^3/\mu L$]
AAR	AST/ALT [U/L]
GPR	GGT [U/L]/platelet count [$\times 10^3/\mu L$]

NLR, neutrophil-to-lymphocyte ratio; d-NLR, derived neutrophil-to-lymphocyte ratio; PLR, platelet-to-lymphocyte ratio; MLR, monocyte-to-lymphocyte ratio; SII, systemic immune inflammation index; SIRI, systemic inflammation response index; AISI, aggregate index of systemic inflammation; PWR, platelet-to-white blood cell ratio; FIB-4, Fibrosis-4 index; APRI, AST to platelet ratio; AAR, AST to ALT ratio; GPR, GGT to platelet ratio index.

4.4. Study Outcome

The primary endpoint of our study was to assess whether blood count-derived inflammatory markers may serve as predictors of liver fibrosis severity in patients with psoriasis vulgaris. Fibrosis severity was assessed using the FIB-4 index according to international consensus, and quantified as follows: mild fibrosis (low risk of significant fibrosis: LR-SF, F0-F1) if the FIB-4 index was lower than 1.3, and moderate-to-severe fibrosis (high risk of significant fibrosis: HR-SF, >F2) if FIB-4 was over 1.3 [9,53,54]. Second, we investigated whether non-invasive fibrosis markers such as APRI, AAR, and GPR were efficient in predicting liver fibrosis in patients with psoriasis vulgaris in comparison with the FIB-4 score.

4.5. Statistical Analysis

The statistical analysis was performed using, and MedCalc Statistic software for Windows, version 22.014. Normality was tested using the Shapiro-Wilk test. Continuous variables were expressed as the median or mean and standard deviation, while for categorical variables, the absolute count (n) and proportions were given. Categorical variables were compared by Chi-square test, while the independent Mann-Whitney test was used for continuous variables. Correlations were evaluated by Spearman's correlation coefficient. The performance of inflammatory scores for predicting liver fibrosis severity was assessed using receiver operating characteristic (ROC) curve analysis and the area under the ROC curves (AUCs). The optimal cut-off values for relevant systemic inflammatory markers were determined using the Youden Index from the ROC curve. The DeLong Z test was used to compare the AUCs of the serum models. Multivariate logistic regression adjusted for sex and age, with variables with $p < 0.1$ in univariate analysis, was performed to identify independent prognostic factors associated with liver fibrosis severity. The Hosmer-Lemeshow test was used to assess the goodness of fit for the logistic regression model. $p < 0.05$ was considered statistically significant throughout all the analyses.

5. Conclusions

In our study group, MLR, PWR, and AISI were identified as being prognostic factors useful for assessing liver fibrosis severity in psoriasis. Additionally, APRI and AAR may be used as additional non-invasive markers to assess liver fibrosis. These findings bring new information and highlight once more the strength between psoriasis, systemic inflammation, and associated comorbidities.

Taking into account the ease and low cost of these ratios, they can be used for a quick and efficient patient risk assessment, guide future diagnostic means, and initial therapeutical decisions.

Author Contributions: Conceptualization O.M.T., S.H.M. and O.S.C.; Formal analysis: O.M.T.; Methodology: O.M.T., C.R.M. and A.C.N.; Resources: C.R.M. and R.A.T.; Validation: O.S.C. and S.H.M.; Visualisation: O.M.T. and R.A.T.; Writing—original draft: O.M.T., C.R.M. and R.A.T.; Writing—revision & editing: O.M.T. and A.C.N.; Supervision: O.S.C. and S.H.M. All authors have read and agreed to the published version of the manuscript.

Funding: This research received no external funding.

Institutional Review Board Statement: The study was conducted in accordance with the Declaration of Helsinki, and approved by the Ethics Committee Mures Clinical County Hospital no. 3770/05.04.2023.

Informed Consent Statement: Informed consent was obtained from all subjects involved in the study.

Data Availability Statement: All data presented can be made available upon request.

Acknowledgments: This article is part of a Ph.D. thesis from the Doctoral School of Medicine and Pharmacy of the University of Medicine, Pharmacy, Science, and Technology George Emil Palade of Targu Mures, titled "The impact of systemic inflammation in modulating disease presentation in psoriasis", which will be presented by Oana Mirela Tiucă by the fall of 2024.

Conflicts of Interest: The authors declare no conflict of interest.

References

1. Damiani, G.; Bragazzi, N.L.; Karimkhani Aksut, C.; Wu, D.; Alicandro, G.; McGonagle, D.; Guo, C.; Dellavalle, R.; Grada, A.; Wong, P.; et al. The Global, Regional, and National Burden of Psoriasis: Results and Insights from the Global Burden of Disease 2019 Study. *Front. Med.* **2021**, *8*, 743180. [CrossRef] [PubMed]
2. Nicolescu, A.C.; Bucur, Ș.; Giurcăneanu, C.; Gheucă-Solovăstru, L.; Constantin, T.; Furtunescu, F.; Ancuța, I.; Constantin, M.M. Prevalence and Characteristics of Psoriasis in Romania—First Study in Overall Population. *J. Pers. Med.* **2021**, *11*, 523. [CrossRef] [PubMed]
3. Armstrong, A.W.; Harskamp, C.T.; Armstrong, E.J. The association between psoriasis and hypertension: A systematic review and meta-analysis of observational studies. *J. Hypertens.* **2013**, *31*, 433–443. [CrossRef] [PubMed]
4. Friedland, R.; Kridin, K.; Cohen, A.D.; Landau, D.; Ben-Amitai, D. Psoriasis and Renal Disorders: A Large-Scale Population-Based Study in Children and Adults. *Dermatology* **2022**, *238*, 904–909. [CrossRef] [PubMed]
5. Ogdie, A.; Grewal, S.K.; Noe, M.H.; Shin, D.B.; Takeshita, J.; Chiesa Fuxench, Z.C.; Carr, R.M.; Gelfand, J.M. Risk of Incident Liver Disease in Patients with Psoriasis, Psoriatic Arthritis, and Rheumatoid Arthritis: A Population-Based Study. *J. Investig. Dermatol.* **2018**, *138*, 760–767. [CrossRef]
6. Meng, F.; Wang, K.; Aoyama, T.; Grivennikov, S.I.; Paik, Y.; Scholten, D.; Cong, M.; Iwaisako, K.; Liu, X.; Zhang, M.; et al. Interleukin-17 Signaling in Inflammatory, Kupffer Cells, and Hepatic Stellate Cells Exacerbates Liver Fibrosis in Mice. *Gastroenterology* **2012**, *143*, 765–776.e3. [CrossRef] [PubMed]
7. Menter, A.; Korman, N.J.; Elmets, C.A.; Feldman, S.R.; Gelfand, J.M.; Gordon, K.B.; Gottlieb, A.B.; Koo, J.Y.; Lebwohl, M.; Lim, H.W.; et al. Guidelines of care for the management of psoriasis and psoriatic arthritis. *J. Am. Acad. Dermatol.* **2009**, *61*, 451–485. [CrossRef] [PubMed]
8. Maybury, C.M.; Samarasekera, E.; Douiri, A.; Barker, J.N.; Smith, C.H. Diagnostic accuracy of noninvasive markers of liver fibrosis in patients with psoriasis taking methotrexate: A systematic review and meta-analysis. *Br. J. Dermatol.* **2014**, *170*, 1237–1247. [CrossRef]
9. Castera, L.; Friedrich-Rust, M.; Loomba, R. Noninvasive Assessment of Liver Disease in Patients with Nonalcoholic Fatty Liver Disease. *Gastroenterology* **2019**, *156*, 1264–1281.e4. [CrossRef]
10. Menter, A.; Gelfand, J.M.; Connor, C.; Armstrong, A.W.; Cordoro, K.M.; Davis, D.M.R.; Elewski, B.E.; Gordon, K.B.; Gottlieb, A.B.; Kaplan, D.H.; et al. Joint American Academy of Dermatology–National Psoriasis Foundation guidelines of care for the management of psoriasis with systemic nonbiologic therapies. *J. Am. Acad. Dermatol.* **2020**, *82*, 1445–1486. [CrossRef]
11. Larmann, J.; Handke, J.; Scholz, A.S.; Dehne, S.; Arens, C.; Gillmann, H.J.; Uhle, F.; Motsch, J.; Weigand, M.A.; Janssen, H. Preoperative neutrophil to lymphocyte ratio and platelet to lymphocyte ratio are associated with major adverse cardiovascular and cerebrovascular events in coronary heart disease patients undergoing non-cardiac surgery. *BMC Cardiovasc. Disord.* **2020**, *20*, 230. [CrossRef] [PubMed]
12. Durmus, E.; Kivrak, T.; Gerin, F.; Sunbul, M.; Sari, I.; Erdogan, O. Neutrophil-to-Lymphocyte Ratio and Platelet-to-Lymphocyte Ratio are Predictors of Heart Failure. *Arq. Bras. Cardiol.* **2015**, *105*, 606–613. [CrossRef]
13. Ye, Z.; Hu, T.; Wang, J.; Xiao, R.; Liao, X.; Liu, M.; Sun, Z. Systemic immune-inflammation index as a potential biomarker of cardiovascular diseases: A systematic review and meta-analysis. *Front. Cardiovasc. Med.* **2022**, *9*, 933913. [CrossRef] [PubMed]
14. Modica, R.; Minotta, R.; Liccardi, A.; Cannavale, G.; Benevento, E.; Colao, A. Evaluation of Neutrophil-to-Lymphocyte Ratio (NLR), Platelet-to-Lymphocyte Ratio (PLR) and Systemic Immune–Inflammation Index (SII) as Potential Biomarkers in Patients with Sporadic Medullary Thyroid Cancer (MTC). *J. Pers. Med.* **2023**, *13*, 953. [CrossRef] [PubMed]
15. Lin, Z.Q.; Ma, C.; Cao, W.Z.; Ning, Z.; Tan, G. Prognostic Significance of NLR, PLR, LMR and Tumor Infiltrating T Lymphocytes in Patients Undergoing Surgical Resection for Hilar Cholangiocarcinoma. *Front. Oncol.* **2022**, *12*, 908907. [CrossRef] [PubMed]
16. Gambardella, C.; Mongardini, F.M.; Paolicelli, M.; Bentivoglio, D.; Cozzolino, G.; Ruggiero, R.; Pizza, A.; Tolone, S.; del Genio, G.; Parisi, S.; et al. Role of Inflammatory Biomarkers (NLR, LMR, PLR) in the Prognostication of Malignancy in Indeterminate Thyroid Nodules. *Int. J. Mol. Sci.* **2023**, *24*, 6466. [CrossRef] [PubMed]
17. Kovács, A.R.; Sulina, A.; Kovács, K.S.; Lukács, L.; Török, P.; Lampé, R. Prognostic Significance of Preoperative NLR, MLR, and PLR Values in Predicting the Outcome of Primary Cytoreductive Surgery in Serous Epithelial Ovarian Cancer. *Diagnostics* **2023**, *13*, 2268. [CrossRef] [PubMed]
18. Maloney, S.; Pavlakis, N.; Itchins, M.; Arena, J.; Mittal, A.; Hudson, A.; Colvin, E.; Sahni, S.; Diakos, C.; Chan, D.; et al. The Prognostic and Predictive Role of the Neutrophil-to-Lymphocyte Ratio (NLR), Platelet-to-Lymphocyte Ratio (PLR), and Lymphocyte-to-Monocyte Ratio (LMR) as Biomarkers in Resected Pancreatic Cancer. *J. Clin. Med.* **2023**, *12*, 1989. [CrossRef]
19. Brito, G.M.C.; Fontenele, A.M.M.; Carneiro, E.C.R.L.; Nogueira, I.A.L.; Cavalcante, T.B.; Vale, A.A.M.; Monteiro, S.C.M.; Filho, N.S. Neutrophil-to-Lymphocyte and Platelet-to-Lymphocyte Ratios in Nondialysis Chronic Kidney Patients. *Int. J. Inflamm.* **2021**, *2021*, 6678960. [CrossRef]
20. Mureșan, A.V.; Russu, E.; Arbănași, E.M.; Kaller, R.; Hosu, I.; Arbănași, E.M.; Voidăzan, S.T. The Predictive Value of NLR, MLR, and PLR in the Outcome of End-Stage Kidney Disease Patients. *Biomedicines* **2022**, *10*, 1272. [CrossRef] [PubMed]
21. Hayran, Y. Elevated neutrophil to lymphocyte ratio as an indicator of secondary erythema nodosum, a retrospective observational study. *Turk. J. Med. Sci.* **2019**, *49*, 624–634. [CrossRef] [PubMed]

22. Rifaioglu, E.N.; Bülbül Şen, B.; Ekiz, Ö.; Cigdem Dogramaci, A. Neutrophil to lymphocyte ratio in Behçet's disease as a marker of disease activity. *Acta Dermatovenerol. Alp. Pannonica Adriat.* **2014**, *23*, 65–67. [PubMed]
23. Korkmaz, C.; Demircioglu, S. The Association of Neutrophil/Lymphocyte and Platelet/Lymphocyte Ratios and Hematological Parameters with Diagnosis, Stages, Extrapulmonary Involvement, Pulmonary Hypertension, Response to Treatment, and Prognosis in Patients with Sarcoidosis. *Can. Respir. J.* **2020**, *2020*, 1696450. [CrossRef] [PubMed]
24. Wang, W.M.; Wu, C.; Gao, Y.M.; Li, F.; Yu, X.L.; Jin, H.Z. Neutrophil to lymphocyte ratio, platelet to lymphocyte ratio, and other hematological parameters in psoriasis patients. *BMC Immunol.* **2021**, *22*, 64. [CrossRef] [PubMed]
25. Yorulmaz, A.; Hayran, Y.; Akpinar, U.; Yalcin, B. Systemic Immune-Inflammation Index (SII) Predicts Increased Severity in Psoriasis and Psoriatic Arthritis. *Curr. Health Sci. J.* **2020**, *46*, 352–357.
26. Aktaş Karabay, E.; Demir, D.; Aksu Çerman, A. Evaluation of monocyte to high-density lipoprotein ratio, lymphocytes, monocytes, and platelets in psoriasis. *An. Bras. Dermatol.* **2020**, *95*, 40–45. [CrossRef]
27. Amalia, L.; Dalimonthe, N.Z. Clinical significance of Platelet-to-White Blood Cell Ratio (PWR) and National Institute of Health Stroke Scale (NIHSS) in acute ischemic stroke. *Heliyon* **2020**, *6*, e05033. [CrossRef]
28. Abdulhadi, B.; Naranjo, M.; Krishnamoorthy, P.; Rangaswami, J. White blood cell count to platelet ratio: A novel biomarker for predicting outcomes in patients on circulatory support devices. *J. Am. Coll. Cardiol.* **2018**, *71*, A810. [CrossRef]
29. Kim, J.H.; Kim, S.E.; Song, D.S.; Kim, H.Y.; Yoon, E.; Kim, T.H.; Jung, Y.K.; Suk, K.T.; Jun, B.G.; Yim, H.J.; et al. Platelet-to-White Blood Cell Ratio Is Associated with Adverse Outcomes in Cirrhotic Patients with Acute Deterioration. *J. Clin. Med.* **2022**, *11*, 2463. [CrossRef]
30. Yu, K.; Du, Z.; Li, Q.; Cheng, Q.; Huang, C.; Shi, G.; Li, N. Comparison of non-invasive models for predicting liver damage in chronic hepatitis B patients. *Gastroenterol. Hepatol.* **2019**, *42*, 281–288. [CrossRef]
31. Ko, D.G.; Park, J.W.; Kim, J.H.; Jung, J.H.; Kim, H.S.; Suk, K.T.; Jang, M.K.; Park, S.H.; Lee, M.S.; Kim, D.J.; et al. Platelet-to-White Blood Cell Ratio: A Feasible Biomarker for Pyogenic Liver Abscess. *Diagnostics* **2022**, *12*, 2556. [CrossRef] [PubMed]
32. Ma, H.L.; Liang, S.; Li, J.; Napierata, L.; Brown, T.; Benoit, S.; Senices, M.; Gill, D.; Dunussi-Joannopoulos, K.; Collins, M.; et al. IL-22 is required for Th17 cell-mediated pathology in a mouse model of psoriasis-like skin inflammation. *J. Clin. Investig.* **2008**, *118*, 597–607. [CrossRef] [PubMed]
33. Chan, J.R.; Blumenschein, W.; Murphy, E.; Diveu, C.; Wiekowski, M.; Abbondanzo, S.; Lucian, L.; Geissler, R.; Brodie, S.; Kimball, A.B.; et al. IL-23 stimulates epidermal hyperplasia via TNF and IL-20R2-dependent mechanisms with implications for psoriasis pathogenesis. *J. Exp. Med.* **2006**, *203*, 2577–2587. [CrossRef] [PubMed]
34. Chiricozzi, A.; Guttman-Yassky, E.; Suarez-Farinas, M.; Nograles, K.E.; Tian, S.; Cardinale, I.; Chimenti, S.; Krueger, J.G. Integrative Responses to IL-17 and TNF-alpha in Human Keratinocytes Account for Key Inflammatory Pathogenic Circuits in Psoriasis. *J. Investig. Dermatol.* **2011**, *131*, 677–687. [CrossRef] [PubMed]
35. Zheng, Y.; Danilenko, D.M.; Valdez, P.; Kasman, I.; Eastham-Anderson, J.; Wu, J.; Ouyang, W. Interleukin-22, a T(H)17 cytokine, mediates IL-23-induced dermal inflammation and acanthosis. *Nature* **2007**, *445*, 648–651. [CrossRef]
36. Arican, O.; Aral, M.; Sasmaz, S.; Ciragil, P. Serum levels of TNF-alpha, IFN-gamma, IL-6, IL-8, IL-12, IL-17 and IL-18 in patients with active psoriasis and correlation with disease severity. *Mediat. Inflamm.* **2005**, *2005*, 273–279. [CrossRef]
37. Tsoi, L.C.; Spain, S.L.; Knight, J.; Ellinghaus, E.; Stuart, P.E.; Capon, F.; Ding, J.; Li, Y.; Tejasvi, T.; Gudjonsson, J.E.; et al. Identification of 15 new psoriasis susceptibility loci highlights the role of innate immunity. *Nat. Genet.* **2012**, *44*, 1341–1348. [CrossRef]
38. Sugimoto, E.; Matsuda, H.; Shibata, S.; Mizuno, Y.; Koyama, A.; Li, L.; Taira, H.; Ito, Y.; Awaji, K.; Yamashita, T.; et al. Impact of Pretreatment Systemic Inflammatory Markers on Treatment Persistence with Biologics and Conventional Systemic Therapy: A Retrospective Study of Patients with Psoriasis Vulgaris and Psoriatic Arthritis. *J. Clin. Med.* **2023**, *12*, 3046. [CrossRef]
39. Asahina, A.; Kubo, N.; Umezawa, Y.; Honda, H.; Yanaba, K.; Nakagawa, H. Neutrophil-lymphocyte ratio, platelet-lymphocyte ratio and mean platelet volume in Japanese patients with psoriasis and psoriatic arthritis: Response to therapy with biologics. *J Dermatol.* **2017**, *44*, 1112–1121. [CrossRef]
40. Annen, S.; Horiguchi, G.; Teramukai, S.; Ichiyama, S.; Ito, M.; Hoashi, T.; Kanda, N.; Saeki, H. Association of Transition of Laboratory Markers with Transition of Disease Activity in Psoriasis Patients Treated with Biologics. *J. Nippon. Med. Sch.* **2022**, *89*, 587–593. [CrossRef]
41. An, I.; Ucmak, D.; Ozturk, M. The effect of biological agent treatment on neutrophil-to-lymphocyte ratio, platelet-to-lymphocyte ratio, mean platelet volume, and C-reactive protein in psoriasis patients. *Adv. Dermatol. Allergol.* **2020**, *37*, 202–206. [CrossRef] [PubMed]
42. Albayrak, H. Neutrophil-to-Lymphocyte Ratio, Neutrophil-to-Monocyte Ratio, Platelet-to-Lymphocyte Ratio, and Systemic Immune-Inflammation Index in Psoriasis Patients: Response to Treatment with Biological Drugs. *J. Clin. Med.* **2023**, *12*, 5452. [CrossRef] [PubMed]
43. Andersen, C.S.B.; Kvist-Hansen, A.; Siewertsen, M.; Enevold, C.; Hansen, P.R.; Kaur-Knudsen, D.; Zachariae, C.; Nielsen, C.H.; Loft, N.; Skov, L. Blood Cell Biomarkers of Inflammation and Cytokine Levels as Predictors of Response to Biologics in Patients with Psoriasis. *Int. J. Mol. Sci.* **2023**, *24*, 6111. [CrossRef] [PubMed]
44. Ataseven, A.; Temiz, S.A.; Eren, G.; Özer, İ.; Dursun, R. Comparison of anti-TNF and IL-inhibitors treatments in patients with psoriasis in terms of response to routine laboratory parameter dynamics. *J. Dermatol. Treat.* **2022**, *33*, 1091–1096. [CrossRef] [PubMed]

45. Taha, M.M.; Al-Asady, Z.T.S. Evaluation of the Effectiveness of Antioxidants and TNF-α in Iraqi Patients with Psoriasis treated with Etanercept. *Res. J. Pharm. Technol.* **2019**, *12*, 665–668. [CrossRef]
46. Olejniczak-Staruch, I.; Narbutt, J.; Bednarski, I.; Woźniacka, A.; Sieniawska, J.; Kraska-Gacka, M.; Śmigielski, J.; Lesiak, A. Interleukin 22 and 6 serum concentrations decrease under long-term biologic therapy in psoriasis. *Postep. Dermatol. Alergol.* **2020**, *37*, 705–711. [CrossRef] [PubMed]
47. Pastore, S.; Mariani, V.; Lulli, D.; Gubinelli, E.; Raskovic, D.; Mariani, S.; Stancato, A.; de Luca, C.; Pecorelli, A.; Valacchi, G.; et al. Glutathione peroxidase activity in the blood cells of psoriatic patients correlates with their responsiveness to Efalizumab. *Free Radic. Res.* **2011**, *45*, 585–599. [CrossRef] [PubMed]
48. Becatti, M.; Urban, M.L.; Taurisano, G.; Mannucci, A.; Barygina, V.; Pescitelli, L.; Prignano, F.; Silvestri, E.; Taddei, N.; Lotti, T.; et al. Secukinumab reduces plasma oxidative stress in psoriasis: A case-based experience. *Dermatol. Ther.* **2018**, *31*, e12675. [CrossRef]
49. Campanati, A.; Orciani, M.; Gorbi, S.; Regoli, F.; Di Primio, R.; Offidani, A. Effect of biologic therapies targeting tumour necrosis factor-α on cutaneous mesenchymal stem cells in psoriasis: Modifications of MSCs in psoriatic patients receiving TNF-α inhibitors. *Br. J. Dermatol.* **2012**, *167*, 68–76. [CrossRef]
50. Ikonomidis, I.; Papadavid, E.; Makavos, G.; Andreadou, I.; Varoudi, M.; Gravanis, K.; Theodoropoulos, K.; Pavlidis, G.; Triantafyllidi, H.; Moutsatsou, P.; et al. Lowering Interleukin-12 Activity Improves Myocardial and Vascular Function Compared with Tumor Necrosis Factor-a Antagonism or Cyclosporine in Psoriasis. *Circ. Cardiovasc. Imaging* **2017**, *10*, e006283. [CrossRef]
51. Elango, T.; Dayalan, H.; Gnanaraj, P.; Malligarjunan, H.; Subramanian, S. Impact of methotrexate on oxidative stress and apoptosis markers in psoriatic patients. *Clin. Exp. Med.* **2014**, *14*, 431–437. [CrossRef] [PubMed]
52. Cheng, H.; Rademaker, M. Monitoring methotrexate-induced liver fibrosis in patients with psoriasis: Utility of transient elastography. *Psoriasis Targets Ther.* **2018**, *8*, 21–29. [CrossRef] [PubMed]
53. Shah, A.G.; Lydecker, A.; Murray, K.; Tetri, B.N.; Contos, M.J.; Sanyal, A.J. Comparison of Noninvasive Markers of Fibrosis in Patients with Nonalcoholic Fatty Liver Disease. *Clin. Gastroenterol. Hepatol.* **2009**, *7*, 1104–1112. [CrossRef] [PubMed]
54. Sterling, R.K.; Lissen, E.; Clumeck, N.; Sola, R.; Correa, M.C.; Montaner, J.; Sulkowski, M.S.; Torriani, F.J.; Dieterich, D.T.; Thomas, D.L.; et al. Development of a simple noninvasive index to predict significant fibrosis in patients with HIV/HCV coinfection. *Hepatology* **2006**, *43*, 1317–1325. [CrossRef] [PubMed]
55. Ülger, Y. Is neutrophil lymphocyte ratio a useful biomarker in predicting fibrosis in chronic hepatitis C infection? *Eastern J. Med.* **2021**, *26*, 123–127. [CrossRef]
56. Kara, M.; Dogru, T.; Genc, H.; Sertoglu, E.; Celebi, G.; Gurel, H.; Kayadibi, H.; Cicek, A.F.; Ercin, C.N.; Sonmez, A. Neutrophil-to-lymphocyte ratio is not a predictor of liver histology in patients with nonalcoholic fatty liver disease. *Eur. J. Gastroenterol. Hepatol.* **2015**, *27*, 1144–1148. [CrossRef]
57. Lu, W.; Zhang, Y.; Zhu, H.; Zhang, T.; Zhang, L.; Gao, N.; Chang, D.; Yin, J.; Zhou, X.; Li, M.; et al. Evaluation and comparison of the diagnostic performance of routine blood tests in predicting liver fibrosis in chronic hepatitis B infection. *Br. J. Biomed. Sci.* **2019**, *76*, 137–142. [CrossRef] [PubMed]
58. Ding, R.; Zhou, X.; Huang, D.; Wang, Y.; Li, X.; Yan, L.; Lu, W.; Yang, Z.; Zhang, Z. Predictive Performances of Blood Parameter Ratios for Liver Inflammation and Advanced Liver Fibrosis in Chronic Hepatitis B Infection. *BioMed Res. Int.* **2021**, *2021*, 6644855. [CrossRef]
59. Sigal, S.; Mitchell, O.; Feldman, D.; Diakow, M. The pathophysiology of thrombocytopenia in chronic liver disease. *Hepatic Med. Evid. Res.* **2016**, *8*, 39–50. [CrossRef]
60. Wai, C. A simple noninvasive index can predict both significant fibrosis and cirrhosis in patients with chronic hepatitis C. *Hepatology* **2003**, *38*, 518–526. [CrossRef]
61. Giannini, E.; Risso, D.; Botta, F.; Chiarbonello, B.; Fasoli, A.; Malfatti, F.; Romagnoli, P.; Testa, E.; Ceppa, P.; Testa, R. Validity and Clinical Utility of the Aspartate Aminotransferase–Alanine Aminotransferase Ratio in Assessing Disease Severity and Prognosis in Patients with Hepatitis C Virus–Related Chronic Liver Disease. *Arch. Intern. Med.* **2003**, *163*, 218–224. [CrossRef] [PubMed]
62. Vallet-Pichard, A.; Mallet, V.; Nalpas, B.; Verkarre, V.; Nalpas, A.; Dhalluin-Venier, V.; Fontaine, H.; Pol, S. FIB-4: An inexpensive and accurate marker of fibrosis in HCV infection. comparison with liver biopsy and fibrotest. *Hepatology* **2007**, *46*, 32–36. [CrossRef] [PubMed]
63. Cross, T.J.S.; Rizzi, P.; Berry, P.A.; Bruce, M.; Portmann, B.; Harrison, P.M. King's Score: An accurate marker of cirrhosis in chronic hepatitis C. *Eur. J. Gastroenterol. Hepatol.* **2009**, *21*, 730–738. [CrossRef] [PubMed]

International Journal of
Molecular Sciences

MDPI

Review

Treatment Strategies in Neutrophilic Dermatoses: A Comprehensive Review

Grisell Starita-Fajardo [1], David Lucena-López [1], María Asunción Ballester-Martínez [2], Montserrat Fernández-Guarino [2] and Andrés González-García [1,3,*]

[1] Systemic Autoimmune Diseases Unit, Department of Internal Medicine, Hospital Universitario Ramón y Cajal, IRYCIS, 28034 Madrid, Spain; grisell.starita@salud.madrid.org (G.S.-F.); david.lucena@salud.madrid.org (D.L.-L.)
[2] Department of Dermatology, Hospital Universitario Ramón y Cajal, IRYCIS, 28034 Madrid, Spain
[3] Faculty of Medicine and Health Sciences, Universidad de Alcalá (UAH), 28801 Alcalá de Henares, Spain
* Correspondence: andres.gonzalez@salud.madrid.org

Abstract: Neutrophilic dermatoses (NDs) are a group of noninfectious disorders characterized by the presence of a sterile neutrophilic infiltrate without vasculitis histopathology. Their physiopathology is not fully understood. The association between neutrophilic dermatoses and autoinflammatory diseases has led some authors to propose that both are part of the same spectrum of diseases. The classification of NDs depends on clinical and histopathological features. This review focuses on the recent developments of treatments in these pathologies.

Keywords: dermatosis; autoinflammatory; immunomodulation; therapy

Citation: Starita-Fajardo, G.; Lucena-López, D.; Ballester-Martínez, M.A.; Fernández-Guarino, M.; González-García, A. Treatment Strategies in Neutrophilic Dermatoses: A Comprehensive Review. *Int. J. Mol. Sci.* **2023**, *24*, 15622. https://doi.org/10.3390/ijms242115622

Academic Editor: Naoko Kanda

Received: 27 September 2023
Revised: 20 October 2023
Accepted: 23 October 2023
Published: 26 October 2023

1. Introduction

The term neutrophilic dermatoses (NDs) was used for the first time in 1964 by Robert Douglas Sweet to describe a case of febrile neutrophilic dermatosis, currently known as Sweet's syndrome.

The most representative entities within this group include pyoderma gangrenosum (PG), Sweet's syndrome (SS), pustular dermatoses predominantly subcorneal, generalized pustular psoriasis (GPP), and those secondary to inflammatory bowel disease (IBD) [1].

In this review, the location of the neutrophil infiltrate (epidermis, dermis, and/or subcutaneous, the clinical presentation, and the chronicity, which make them unique from the rest, are used to classify each entity [2]. The first classification of ND was defined by Wallach and Vignon-Pennamen [3]. Given its initial complexity, it was reformulated, prioritizing the location of the neutrophilic infiltrate [4].

The pathogenesis of ND is not clearly understood and has been related to abnormal neutrophil function, inflammasome activation, the malignant transformation of neutrophils that infiltrate the dermis, as well as genetic predisposition [5].

There are a wide variety of inflammatory markers and cytokines expressed, among which are CD3 and CD163, IL-1 (α and β), IFN-γ, IL-2, IL-6, IL-8, IL-17, myeloperoxidase, and TNF-α [6].

A unique case is represented by GPP, whose etiology seems to depend on a loss of function in IL36RN, the gene that encodes IL-36Ra. The secretion of IL-36 by keratinocytes or inflammatory cells and the stimulation of autocrine and paracrine pathways trigger an inflammatory response mediated by cytokines that play a key role in the development of this disease: CXCL1, CXCL2, CCL20, IL-8, IL-12, IL-1b, IL-23, IL-6, and TNF-a.

Subsequently, because of the release of these cytokines, the activation of T cells occurs, which produces secretions of IL-22, IL-17, and IFN-c [7].

The treatment of ND varies according to each subtype. The treatment is based in controlling the underlying disease, if found, using glucocorticoids. In addition, a wide variety of alternatives, such as immunosuppressive agents and antimetabolites, as well as azathioprine, cyclosporine, mycophenolate, and cyclophosphamide, could be added in the case of an absence of response. Biological treatment varies according to the desired therapeutic target, as anti-TNF-α, as well as anti-IL 12/IL-23, anti-IL-17, anti-IL-1, anti-IL-1β, and anti-IL-36, among others, can be used [1].

The objective of this article is to summarize the therapeutic novelties of the main syndromes that include neutrophilic dermatoses.

2. Sweet's Syndrome

2.1. Introduction

As previously mentioned, Sweet's syndrome was first described in 1964 by Dr. Robert Douglas Sweet, who used the term "acute febrile neutrophilic dermatosis" to describe eight cases of women with systemic symptoms including fever, leukocytosis, and painful plaques with an extensive neutrophilic infiltrate on the histopathology. In all cases, infections had been ruled out; all of them also exhibited a good response to treatment with steroids [1,5].

SS is characterized by erythematous papules or plaques that can occur on the trunk, upper extremities, head, and neck. It is characteristically accompanied by fever and neutrophilia. It predominantly affects the female sex and can occur at any age. SS could be idiopathic or secondary to other pathologies, as well as infections, inflammatory bowel disease, endocrinopathies, autoimmune diseases, and tumors, among others. It could also occur with drugs, such as antibiotics, retinoids, antiepileptics, and anti-TNF-α.

Histologically, it presents with a dense neutrophilic infiltrate in the superficial dermis, which may affect the subcutaneous portion.

2.2. Pathogenesis

The pathogenesis is not exactly known; currently, the postulated hypothesis is that an external or internal agent triggers an activating signal with the consequent release of proinflammatory cytokines, among which are IL-1, IL-6, and IL-8, causing neutrophilic migration to the dermal region [1–3].

In the case of SS, it is crucial to influence the underlying pathology or disorder as the possible causative agent.

2.3. Treatment

2.3.1. Topical Therapy

In localized lesions, topical or intralesional glucocorticoids could be used.

2.3.2. Systemic Treatment

In addition, targeted therapy based on glucocorticoids is usually necessary, such as the use of prednisolone, at a dose of 0.5 to 1 mg/kg/day, with a progressive decrease over 4–6 weeks [2]. Our approach is to avoid higher doses of glucocorticoids, and to try to combine another immunosuppressant whenever the disease needs to be controlled. In this scenario, second-line treatments, such as dapsone (100–200 mg/24 h) and colchicine (1.5 mg/24 h), are useful in monotherapy and in combination, with the aim being to decrease the burden of chronic treatment with glucocorticosteroids [1,2]. The evidence regarding biological treatments in SS is limited, and mostly represented by case reports and a few open studies. Likewise, a case of rheumatoid arthritis with SS refractory to initial treatment with prednisone, infliximab, rituximab, methotrexate, abatacept, tocilizumab, and golimumab is described in the literature, which finally responded to therapy with baricitinib [8].

In addition, there is one reported case of a 12-year-old girl diagnosed with CANDLE syndrome (recurrent fever, visceral inflammation, lipodystrophy, and fixed skin lesions) who presented a complete response to tofacitinib [9]. Both cases lead us to consider the possible role of JAK inhibitors in SS.

A special case is SS associated with inflammatory bowel disease, where TNF-α inhibitors, including etanercept, infliximab, and adalimumab, have demonstrated efficacy. Likewise, the role of ustekinumab in Crohn's disease has been shown, leading to remission in a patient with secondary SS [10–13]. See Table 1.

Table 1. Biological agents in the treatment of Sweet's syndrome.

Biological Agent	Dosage	Reference
Adalimumab	40 mg every other week (alone or combined with systemic steroids)	[14]
Infliximab	5 mg/kg at weeks 0, 2, and 6, and every 6 to 8 weeks thereafter (alone or combined with topical or systemic steroids)	[11,12]
Ustekinumab	90 mg every 8 weeks	[13]
Anakinra	100 mg/day subcutaneously (combined with systemic steroids)	[15]
Rituximab	Rheumatoid arthritis protocol, (1000 mg at days 1 and 15) or 375 mg/m2 body surface, 2 additional cycles at 6 months and 18 months after the initial dose (combined with systemic steroids)	[14,16,17]

Refractory cases usually require high doses of methylprednisolone (250 mg/24 h for a period of 3–5 days). Rituximab and anakinra are also postulated as favorable alternatives [2,14–17].

3. Pyoderma Gangrenosum

3.1. Introduction

This entity was described in 1916 by Brocq, and was later renamed in 1930 by Brunsting, Goeckerman, and O'Leary [18,19]. The prevalence is 5.8 cases per 100,000 inhabitants, predominantly in the female sex.

Pyoderma gangrenosum is frequently shown in association with systemic pathology, including inflammatory bowel disease, rheumatoid arthritis, and hematological malignancies. PG is closely related to exposure to drugs, among which colony-stimulating factors, levamisole, cocaine, and immunomodulatory agents stand out [1–3].

There are different types of PG; approximately 85% are classified as classic ulcerative, while the other 15% include bullous, vegetative, pustular, peristomal, and superficial granulomatous variants.

The most common is the ulcerative subtype, which classically presents as single or multiple lesions. It could be a nodule or pustule that rapidly expands to form a painful purplish ulcer with a fibrinous bottom and ulcerative edge. It can occur anywhere in the body and presents pathergy [1–3,5].

It is important to emphasize the increase in morbidity and mortality of patients with PG compared with controls matched by age and sex [20,21].

3.2. Pathogenesis

The etiopathogenesis underlying this entity is unknown. It is believed to be based on a dysregulation of innate and acquired immunity. There is an alteration in the response of the immune system to superantigens as well as neutrophil, TNF-α, IL-12/IL-23 dysfunction, and genetic predisposition. The role played by neutrophils in this entity is conditioned by defects in chemotaxis, phagocytosis, and bactericidal ability [1,22].

Other mechanisms implied in the etiology of PG have been described. Recent studies have focused on the role of lymphocytes and biomarkers. A clonal expression of T lymphocytes has been observed in intralesional and peripheral blood, mainly for CD3+ and CD163 macrophages [22]. In addition, the overexpression of IL-8, IL-16, IL-18, IL-17, IL-23, MMP (metalloproteinases) 2, 9, and TNF-α, and deregulation between effector T-reg and Th17 cells, has also been demonstrated.

Although its role is not well defined, the expression of IL-1β in PG lesions suggests an autoinflammatory basis with consequent activation of the inflammasome. Additionally, genetics is an essential factor contributing to syndromes that associate PG and autoinflammatory phenomena, as has been verified with mutation in the Proline-Serine-Threonine Phosphatase Interactive Protein (PSTPIP)-1 gene that encodes for the CD2-binding protein 1, located on chromosome 15q, which is involved in PG and associated autoinflammatory syndromes such as PAPA syndrome (pyogenic sterile arthritis, PG, and cystic acne) and PASH syndrome (PG, acne, and suppurative hidradenitis) [22,23].

3.3. *Treatment*

3.3.1. Topical Treatment

Regarding treatment, the first line is based on topical treatment, with both analgesia and topical corticosteroids or tracrolimus [24].

3.3.2. Systemic Treatment

Glucocorticoids

Prednisone is usually administered at a dose of 0.5–1 mg/kg/day up to 2 mg/kg/day, with a gradual decrease between 4 and 6 weeks, and can be prolonged until completion at 4–6 months. Some authors recommend methylprednisolone pulses (250–1000 mg) for 3–5 consecutive days with consequent transition to the oral route, thus achieving a faster effect.

Immunosuppressants

The commencement of corticosteroid-sparing drugs should be performed as quickly as possible, because high doses of prednisone are associated with high mortality rates [25]. Among them, oral cyclosporine has emerged as the main immunosuppressant at doses of 2–3 to 4–5 mg/kg/day, and could be used both alone and in combination with glucocorticoids. The choice of using cyclosporine against corticosteroids depends on the patient's comorbidities. Pre-existing conditions that favor the use of corticosteroids over cyclosporine include renal failure or oncology history. However, patients with obesity, diabetes mellitus, osteoporosis, or peptic ulcer will benefit from cyclosporine [26]. In the same way, during the reduction in corticosteroids, dapsone 50–200 mg, azathioprine 100–300 mg/day, methotrexate 10–30 mg/week, cyclophosphamide 1.5–3.0 mg/kg/day, mycophenolate mofetil 2–3 g/day, mercaptopurine, melphalan, thalidomide, and IVIG could be used. In addition, there are case series described in patients with PG refractory to conventional treatment who responded to the association of glucocorticoids with tracrolimus [27,28].

TNF-α Inhibitors

Infliximab, adalimumab, etanercept, certolizumab, and golimumab have recognized efficacy in refractory PG and are associated with IBD [26], according to a semi-systematic review published by Ben Abdallah et al. After analyzing 222 articles that included 356 patients with PG treated with TNF-α inhibitors, an 87% response rate and 67% complete remission were described, without finding significant differences between different drugs in terms of effectiveness [23].

Infliximab

In a double-blind randomized clinical trial, Brooklyn et al. compared infliximab with a placebo, for which 30 patients with PG and IBD were recruited. Subjects were randomized to receive infliximab 5 mg/kg for 2 weeks. After two weeks of treatment, a response rate of 46% was observed in the infliximab group vs. 6% in the placebo group. Subsequently, given the obtained results, an open label trial was carried out that included the rest of the untreated patients; it was observed that at week 6, 90% had presented remission, with complete resolution in 21% of the patients treated with infliximab [29]. In the review published by Pascal Juillerat et al., wherein 22 articles with 85 patients with a diagnosis of PG associated with IBD being treated with infliximab were analyzed, the efficacy of the treatment in cases of corticosteroid resistance and ulcerative phenotype was concluded [30]. Arguelles-Arias et al. also carried out a retrospective analysis of a cohort of subjects with PG, in which they showed response rates of 92% and 100% with infliximab and adalimumab, respectively [31]. In total, 58 cases of PG without IBD treated with anti-TNF-α have been reported in the literature, of which 41% were idiopathic PG, 17% were associated with rheumatoid arthritis, 10% were post-surgical/traumatic, 7% were associated with hidradenitis suppurativa, 4% were associated with monoclonal gammopathy, and 3.5% were related to cocaine use (levimasol) [32]. There is robust evidence supporting the use of infliximab in PG, both associated with and unrelated to IBD [29–32]. See Table 2.

Table 2. Biological agents in the treatment of pyoderma gangrenosum.

Biological Agent	Dosage	Reference
Adalimumab	Induction dose of 160 mg at week 0, 80 mg at week 1, and 40 mg every 2 weeks.	[33–35]
Infliximab	5 mg/kg at weeks 0, 2, and 6, and every 6 to 8 weeks thereafter (alone or combined with topical or systemic steroids)	[29–32]
Certolizumab pegol	400 mg every other week for the first three injections, followed by 400 mg every 4 weeks (combined with systemic steroids)	[23,36]
Etanercept	50 mg every 2 weeks	[32]
Golimumab	200 mg at week 0, 100 mg at week 2, and every 4 weeks thereafter (combined with topical or systemic steroids)	[37]
Ustekinumab	90 mg every 8 weeks or at week 0, week 4, week 8, and every 8 weeks for a minimum of 12 months. Usually administered in the absence of concomitant therapy	[38–41]
Secukinumab	300 mg subcutaneously initially and later at weeks 0, 1, 2, 3, and 4, followed by a monthly maintenance dose	[42,43]
Canakinumab	150 mg of canakimumab subcutaneously at week 0, with a possible extra dose after two weeks in cases of refractoriness, as well as an optional dose of 150–300mg at week 8	[44]
Anakinra	100 mg daily subcutaneously, in combination or not with glucocorticoids, which can be increased to 200 mg daily (2mg/kg day) in cases of inadequate clinical response, or 4 weeks of loading at 2 mg/kg daily, followed by 100 mg once daily	[45–48]

Adalimumab

The use of adalimumab has been shown to be effective in cases of recalcitrant PG, as demonstrated in some cases reported in the literature [33,34]. Similarly, the case of a patient diagnosed with rheumatoid arthritis treated with methotrexate and etanercept, who developed refractory PG after 2 months of orthopedic surgery, has recently been published [35]. Initially, it was decided to add prednisone, despite which remission was not achieved; thus, it was decided to change etanercept to adalimumab, achieving practical resolution of the lesions after 25 weeks of treatment.

As previously mentioned, Rousset L. et al. described 14 cases of patients with PG not associated with IBD treated with adalimumab, of whom 64% presented complete remission—figures similar to those obtained after treatment with infliximab [32]. Herberger et al. analyzed 52 patients with PG who received treatment with biologics or intravenous immunoglobulins; it was observed that up to 57.1% (16/28) of the patients treated with adalimumab experienced complete remission or improvement of the lesions [38]. Lastly, the use of adalimumab has also been described in autoinflammatory pathologies such as PASH and PAPA syndrome, with the adequate response and resolution of PG [49,50].

Etanercept

Etanercept represents a useful option in cases of recalcitrant PG. According to the series of cases collected by Rousset L. et al., 47% (9/19) of patients presented complete remission after treatment with etanercept [32]. Similarly, Herberger et al. conducted a retrospective cohort study in patients with a diagnosis of PG not associated with IBD, in which clinical improvement was evidenced in 71.4% (5/7) of patients treated with etanercept [38].

Golimumab

The evidence available in the literature regarding the use of golimumab in PG refers to a few isolated cases. Diotavelli F. et al. published the case of a 68-year-old subject with a history of ulcerative colitis, who received treatment with infliximab and adalimumab, and then suffered an episode of rectocolitis and the appearance of an ulcer in the distal third of the left leg. After performing a biopsy and screening for infectious disease, treatment with glucocorticoids and golimumab was started, with excellent clinical evolution [37].

Certolizumab

The use of certolizumab in PG is limited to specific cases, as we previously observed in the series of cases reported by Rousset L. et al., which added a subject who received treatment with certolizumab with an adequate response and disappearance of lesions [32] Similarly, a case of a patient with Crohn's disease with significant skin involvement due to disseminated PG, refractory to multiple lines of treatment, was reported; they received certolizumab with systemic glucocorticoids and tacrolimus, obtaining response and resolution of lesions after 11 months of treatment [36].

IL-1 Inhibitors

Anakinra

Anakinra acts by inhibiting IL-1 α and β; it plays a fundamental role in the treatment of monogenic autoinflammatory syndromes, such as CAPS (cryopyrin-associated periodic syndromes) and Still's disease in adults [51]. If we delve into the pathophysiology of PG, the expression of IL-1β and its receptor has been observed in PG lesions, hence its use in this pathology [1,22,26]. Based on these data, anakinra could play a role in recalcitrant PG and autoinflammatory syndromes, such as PASH and PAPA syndrome, with adequate clinical responses to treatment [45–48,52]. The dose used was 100 mg daily subcutaneously, in combination or not with glucocorticoids, which can be increased to 200 mg daily (2 mg/kg day) in the case of an inadequate clinical response.

Canakinumab

The use of canakimumab is based on the inhibition of IL-1β, widely used in CAPS and adult-onset Still's disease [51]. Regarding the evidence supporting its use, a clinical trial published by Kolios A.G. et al. presented the selection of five subjects diagnosed with steroid-refractory PG. The intervention consisted of receiving 150 mg of canakimumab subcutaneously at week 0, with a possible extra dose after two weeks in case of refractoriness, as well as an optional dose of 150–300 mg at week 8 based on clinical assessment. At week 16, 80% of the patients presented improvements and 60% exhibited complete remission [44].

IL-17A Inhibitors

Secukinumab

There are no clinical trials or case series that support the use of secukinumab; therefore, its evidence is relegated to reports of isolated clinical cases. The PG subtype that has presented a favorable response in the reported cases is ulcerative, one of which is post-surgical. Usually, they are patients who have presented refractoriness to conventional treatment lines, in which it is used as an off-label drug. The dose used in both clinical cases was 300 mg subcutaneously initially, and later at weeks 0, 1, 2, 3, and 4, followed by a monthly maintenance dose [42,43].

IL-23 Inhibitors

Ustekinumab

Ustekinumab is used in the management of PG, including severe and recalcitrant cases, at a dose of 90 mg every 8 weeks or at week 0, week 4, week 8, and every following 8 weeks for a minimum of 12 months. It is usually administered in the absence of concomitant therapy [38–41]. It could be an option than may control both PG and Crohn disease. As we have seen, it is an interesting option in cases of intolerance, contraindication, or resistance to TNF-α inhibitors or steroids [53].

Anti-IL-17 Receptor

Brodalumab

Two cases are described, both with coexistent hidradenitis suppurativa, in which a weekly subcutaneous dose of 210 mg/1.5 mg was used as HS treatment, achieving practical resolution of the PG lesions [54].

Anti-IL-6 Receptor

Tocilizumab

As we already know, IL-6 plays a fundamental role in the inflammatory cascade; hence, its blocking can have favorable effects in multiple pathologies dependent on its activation. Two cases of favorable response to tocilizumab are described in the literature. The first describes a patient with rheumatoid arthritis and interstitial lung disease who was diagnosed with PG. Initially, treatment with glucocorticoids was established at a dose of 0.5 mg/kg/day with poor response. Subsequently, given the contraindication for the use of anti-TNF due to the pulmonary involvement, the use of tocilizumab was chosen, with an initial dose of 162 mg subcutaneously every two weeks. Finally, the patient presented adequate clinical evolution after IL-6 blockade with practical resolution of the lesions [55]. The second case was a patient with a longstanding history of PG refractory to multiple lines of treatment who was recently diagnosed with Takayasu's arteritis. Given this situation, the decision was made to start tocilizumab, with a favorable response: control of the disease and healing of lesions [56].

Anti-IL-23

Tildrakizumab

There are three cases in the literature in which tildrakizumab has been used as a treatment for PG. The cases described in these reports were of ulcerative PG and vegetative PG subtype. The patients had coexisting entities such as polymyalgia rheumatica and PASH. The initial dose used was 100 mg subcutaneously in weeks 0 and 4, and then later every 12 weeks; after the start of the treatment, it was possible to reduce the concomitant immunosuppressive treatment as well as heal the lesions [57–59].

4. Hidradenitis Suppurativa

4.1. Introduction

Hidradenitis suppurativa (HS) was initially described in 1839 by the French surgeon Verneuil [60]. It is a chronic, recurrent, and debilitating inflammatory disease that usually presents after puberty with deep, inflamed, and painful lesions, spreading exclusively to body areas with the presence of apocrine glands, the most affected regions being the axillary, anogenital, and inguinal regions [61].

Regarding its epidemiology, despite the fact that the real prevalence is unknown, it is estimated that it can be between 0.00033% and 4.10%, with a predominance in the female sex and the African American race. There are no exact data on the actual incidence, although according to a retrospective study it could be 11.4 cases per 100,000 inhabitants, with twice the number of cases in women. The age distribution is situated between 18 and 44 years.

Multiple comorbidities are associated with HS, including obesity and smoking. In addition, there is a higher prevalence of psoriasis among patients suffering from this entity. Approximately 40% of HS patients have an affected family member, implying a genetic predisposition.

4.2. Pathogenesis

In relation to its etiopathogenesis, the primary event consists of follicular hyperkeratosis that, consequently, produces a rupture of the hair follicle and inflammation of the apocrine glands. Both interleukin IL-17 and TNF-α play fundamental roles. Elevated levels of TNF-α in the skin and serum IL-17 correlate with the severity of the disease. The involvement of sex hormones in this pathology is not exactly known [62].

4.3. Classification

Treatment depends on the severity of the disease, which is graded according to the Hurley scale:

- Hurley I—Abscesses, single or multiple, without fistulous tracts or scarring;
- Hurley II—Abscesses separated from each other and recurrent with fistulous tracts and scarring;
- Hurley III—Multiple abscesses with fistulous tracts and abundant scarring [63].

4.4. Treatment

4.4.1. Non-Pharmacological Treatments

Therapeutic options vary from pharmacological therapy to surgical interventions. Among non-pharmacological interventions, lifestyle changes stand out. Cessation of smoking seems to have potentiating effects in terms of reducing the severity of the disease [64]. In the systematic review carried out by Weber et al., which included a total of 2829 patients, a significant but weak improvement was observed in the patients who lost weight and changed their diet. The same occurred with those who were supplemented with oral vitamin D and zinc [65].

4.4.2. Topical Treatment

Topical therapy is the first-line therapy in localized forms. Its use is also recognized as a complement to systemic therapy in more complex forms. It consists of the use of antiseptics, topical antibiotics, keratolytics, and/or intralesional corticosteroids.

4.4.3. Systemic Treatment

Antibiotics

Regarding systemic treatment, we must emphasize the role of antibiotics. Among them, in the first line, we find oral tetracyclines, which are very useful because of their anti-inflammatory effects. Subsequently, in the second and third lines, we find clindamycin–rifampicin and metronidazole/moxifloxacin/rifampicin, respectively. There is also a report of the use of ertapenem in cases refractory to other lines of antibiotic therapy, with an adequate response.

The use of dapsone should be relegated to third-line treatments, especially in those patients with moderate involvement (Hurley I–II) if the first- and second-line treatments have failed. The dose used varies between 25 and 200 mg daily, and it is recommended for at least 3 months [66].

There is little evidence about the use of zinc in patients with Hurley stage I and II; despite this, it seems that its key role in innate immunity could be favorable in certain cases [67].

Retinoids

Retinoids are also a fundamental part of the therapeutic arsenal for this pathology. They are usually relegated to the second or third line, when antibiotics have failed. The best known is acitretin, at doses of 0.2 to 0.88 mg/kg per day. It seems that there are many factors that predispose one to a better response with this drug, among which are a family history of HS, elevated levels of activity, and a history of acne conglobata [68–70]. In the case of isotretinoin, evidence about its use is contradictory; usually, the dose used is 0.5 to 1.2 mg/kg [69,70].

Biological Treatment

In recent years, the use of biological therapy has increased. Immunomodulation is essential in refractory or severe cases. Treatments are based on IL-1 (anakinra), IL-12/23 (ustekinumab), IL-17 (secukinumab), and the TNF-alpha (infliximab, adalimumab) blockade. To date, only adalimumab has been approved for first-line therapy, and infliximab for the second line [66].

TNF-α inhibitors

Adalimumab

Adalimumab is a recombinant human monoclonal antibody against TNF-α effective for moderate and severe cases. The most relevant clinical trials in relation to its effectiveness are PIONEER I and II [71], which included a total of 633 patients who were randomized to receive placebo or adalimumab. The design was similar in both trials, the difference being that in the second trial, concomitant treatment with oral tetracyclines was allowed. The primary endpoint was clinical response, defined as a greater than 50% reduction in lesions, this being significantly greater in adalimumab-treated patients compared with placebo (41.8 vs. 26% in PIONEER I and 58.9 vs. 27.6% in PIONEER II). Based on these results, adalimumab was approved by the FDA for moderate to severe HS.

Infliximab

Infliximab is a monoclonal chimeric antibody against TNF-α, indicated as the second-line treatment in moderate–severe cases refractory to adalimumab. Its use in HS has not been specifically approved in this entity; despite this, the European guidelines recommend a dose of 5 mg/kg body weight administered on weeks 0, 2 and 6, and then regularly every 8 weeks [68].

IL-1 inhibitors

Anakinra

Anakinra is a recombinant human IL-1 receptor antagonist that blocks the inflammatory effects of IL-1. Its efficacy has been demonstrated in two clinical trials. The first was a randomized clinical trial in 20 patients with Hurley stage II/II, in which the group randomized to receive anakinra presented clinically significant responses of 78%, while in the placebo group, this was 30% [72]. Similarly, Leslie et al. carried out an open clinical trial with five patients diagnosed with HS in the moderate–severe phase who received treatment with anakinra for 16 weeks, with an objective decrease in activity. The dose usually administered is 100 mg/day subcutaneously [73]. The HS ALLIANCE group currently recommends it as a third-line therapy in cases of the failure of TNF-alpha inhibitors [74].

IL-23 inhibitors

Ustekinumab

Ustekinumab is a human IgG1 class monoclonal antibody that modulates IL-12 and IL-23 signaling. Regarding evidence of its use, a cohort of 17 patients with Hurley stage II–III HS received 45 mg s.c. at weeks 0, 4, 16, and 28. Of the subjects included, 82% presented a great clinical improvement [75]. The North American and European guidelines consider it in cases of refractoriness to previous lines [68,76].

L-23 inhibitors

Secukinumab

Secukinumab is a human monoclonal antibody directed against IL-17A. There seems to be an increase in IL-17A in the blood of patients with HS, related to the severity of the disease. Current clinical guidelines have not mentioned the use of secukinumab in this entity. However, there are several trials that have reported its use [77,78], including SUNSHINE and SUNRISE, phase 3 multicenter randomized clinical trials with a total of 541 and 543 patients, respectively. The included cases were patients with moderate–severe HS who were randomized to receive secukinumab 300 mg s.c. every 2 weeks or every 4 weeks, or a placebo. The primary endpoint was clinically significant improvement, defined as a more than 50% improvement in lesions. Of the patients randomized to secukinumab, it was verified in both trials that the most effective regimen was every 2 weeks. Despite this, it is necessary to continue investigating the indication in this entity [78]. See Table 3.

Table 3. Biological agents in the treatment of Hidradenitis suppurativa.

Biological Agent	Dosage	Reference
Adalimumab	80 mg s.c. first week, 40 mg s.c. second week	[68,71]
Infliximab	5 mg/kg body weight is administered on week 0, 2, 6, and then regularly every 8 weeks	[68]
Anakinra	100 mg/day subcutaneously	[72–74]
Ustekinumab	45 mg s.c. at weeks 0, 4, 16, and 28	[68,75]
Secukinumab	300 mg s.c. every 2 weeks, every 4 weeks	[77,78]

Regarding immunosuppressive treatment, the following drugs are distinguished.

4.4.4. Glucocorticoids

The European, North American, and HS ALLIANCE clinical guidelines indicate glucocorticoids as a treatment in severe cases, or in order to perform bridging therapy with another drug [68,74,76]. The North American and European guidelines recommend a dose of 0.5–0.7 mg/kg oral prednisolone. Prolonged treatments are not recommended due to their potential side effects [68,76].

4.4.5. Immunosuppressants

Cyclosporin A

Evidence about the effectiveness of cyclosporin Ais scarce [79,80]. The clinical guidelines recommend cyclosporine in cases of first-, second-, or third-line failure. The doses usually used are 2–6 mg/kg once daily for various durations (5 to 30 weeks) [66,68,79,80].

4.4.6. Hormone Therapy

Hormone therapy is one option to consider; androgens promote the occlusion of the hair follicle through a proliferation of keratinocytes, giving rise to acanthosis and keratosis follicularis. The predominance in females—changes with menstruation, a worsening in the menopause, and improvements during pregnancy—make this theory plausible [78,81].

Among other treatments, we find metformin, which could be beneficial in patients with polycystic ovaries and diabetes mellitus. The North American guidelines recommend a dose of 500 mg two or three times a day [69,76,82].

Finasteride can also be considered; it could be useful via its action of inhibiting the androgen-mediated exacerbation of HS. The North American guidelines recommend doses of 1.25 to 5 mg/d, which have been reported as effective in several trials. It can be used both in monotherapy in moderate–severe cases and in additional therapy in severe cases [76,83].

4.4.7. Other Therapies

Finally, it is worth mentioning spironolactone. According to the North American guidelines, patients who used spironolactone at doses of 100–150 mg daily showed clinical improvements after 3–6 months of treatment [76].

Among experimental therapies, the role of the botulinum toxin should be highlighted. Although the underlying mechanism is not clear, it seems to be a plausible option for patients with extensive Hurley III involvement [84,85].

The surgical option should be considered in patients with severe involvement with chronic lesions that do not respond to conventional therapy. Amongst the different surgical options, we find radical surgical excision, deroofing, drainage, carbon dioxide laser therapy, and YAG laser therapy [64,74,76].

5. Generalized Pustular Psoriasis

5.1. Introduction

GPP is a relatively rare variant of psoriasis, characterized by the appearance of erythematous plaques with neutrophilic, sterile pustular lesions, associated with systemic symptoms; the presence of fever, malaise, and elevation of inflammatory biomarkers is frequent and usually implies increases in morbidity and mortality [85].

The exact prevalence of GPP is unknown; however, it is considered a rare disease. It can occur in all races, and a certain preponderance in women has been reported. GPP presents as flares that require long-term control of the disease; these could be precipitated by external factors such as smoking, infections, pregnancy, and drugs. A paradoxical reaction to treatment with ustekinumab and TNF-α inhibitors has been described [86]. The low prevalence of this entity makes the diagnosis difficult. Likewise, there is scant evidence regarding the optimal management of this pathology [87].

5.2. Pathogenesis

The new advances in the pathophysiology of this disease have broadened the horizons of possible therapeutic targets for GPP:

- Mutations in IL36RN (gene that encodes the interleukin-36 receptor antagonist) have been identified in cases of GPP. These loss-of-function mutations result in the hyperactivation of IL-36 signaling. This induces neutrophil epidermal accumulation and the formation of pustules mediated by the production of inflammatory cytokines;
- Proinflammatory functions of IL-36 can be potentiated by a positive feedback loop with the IL-17/IL-23 axis. The sustained activation of IL-1 and IL-36 in GPP suggests that the IL-1/IL-36 inflammatory axis is the main physiopathological mechanism in GPP. IL-1 inhibition produces a partial response in patients with this entity, suggesting that IL-1 by itself may not play a central role in GPP; instead, IL-1 may act in a positive loop with IL-36;
- Mutations in caspase recruitment domain family member 14 (CARD14) and mutations in the adapter protein family 1 (AP1S3) have also been associated with pustular psoriasis [88].

5.3. Treatment

Treatment options include topical therapies, phototherapy, and systemic therapies.

5.3.1. Phototherapy

Many phototherapy studies are case reports, and no randomized controlled trials (RCTs) have been conducted to date. They should be used with caution, and the dose should be adapted progressively, watching the skin for reactions after each irradiation. Any recommendations should be categorized as an expert opinion.

5.3.2. Topical Therapies

Calcipotriene and tacrolimus have been used in monotherapies, and also combined with systemic therapies to treat severe disease [89].

5.3.3. Retinoids

In a retrospective study that included 10 patients with GPP, acitretin resulted in a good but slow response, defined as the absence of new pustules within 3 days of treatment, and clearance of the majority of skin lesions within 4–6 weeks. However, it is important to note that a relapse could be observed upon acitretin withdrawal [90].

5.3.4. Dapsone

Dapsone is not recommended for use as a first-line drug in cases of flares due to the slow onset of action. However, it could be considered as an alternative treatment when there is a poor response to first-line drugs. We initiated 50–100 mg of dapsone in two to three divided doses per day [85,89].

5.3.5. Immunosuppressants

Cyclosporine

Because of its ability to yield immediate symptomatic relief, cyclosporine is usually considered as a first-line agent. The general approach is to initiate with cyclosporine 2.5–5.0 mg/kg per day (twice daily), and then adjust the dose based on symptoms [91].

Methotrexate

No RCTs have been performed, probably because of the small number of cases and the severity of disease, which makes large-scale comparisons difficult [92]. We recommend the use of methotrexate in patients with joint involvement, or in cases of refractoriness to the first-line treatment.

Glucocorticoids

Steroids by themselves could induce the formation of pustules, which is why we do not recommended them as a first-line therapy, although they could be of great help for use as an adjuvant therapy in cases of severe flares with systemic symptoms [89].

Mycophenolate mofetil

In a case study, improvements in skin lesions were described in one patient after seven days of treatment with mycophenolate mofetil; these were sustained for 4 months [93].

5.3.6. Biological Treatment

TNF-α Inhibitors

Many case reports describe the efficacy of TNF-α inhibitors. However, a paradoxical reaction after administration has been reported. The physiopathology of this event is not fully understood. See Table 4.

Table 4. Biological agents in the treatment of generalized pustular psoriasis.

Biological Agent	Dosage	Reference
Etanercept	50 mg of etanercept twice weekly subcutaneously	[94]
Infliximab	5 mg/kg body weight is administered on week 0, 2, 6, and then regularly every 8 weeks	[95]
Adalimumab	Dose of 80 mg is given s.c. in adults, and after the second week, a dose of 40 mg is given s.c. every 2 weeks. If the efficacy is insufficient, the dose may be increased to 80 mg/administration	[89]
Brodalumab	s.c. injections of 210 mg at weeks 0, 1, 2 and then every 2 weeks thereafter	[89,96]
Secukinumab	Weekly s.c. injections of 300 mg on weeks 0, 1, 2, 3, and 4, and then every 4 weeks thereafter (may be decreased to 150 mg)	[89]
Ixekizumab	s.c. injections of 160 mg at week 0, followed by 80 mg at weeks 2, 4, 6, 8, 10, and 12, then 80 mg every 4 weeks thereafter	[89]
Guselkumab	100 mg dose subcutaneously on weeks 0 and 4, followed by 100 mg every 8 weeks	[97]
Risankizumab	150 mg subcutaneously plus two additional samples at weeks 4 and 16	[98]
Anakinra	100 mg daily subcutaneously	[99,100]
Canakinumab	150 mg subcutaneously per month	[100]
Gevokizumab	60 mg subcutaneously every 4 weeks for a total of three injections (12 weeks)	[101]
Spesolimab	Single intravenous dose of 10 mg/kg	[102]

Infliximab

In a retrospective study, the administration of infliximab in a standard regimen (intravenous infusion at weeks 0, 2, and 6, and subsequently every 4 weeks) demonstrated flare control in four patients after 24–48 h of the infusion. Additionally, in an open-label study that included 10 patients with GPP flares, the time to pustular clearance ranged from 1 to 8 days [103].

Adalimumab

Adalimumab was described as effective and well tolerated for up to 52 weeks in 10 Japanese patients. Time to remission was variable, from 1 to 4 weeks [89].

Etanercept

A case series that included six patients with GPP showed a reduction in inflammatory biomarkers and clinical improvement [103].

IL-17A Inhibitors

Brodalumab

In an open-label, multicenter, long-term, phase III study, patients showed improved clinical status or remission after 12 weeks of treatment. By week 52, 91.7% were in clinical remission or had improved clinical status with the administration of brodalumab, an IL-17 receptor antagonist [96].

Secukinumab

Secukinumab is a monoclonal antibody that targets IL-17A, which demonstrated efficacy in a phase III study that included 12 patients with GPP in Japan. It was used as a monotherapy or in combination with other immunosuppressant drugs, and resulted in 9/12 patients (75%) achieving a Clinical Global Impression (CGI) score of "very much improved" at week 12, along with 7/12 patients (58.3%) achieving this at week 52 [89,94];

Ixekizumab

Another IL-17A antagonist, similar to secukinumab, is ixekizumab; efficacy has been demonstrated in patients with GPP in three phase III, open-label, multicenter studies, which included Japanese patients with GPP [89,104].

Anti IL-23 and IL-23/IL-12 Inhibitors

Guselkumab

Guselkumab is an IL-23 inhibitor that showed efficacy in a phase III, multicenter, open-label study in Japan that included 10 patients with GPP. In total, 50% of the patients showed improvement after one week of the administration of guselkumab [97].

Risankizumab

Risankizumab targets the p19 subunit of IL-23 and was approved in Japan for the treatment of patients with GPP [98,105].

Anti IL-1β and IL-1R Inhibitors

Anakinra

Anakinra is a recombinant IL-1 receptor antagonist, showing efficacy in reducing symptoms, normalizing inflammatory biomarkers, and stopping pustule formations in a patient with GPP and IL36RN mutation after 5 month of treatment [99].

Canakinumab

A monoclonal antibody that targets IL-1β, canakinumab, was used in a patient intolerant to anakinra, resulting in complete skin clearance and the improvement of systemic symptoms [100].

Gevokizumab

Gevokizumab blocks the activation of IL-1β receptors and has shown promising results in an open-label study in two patients with severe and refractory GPP [101].

IL-36 Pathway Inhibitor

Spesolimab

Spesolimab is a selective, humanized antibody against the IL-36 receptor that blocks its activation and suppresses the inflammatory response. In a phase II, multicenter, randomized, double-blind, placebo-controlled trial, patients treated with a single intravenous 10 mg/kg dose of spesolimab were more likely to achieve remission, defined by the clearance of pustular lesions within one week, than those in the placebo group [102].

5.4. Other Therapies

Therapeutic granulocyte and monocyte apheresis (GMA) is an extracorporeal circulation therapy that inhibits and removes neutrophils, macrophages, and monocytes, which accumulate in inflamed tissues. This therapy has shown efficacy in GPP only in case reports, case series, and reviews. No RCTs have been performed [89].

The majority of treatments discussed previously do not have a prescribing label for GPP, except in Japan, where TNF-α-blocking agents, IL-17/IL-17R inhibitors, and IL-23 inhibitors are approved for use against this disease. Brodalumab is also officially accepted in Taiwan and Thailand [96]. Recently, in September and October 2022, spesolimab was approved in Japan and the EU, respectively, for the treatment of acute symptoms in GPP [102]. Prospective studies are needed to review the outcomes and standardize the treatment of GPP.

6. Conclusions

In our review, we found that there are certain limitations when it comes to establishing action protocols in each disease, mainly due to the low quality of scientific evidence at present. Most of the publications are based on case reports. There are few randomized, controlled clinical trials; in most cases, the existing publications have small sample sizes, due to low prevalence rates. Likewise, in many cases, the drugs used for the treatment of neutrophilic dermatoses tend to have been developed recently, which is why we believe that it is essential to subsequently elucidate the pathophysiology and molecular pathways to extend the follow-up times of these patients and to closely monitor both the evolution and the side effects, in order to construct standardized treatment algorithms in the future.

Author Contributions: Conceptualization, G.S.-F. and D.L.-L.; methodology, G.S.-F. and D.L.-L.; writing—original draft preparation, G.S.-F. and D.L.-L.; writing—review and editing, G.S.-F.; visualization, G.S.-F. and D.L.-L.; supervision, A.G.-G., M.A.B.-M. and M.F.-G. All authors have read and agreed to the published version of the manuscript.

Funding: This research received no external funding.

Conflicts of Interest: The authors declare no conflict of interest.

References

1. Molinelli, E.; Brisigotti, V.; Paolinelli, M.; Offidani, A. Novel Therapeutic Approaches and Targets for the Treatment of Neutrophilic Dermatoses, Management of Patients with Neutrophilic Dermatoses and Future Directions in the Era of Biologic Treatment. *Curr. Pharm. Biotechnol.* **2021**, *22*, 46–58. [CrossRef] [PubMed]
2. Weiss, E.H.; Ko, C.J.; Leung, T.H.; Micheletti, R.G.; Mostaghimi, A.; Ramachandran, S.M.; Rosenbach, M.; Nelson, C.A. Neutrophilic Dermatoses: A Clinical Update. *Curr. Derm. Rep.* **2022**, *11*, 89–102. [CrossRef] [PubMed]
3. Wallach, D. Neutrophilic dermatoses: An overview. *Clin. Dermatol.* **2000**, *18*, 229–231. [CrossRef] [PubMed]
4. McGonagle, D.; McDermott, M.F. A proposed classification of the immunological diseases. *PLoS Med.* **2006**, *3*, e297. [CrossRef]
5. Nelson, C.A.; Stephen, S.; Ashchyan, H.J.; James, W.D.; Micheletti, R.G.; Rosenbach, M. Neutrophilic dermatoses. *J. Am. Acad. Dermatol.* **2018**, *79*, 987–1006. [CrossRef]
6. Marzano, A.V.; Cugno, M.; Trevisan, V.; Fanoni, D.; Venegoni, L.; Berti, E.; Crosti, C. Role of infammatory cells, cytokines and matrix metalloproteinases in neutrophil-mediated skin diseases. *Clin. Exp. Immunol.* **2010**, *162*, 100–107. [CrossRef]
7. Sugiura, K. Role of Interleukin 36 in Generalised Pustular Psoriasis and Beyond. *Dermatol. Ther.* **2022**, *12*, 315–328. [CrossRef]
8. Nousari, Y.; Wu, B.C.; Valenzuela, G. Successful use of baricitinib in the treatment of refractory rheumatoid arthritis-associated Sweet syndrome. *Clin. Exp. Dermatol.* **2021**, *46*, 1330–1332. [CrossRef]
9. Patel, P.N.; Hunt, R.; Pettigrew, Z.J.; Shirley, J.B.; Vogel, T.P.; de Guzman, M.M. Successful treatment of chronic atypical neutrophilic dermatosis with lipodystrophy and elevated temperature (CANDLE) syndrome with tofacitinib. *Pediatr. Dermatol.* **2021**, *38*, 528–529. [CrossRef]
10. Marzano, A.V.; Ishak, R.S.; Saibeni, S.; Crosti, C.; Meroni, P.L.; Cugno, M. Autoinflammatory skin disorders in inflammatory bowel diseases, pyoderma gangrenosum and Sweet's syndrome: A comprehensive review and disease classification criteria. *Clin. Rev. Allergy Immunol.* **2013**, *45*, 202–210. [CrossRef]
11. Foster, E.N.; Nguyen, K.K.; Sheikh, R.A.; Prindiville, T.P. Crohn's disease associated with Sweet's syndrome and Sjögren's syndrome treated with infliximab. *Clin. Dev. Immunol.* **2005**, *12*, 145–149. [CrossRef] [PubMed]
12. Moreno Márquez, C.; Maldonado Pérez, B.; Castro Laria, L. Infliximab as Rescue Treatment in Sweet's Syndrome Related to Corticodependent Ulcerative Colitis. *J. Crohn's Colitis* **2018**, *12*, 755–756. [CrossRef] [PubMed]
13. Hu, K.A.; Shen, J.; Rieger, K.; Wei, M.T.; Gubatan, J. Subcutaneous Sweet Syndrome Successfully Treated with Ustekinumab in a Patient with Ulcerative Colitis. *ACG Case Rep. J.* **2022**, *9*, e00881. [CrossRef] [PubMed]
14. Hashemi, S.M.; Fazeli, S.A.; Vahedi, A.; Golabchifard, R. Rituximab for refractory subcutaneous Sweet's syndrome in chronic lymphocytic leukemia: A case report. *Mol. Clin. Oncol.* **2016**, *4*, 436–440. [CrossRef] [PubMed]
15. Shahid, Z.; Kalayanamitra, R.; Patel, R.; Groff, A.; Jain, R. Refractory Sweet Syndrome Treated with Anakinra. *Cureus* **2019**, *11*, e4536. [CrossRef]
16. Seminario-Vidal, L.; Guerrero, C.; Sami, N. Refractory Sweet's syndrome successfully treated with rituximab. *JAAD Case Rep.* **2015**, *1*, 123–125. [CrossRef]
17. Vitale, A.; Barneschi, S.; Mourabi, M.; Frediani, B.; Cantarini, L. Effectiveness of rituximab in bullous Sweet's syndrome. *Int. J. Dermatol.* **2022**, *61*, e485–e486. [CrossRef]
18. Brunsting, L.A.; Goeckerman, W.H.; O'Leary, P.A. Pyoderma (echthyma) gangrenosum: Clinical and experimental observations in five cases occurring in adults. *Arch. Dermatol.* **1982**, *118*, 743–768. [CrossRef]
19. Brocq, A. New contribution to the study of geometric phagedenism. *Ann Dermatol Syphiligr* **1916**, *9*, 1–39.

20. Ben Abdallah, H.; Bech, R.; Fogh, K.; Olesen, A.B.; Vestergaard, C. Comorbidities, mortality and survival in patients with pyoderma gangrenosum: A Danish nationwide registry-nested case-control study. *Br. J. Dermatol.* **2021**, *185*, 1169–1175. [CrossRef]
21. Ormerod, A.D. Epidemiology, comorbidities and mortality of pyoderma gangrenosum: New insights. *Br. J.Dermatol.* **2021**, *185*, 1089–1090. [CrossRef] [PubMed]
22. Braswell, S.F.; Kostopoulos, T.C.; Ortega-Loayza, A.G. Pathophysiology of pyoderma gangrenosum (PG): An updated review. *J. Am. Acad. Dermatol.* **2015**, *73*, 691–698. [CrossRef] [PubMed]
23. Ben Abdallah, H.; Fogh, K.; Bech, R. Pyoderma gangrenosum and tumour necrosis factor alpha inhibitors: A semi-systematic review. *Int. Wound J.* **2019**, *16*, 511–521. [CrossRef]
24. George, C.; Deroide, F.; Rustin, M. Pyoderma gangrenosum—A guide to diagnosis and management. *Clin. Med.* **2019**, *19*, 224–228. [CrossRef]
25. Schøsler, L.; Fogh, K.; Bech, R. Pyoderma Gangrenosum: A Retrospective Study of Clinical Charac-teristics, Comorbidities, Response to Treatment and Mortality Related to Prednisone Dose. *Acta Derm. Venereol.* **2021**, *101*, adv00431. [CrossRef] [PubMed]
26. Maronese, C.A.; Pimentel, M.A.; Li, M.M.; Genovese, G.; Ortega-Loayza, A.G.; Marzano, A.V. Pyoderma Gangrenosum: An Updated Literature Review on Established and Emerging Pharmacological Treatments. *Am. J. Clin. Dermatol.* **2022**, *23*, 615–634. [CrossRef]
27. Sadati, M.S.; Dastgheib, L.; Afaki, E. Recalcitrant cases of pyoderma gangrenosum, responding dramatically to systemic tacrolimus. *G. Ital. Di Dermatol. E'Venereol. OrganoUff. Soc. Ital. Di Dermatol. E Sifilogr.* **2017**, *152*, 308–310. [CrossRef]
28. Abu-Elmagd, K.; Jegasothy, B.V.; Ackerman, C.D.; Thomson, A.W.; Rilo, H.; Nikolaidis, N.; Van Thiel, D.; Fung, J.J.; Todo, S.; Starzl, T.E. Efficacy of FK 506 in the treatment of recalcitrant pyoderma gangrenosum. *Transpl. Proc.* **1991**, *23*, 3328–3329.
29. Brooklyn, T.N.; Dunnill, M.G.; Shetty, A.; Bowden, J.J.; Williams, J.D.; Griffiths, C.E.; Forbes, A.; Greenwood, R.; Probert, C.S. Infliximab for the treatment of pyoderma gangrenosum: A randomised, double blind, placebo controlled trial. *Gut* **2006**, *55*, 505–509. [CrossRef]
30. Juillerat, P.; Christen-Zäch, S.; Troillet, F.X.; Gallot-Lavallée, S.; Pannizzon, R.G.; Michetti, P. Infliximab for the treatment of disseminated pyoderma gangrenosum associated with ulcerative colitis. Case report and literature review. *Dermatology* **2007**, *215*, 245–251. [CrossRef]
31. Argüelles-Arias, F.; Castro-Laria, L.; Lobatón, T.; Aguas-Peris, M.; Rojas-Feria, M.; Barreiro-de Acosta, M.; Soto-Escribano, P.; Calvo-Moya, M.; Ginard-Vicens, D.; Chaparro-Sánchez, M.; et al. Characteristics and treatment of pyoderma gangrenosum in inflammatory bowel disease. *Dig. Dis. Sci.* **2013**, *58*, 2949–2954. [CrossRef]
32. Rousset, L.; de Masson, A.; Begon, E.; Villani, A.; Battistella, M.; Rybojad, M.; Jachiet, M.; Bagot, M.; Bouaziz, J.D.; Lepelletier, C. Tumor necrosis factor-α inhibitors for the treatment of pyoderma gangrenosum not associated with inflammatory bowel diseases: A multicenter retrospective study. *J. Am. Acad. Dermatol.* **2019**, *80*, 1141–1143. [CrossRef] [PubMed]
33. Campanati, A.; Brisigotti, V.; Ganzetti, G.; Molinelli, E.; Giuliodori, K.; Consales, V.; Racchini, S.; Bendia, E.; Offidani, A. Finally, recurrent pyoderma gangrenosum treated with Adalimumab: Case report and review of the literature. *J. Eur. Acad. Dermatol. Venereol.* **2015**, *29*, 1245–1247. [CrossRef] [PubMed]
34. Sagami, S.; Ueno, Y.; Tanaka, S.; Nagai, K.; Hayashi, R.; Chayama, K. Successful Use of Adalimumab for Treating Pyoderma Gangrenosum with Ulcerative Colitis under Corticosteroid-tapering Conditions. *Intern. Med.* **2015**, *54*, 2167–2172. [CrossRef] [PubMed]
35. Ohmura, S.I.; Homma, Y.; Hanai, S.; Otsuki, Y.; Miyamoto, T. Successful switching treatment of adalimumab for refractory pyoderma gangrenosum in a patient with rheumatoid arthritis with prior use of tumour necrosis factor inhibitors: A case report and review of the literature. *Mod. Rheumatol. Case Rep.* **2023**, *7*, 9–13. [CrossRef] [PubMed]
36. Hurabielle, C.; Schneider, P.; Baudry, C.; Bagot, M.; Allez, M.; Viguier, M. Certolizumab pegol—A new therapeutic option for refractory disseminated pyoderma gangrenosum associated with Crohn's disease. *J. Dermatolog. Treat.* **2016**, *27*, 67–69. [CrossRef] [PubMed]
37. Diotallevi, F.; Campanati, A.; Radi, G.; Brisigotti, V.; Molinelli, E.; Brancorsini, D.; Offidani, A. Pyoderma gangrenosum successfully treated with golimumab: Case report and review of the literature. *Dermatol. Ther.* **2019**, *32*, e12928. [CrossRef]
38. Herberger, K.; Dissemond, J.; Brüggestrat, S.; Sorbe, C.; Augustin, M. Biologics and immunoglobulins in the treatment of pyoderma gangrenosum—Analysis of 52 patients. *J. Dtsch. Dermatol. Ges.* **2019**, *17*, 32–41. [CrossRef]
39. Guenova, E.; Teske, A.; Fehrenbacher, B.; Hoerber, S.; Adamczyk, A.; Schaller, M.; Hoetzenecker, W.; Biedermann, T. Interleukin 23 expression in pyoderma gangrenosum and targeted therapy with ustekinumab. *Arch. Dermatol.* **2011**, *147*, 1203–1205. [CrossRef]
40. Goldminz, A.M. High-dose ustekinumab for the treatment of severe, recalcitrant pyoderma gangrenosum. *Dermatol. Ther.* **2016**, *29*, 482–483.
41. Nunes, G.; Patita, M.; Fernandes, V. Refractory Pyoderma Gangrenosum in a Patient with Crohn's Disease: Complete Response to Ustekinumab. *J. Crohn's Colitis* **2019**, *13*, 812–813. [CrossRef] [PubMed]
42. McPhie, M.L.; Kirchhof, M.G. Pyoderma gangrenosum treated with secukinumab: A case report. *SAGE Open Med. Case Rep.* **2020**, *8*, 2050313X20940430. [CrossRef] [PubMed]
43. Moreno García, M.; Madrid González, M.; Prada Lobato, J.M. Secukinumab for pyoderma gangrenosum: A case report. Secukinumab en pioderma gangrenoso: Descripción de un caso. *Med. Clin.* **2019**, *152*, 246. [CrossRef]

44. Kolios, A.G.; Maul, J.T.; Meier, B.; Kerl, K.; Traidl-Hoffmann, C.; Hertl, M.; Zillikens, D.; Röcken, M.; Ring, J.; Facchiano, A.; et al. Canakinumab in adults with steroid-refractory pyoderma gangrenosum. *Br. J. Dermatol.* **2015**, *173*, 1216–1223. [CrossRef] [PubMed]
45. O'Connor, C.; Gallagher, C.; Hollywood, A.; Paul, L.; O'Connell, M. Anakinra for recalcitrant pyoderma gangrenosum. *Clin. Exp. Dermatol.* **2021**, *46*, 1558–1560. [CrossRef] [PubMed]
46. Rousset, P.; Dugourd, P.M.; Lanteri, A.; Montaudié, H.; Passeron, T. Successful treatment of pyoderma gangrenosum associated with IgA gammopathy with the IL-1 receptor antagonist anakinra. *J. Eur. Acad. Dermatol. Venereol.* **2021**, *35*, e447–e450. [CrossRef] [PubMed]
47. Jennings, L.; Molloy, O.; Quinlan, C.; Kelly, G.; O'Kane, M. Treatment of pyoderma gangrenosum, acne, suppurative hidradenitis (PASH) with weight-based anakinra dosing in a Hepatitis B carrier. *Int. J. Dermatol.* **2017**, *56*, e128–e129. [CrossRef]
48. Brenner, M.; Ruzicka, T.; Plewig, G.; Thomas, P.; Herzer, P. Targeted treatment of pyoderma gangrenosum in PAPA (pyogenic arthritis, pyoderma gangrenosum and acne) syndrome with the recombinant human interleukin-1 receptor antagonist anakinra. *Br. J. Dermatol.* **2009**, *161*, 1199–1201. [CrossRef]
49. De Wet, J.; Jordaan, H.F.; Kannenberg, S.M.; Tod, B.; Glanzmann, B.; Visser, W.I. Pyoderma gangrenosum, acne, and suppurative hidradenitis syndrome in end-stage renal disease successfully treated with adalimumab. *Dermatol. Online J.* **2017**, *23*, 13030/qt82d4m2zw. [CrossRef]
50. Sood, A.K.; McShane, D.B.; Googe, P.B.; Wu, E.Y. Successfull treatment of PAPA syndrome with Dual adalimumab and tacrolimus therapy. *J. Clin. Immunol.* **2019**, *39*, 832–835. [CrossRef]
51. Arnold, D.D.; Yalamanoglu, A.; Boyman, O. Systematic Review of Safety and Efficacy of IL-1-Targeted Biologics in Treating Immune-Mediated Disorders. *Front Immunol.* **2022**, *13*, 888392. [CrossRef] [PubMed]
52. Hsiao, J.L.; Antaya, R.J.; Berger, T.; Maurer, T.; Shinkai, K.; Leslie, K.S. Hidradenitis suppurativa and concomitant pyoderma gangrenosum: A case series and literature review. *Arch. Dermatol.* **2010**, *146*, 1265–1270. [CrossRef] [PubMed]
53. De Risi-Pugliese, T.; Seksik, P.; Bouaziz, J.D.; Chasset, F.; Moguelet, P.; Gornet, J.M.; Bourrier, A.; Amiot, A.; Beaugerie, L.; Francès, C. Ustekinumab treatment for neutrophilic dermatoses associated with Crohn's disease: A multicenter retrospective study. *J. Am. Acad. Dermatol.* **2019**, *80*, 781–784. [CrossRef] [PubMed]
54. Tee, M.W.; Avarbock, A.B.; Ungar, J.; Frew, J.W. Rapid resolution of pyoderma gangrenosum with brodalumab therapy. *JAAD Case Rep.* **2020**, *6*, 1167–1169. [CrossRef]
55. Lee, W.S.; Choi, Y.J.; Yoo, W.H. Use of tocilizumab in a patient with pyoderma gangrenosum and rheumatoid arthritis. *J. Eur. Acad Dermatol. Venereol.* **2017**, *31*, e75–e77. [CrossRef]
56. Choong, D.J.; Ng, J.L.; Vinciullo, C. Pyoderma gangrenosum associated with Takayasu's arteritis in a young Caucasian woman and response to biologic therapy with tocilizumab. *JAAD Case Rep.* **2021**, *9*, 4–6. [CrossRef]
57. John, J.M.; Sinclair, R.D. Tildrakizumab for treatment of refractory pyoderma gangrenosum of the penis and polymyalgia rheumatica: Killing two birds with one stone. *Australas. J. Dermatol.* **2020**, *61*, 170–171. [CrossRef]
58. Leow, L.J.; Zubrzycki, N. Recalcitrant Ulcerative Pyoderma Gangrenosum of the Leg Responsive to Tildrakizumab: A Case Report. *Clin. Cosmet. Investig. Dermatol.* **2022**, *15*, 1729–1736. [CrossRef]
59. Kok, Y.; Nicolopoulos, J.; Varigos, G.; Howard, A.; Dolianitis, C. Tildrakizumab in the treatment of PASH syndrome: A potential novel therapeutic target. *Australas. J. Dermatol.* **2020**, *61*, e373–e374. [CrossRef]
60. Verneuil, A. Etudes sur les tumeurs de la peau; de quelques maladies des glandes sudoripares. *Arch. Gen. Med.* **1854**, *4*, 447–468.
61. Fimmel, S.; Zouboulis, C.C. Comorbidities of hidradenitis suppurativa (acne inversa). *Derm.-Endocrinol.* **2010**, *2*, 9–16. [CrossRef] [PubMed]
62. Goldburg, S.R.; Strober, B.E.; Payette, M.J. Hidradenitis suppurativa: Epidemiology, clinical presentation, and pathogenesis. *J. Am. Acad. Dermatol.* **2020**, *82*, 1045–1058. [CrossRef] [PubMed]
63. Martorell, A.; García-Martínez, F.J.; Jiménez-Gallo, D.; Pascual, J.C.; Pereyra-Rodriguez, J.; Salgado, L.; Vilarrasa, E. An Update on Hidradenitis Suppurativa (Part I): Epidemiology, Clinical Aspects, and Definition of Disease Severity. *Actas Dermosifiliogr.* **2015**, *106*, 703–715. [CrossRef] [PubMed]
64. Gulliver, W.; Zouboulis, C.C.; Prens, E.; Jemec, G.B.; Tzellos, T. Evidence-based approach to the treatment of hidradenitis suppurativa/acne inversa, based on the European guidelines for hidradenitis suppurativa. *Rev. Endocr. Metab. Disord.* **2016**, *17*, 343–351. [CrossRef]
65. Weber, I.; Giefer, J.; Martin, K.L. Effects of Exercise and Dietary Modifications on Hidradenitis Suppurativa: A Systematic Review. *Am. J. Clin. Dermatol.* **2023**, *24*, 343–357. [CrossRef]
66. Lewandowski, M.; Świerczewska, Z.; Barańska-Rybak, W. Hidradenitis suppurativa: A review of current treatment options. *Int. J. Dermatol.* **2022**, *61*, 1152–1164. [CrossRef]
67. Brocard, A.; Knol, A.C.; Khammari, A.; Dréno, B. Hidradenitis suppurativa and zinc: A new therapeutic approach. A pilot study. *Dermatology* **2007**, *214*, 325–327. [CrossRef]
68. Zouboulis, C.C.; Desai, N.; Emtestam, L.; Hunger, R.E.; Ioannides, D.; Juhász, I.; Lapins, J.; Matusiak, L.; Prens, E.P.; Revuz, J.; et al. European S1 guideline for the treatment of hidradenitis suppurativa/acne inversa. *J. Eur. Acad. Dermatol. Venereol.* **2015**, *29*, 619–644. [CrossRef]

69. Ingram, J.R.; Collier, F.; Brown, D.; Burton, T.; Burton, J.; Chin, M.F.; Desai, N.; Goodacre, T.E.E.; Piguet, V.; Pink, A.E.; et al. British Association of Dermatologists guidelines for the management of hidradenitis suppurativa (acne inversa) 2018. *Br. J. Dermatol.* **2019**, *180*, 1009–1017. [CrossRef]
70. Sánchez-Díaz, M.; Díaz-Calvillo, P.; Rodríguez-Pozo, J.Á.; Arias-Santiago, S.; Molina-Leyva, A. Effectiveness and Safety of Acitretin for the Treatment of Hidradenitis Suppurativa, Predictors of Clinical Response: A Cohort Study. *Dermatology* **2023**, *239*, 52–59. [CrossRef]
71. Kimball, A.B.; Okun, M.M.; Williams, D.A.; Gottlieb, A.B.; Papp, K.A.; Zouboulis, C.C.; Armstrong, A.W.; Kerdel, F.; Gold, M.H.; Forman, S.B.; et al. Two phase 3 trials of adalimumab for hidradenitis suppurativa. *N. Engl. J. Med.* **2016**, *375*, 422–434. [CrossRef] [PubMed]
72. Tzanetakou, V.; Kanni, T.; Giatrakou, S.; Katoulis, A.; Papadavid, E.; Netea, M.G.; Dinarello, C.A.; van der Meer, J.W.M.; Rigopoulos, D.; Giamarellos-Bourboulis, E.J. Safety and efficacy of anakinra in severe hidradenitis suppurativa a randomized clinical trial. *JAMA Dermatol.* **2016**, *152*, 52–59. [CrossRef] [PubMed]
73. Leslie, K.S.; Tripathi, S.V.; Nguyen, T.V.; Pauli, M.; Rosenblum, M.D. An open-label study of anakinra for the treatment of moderate to severe hidradenitis suppurativa. *J. Am. Acad. Dermatol.* **2014**, *70*, 243–251. [CrossRef] [PubMed]
74. Zouboulis, C.C.; Bechara, F.G.; Dickinson-Blok, J.L.; Gulliver, W.I.; Horváth, B.; Hughes, R.; Kimball, A.B.; Kirby, B.; Martorell, A.; Podda, M.; et al. Hidradenitis suppurativa/acne inversa: A practical framework for treatment optimization—Systematic review and recommendations from the HS ALLIANCE working group. *J. Eur. Acad. Dermatol. Venereol.* **2019**, *33*, 19–31. [CrossRef] [PubMed]
75. Blok, J.L.; Li, K.; Brodmerkel, C.; Horvátovich, P.; Jonkman, M.F.; Horváth, B. Ustekinumab in hidradenitis suppurativa: Clinical results and a search for potential biomarkers in serum. *Br. J. Dermatol.* **2016**, *174*, 839–846. [CrossRef]
76. Alikhan, A.; Sayed, C.; Alavi, A.; Alhusayen, R.; Brassard, A.; Burkhart, C.; Crowell, K.; Eisen, D.B.; Gottlieb, A.B.; Hamzavi, I.; et al. North American clinical management guidelines for hidradenitis suppurativa: A publication from the United States and Canadian Hidradenitis Suppurativa Foundations: Part II: Topical, intralesional, and systemic medical management. *J. Am. Acad. Dermatol.* **2019**, *81*, 91–101. [CrossRef]
77. Casseres, R.G.; Prussick, L.; Zancanaro, P.; Rothstein, B.; Joshipura, D.; Saraiya, A.; Turkowski, Y.; Au, S.C.; Alomran, A.; Abdat, R.; et al. Secukinumab in the treatment of moderate to severe hidradenitis suppurativa: Results of an open-label trial. *J. Am. Acad. Dermatol.* **2020**, *82*, 1524–1526. [CrossRef]
78. Kimball, A.B.; Jemec, G.B.E.; Alavi, A.; Reguiai, Z.; Gottlieb, A.B.; Bechara, F.G.; Paul, C.; Giamarellos Bourboulis, E.J.; Villani, A.P.; Schwinn, A. Secukinumab in moderate-to-severe hidradenitis suppurativa (SUNSHINE and SUNRISE): Week 16 and week 52 results of two identical, multicentre, randomised, placebo-controlled, double-blind phase 3 trials. *Lancet* **2023**, *401*, 747–761. [CrossRef]
79. Gupta, A.K.; Ellis, C.N.; Nickoloff, B.J.; Goldfarb, M.T.; Ho, V.C.; Rocher, L.L.; Griffiths, C.E.; Cooper, K.D.; Voorhees, J.J. Oral cyclosporine in the treatment of inflammatory and noninflammatory dermatoses: A clinical and immunopathologic analysis. *Arch. Dermatol.* **1990**, *126*, 339–350. [CrossRef]
80. Rose, R.F.; Goodfield, M.J.; Clark, S.M. Treatment of recalcitrant hidradenitis suppurativa with oral ciclosporin. *Clin. Exp. Dermatol.* **2006**, *31*, 154–155. [CrossRef]
81. Karagiannidis, I.; Nikolakis, G.; Zouboulis, C.C. Endocrinologic aspects of hidradenitis suppurativa. *Dermatol. Clin.* **2016**, *34*, 45–49. [CrossRef] [PubMed]
82. Alavi, A.; Lynde, C.; Alhusayen, R.; Bourcier, M.; Delorme, I.; George, R.; Gooderham, M.; Gulliver, W.; Kalia, S.; Marcoux, D.; et al. Approach to the management of patients with hidradenitis suppurativa: Consensus document. *J. Cutan. Med. Surg.* **2017**, *21*, 513–524. [CrossRef] [PubMed]
83. Joseph, M.A.; Jayaseelan, E.; Ganapathi, B.; Stephen, J. Hidradenitis suppurativa treated with finasteride. *J. Dermatolog. Treat.* **2005**, *16*, 75–78. [CrossRef]
84. Grimstad, Ø.; Kvammen, B.Ø.; Swartling, C. Botulinum toxin type B for hidradenitis suppurativa: A randomised, double-blind, placebo-controlled pilot study. *Am. J. Clin. Dermatol.* **2020**, *21*, 741–748. [CrossRef]
85. Choon, S.E.; Lai, N.M.; Mohammad, N.A.; Nanu, N.M.; Tey, K.E.; Chew, S.F. Clinical profile, morbidity, and outcome of adult-onset generalized pustular psoriasis: Analysis of 102 cases seen in a tertiary hospital in Johor, Malaysia. *Int. J. Dermatol.* **2014**, *53*, 676. [CrossRef] [PubMed]
86. Ciccarelli, F.; De Martinis, M.; Sirufo, M.M.; Ginaldi, L. Psoriasis induced by anti-tumor necrosis factor alpha agents: A comprehensive review of the literature. *Acta Dermatovenerol. Croat.* **2016**, *24*, 169–174.
87. Menter, A.; Van Voorhees, A.S.; Hsu, S. Pustular Psoriasis: A Narrative Review of Recent Developments in Pathophysiology and Therapeutic Options. *Dermatol. Ther.* **2021**, *11*, 1917–1929. [CrossRef]
88. Takeichi, T.; Akiyama, M. Generalized pustular psoriasis: Clinical management and update on autoinflammatory aspects. *Am. J. Clin. Dermatol.* **2020**, *21*, 227–236. [CrossRef]
89. Fujita, H.; Terui, T.; Hayama, K.; Akiyama, M.; Ikeda, S.; Mabuchi, T.; Ozawa, A.; Kanekura, T.; Kurosawa, M.; Komine, M.; et al. Japanese guidelines for the management and treatment of generalized pustular psoriasis: The new pathogenesis and treatment of GPP. *J. Dermatol.* **2018**, *45*, 1235. [CrossRef]
90. Kang, S.; Li, X.Y.; Voorhees, J.J. Pharmacology and molecular action of retinoids and vitamin D in skin. *J. Investig. Dermatol. Symp. Proc.* **1996**, *1*, 15–21.

91. Hong, S.B.; Kim, N.I. Generalized pustular psoriasis following withdrawal of short-term cyclosporin therapy for psoriatic arthritis. *J. Eur. Acad. Dermatol. Venereol.* **2005**, *19*, 522. [CrossRef]
92. Haustein, U.F.; Rytter, M. Methotrexate in psoriasis: 26 years' experience with low-dose long-term treatment. *J. Eur. Acad. Dermatol. Venereol.* **2000**, *14*, 382–388. [CrossRef]
93. Ji, Y.Z.; Geng, L.; Ma, X.H.; Wu, Y.; Zhou, H.B.; Li, B.; Xiao, T.; Chen, H.D. Severe generalized pustular psoriasis treated with mycophenolate mofetil. *J. Dermatol.* **2011**, *38*, 603–605. [CrossRef]
94. Imafuku, S.; Honma, M.; Okubo, Y.; Komine, M.; Ohtsuki, M.; Morita, A.; Seko, N.; Kawashima, N.; Ito, S.; Shima, T.; et al. Efficacy and safety of secukinumab in patients with generalized pustular psoriasis: A 52-week analysis from phase III openlabel multicenter Japanese study. *J. Dermatol.* **2016**, *43*, 1011–1017. [CrossRef] [PubMed]
95. Routhouska, S.B.; Sheth, P.B.; Korman, N.J. Long-term management of generalized pustular psoriasis with infliximab: Case series. *J. Cutan. Med. Surg.* **2008**, *12*, 184–188. [CrossRef] [PubMed]
96. Yamasaki, K.; Nakagawa, H.; Kubo, Y.; Ootaki, K. Japanese Brodalumab Study Group. Efficacy and safety of brodalumab in patients with generalized pustular psoriasis and psoriatic erythroderma: Results from a 52-week, open-label study. *Br. J. Dermatol.* **2017**, *176*, 741–751. [CrossRef] [PubMed]
97. Sano, S.; Kubo, H.; Morishima, H.; Goto, R.; Zheng, R.; Nakagawa, H. Guselkumab, a human interleukin-23 monoclonal antibody in Japanese patients with generalized pustular psoriasis and erythrodermic psoriasis: Efficacy and safety analyses of a 52-week, phase 3, multicenter, open-label study. *J. Dermatol.* **2018**, *45*, 529–539. [CrossRef]
98. Song, E.J. Generalized Pustular Psoriasis Treated with Risankizumab. *Cutis* **2023**, *111*, 96–98. [CrossRef]
99. Hüffmeier, U.; Wätzold, M.; Mohr, J.; Schön, M.P.; Mössner, R. Successful therapy with anakinra in a patient with generalized pustular psoriasis carrying IL36RN mutations. *Br. J. Dermatol.* **2014**, *170*, 202–204. [CrossRef]
100. Skendros, P.; Papagoras, C.; Lefaki, I.; Giatromanolaki, A.; Kotsianidis, I.; Speletas, M.; Bocly, V.; Theodorou, I.; Dalla, V.; Ritis, K. Successful response in a case of severe pustular psoriasis after interleukin-1beta inhibition. *Br. J. Dermatol.* **2017**, *176*, 212–215. [CrossRef]
101. Mansouri, B.; Richards, L.; Menter, A. Treatment of two patients with generalized pustular psoriasis with the interleukin-1β inhibitor gevokizumab. *Br. J. Dermatol.* **2015**, *173*, 239–241. [CrossRef] [PubMed]
102. Bachelez, H.; Choon, S.E.; Marrakchi, S.; Burden, A.D.; Tsai, T.F.; Morita, A.; Navarini, A.A.; Zheng, M.; Xu, J.; Turki, H.; et al. Trial of Spesolimab for Generalized Pustular Psoriasis. *N. Engl. J. Med.* **2021**, *385*, 2431. [CrossRef] [PubMed]
103. Esposito, M.; Mazzotta, A.; Casciello, C.; Chimenti, S. Etanercept at different dosages in the treatment of generalized pustular psoriasis: A case series. *Dermatology* **2008**, *216*, 355–360. [CrossRef] [PubMed]
104. Saeki, H.; Nakagawa, H.; Nakajo, K.; Ishii, T.; Morisaki, Y.; Aoki, T.; Cameron, G.S.; Osuntokun, O.O. Efficacy and safety of ixekizumab treatment for Japanese patients with moderate to severe plaque psoriasis, erythrodermic psoriasis and generalized pustular psoriasis: Results from a 52-week, open-label, phase 3 study (UNCOVER-J). *J. Dermatol.* **2017**, *44*, 355–362. [CrossRef]
105. Yamanaka, K.; Okubo, Y.; Yasuda, I.; Saito, N.; Messina, I.; Morita, A. Efficacy and safety of risankizumab in Japanese patients with generalized pustular psoriasis or erythrodermic psoriasis: Primary analysis and 180-week follow-up results from the phase 3, multicenter IMMspire study. *J. Dermatol.* **2023**, *50*, 195–202. [CrossRef]

International Journal of
Molecular Sciences

MDPI

Article

Comprehensive Physicochemical Characterization, In Vitro Membrane Permeation, and In Vitro Human Skin Cell Culture of a Novel TOPK Inhibitor, HI-TOPK-032

Basanth Babu Eedara [1], Bhagyashree Manivannan [1], Wafaa Alabsi [2,3], Bo Sun [2], Clara Curiel-Lewandrowski [4,5,6], Tianshun Zhang [7], Ann M. Bode [7] and Heidi M. Mansour [1,8,9,*]

1 Center for Translational Science, Florida International University, Port St. Lucie, FL 34987, USA; babubasanth@gmail.com (B.B.E.); bmanivan@fiu.edu (B.M.)
2 Skaggs Pharmaceutical Sciences Center, College of Pharmacy, The University of Arizona, Tucson, AZ 85721, USA; wafaaalabsi@arizona.edu (W.A.); bsun168@arizona.edu (B.S.)
3 Department of Chemistry and Biochemistry, The University of Arizona, Tucson, AZ 85721, USA
4 Skin Cancer Institute, The University of Arizona Cancer Center, Tucson, AZ 85724, USA; ccuriel@arizona.edu
5 University of Arizona Cancer Center, University of Arizona, Tucson, AZ 85724, USA
6 Department of Medicine, Division of Dermatology, College of Medicine, The University of Arizona, Tucson, AZ 85724, USA
7 The Hormel Institute, University of Minnesota, Austin, MN 55912, USA; zhan4145@umn.edu (T.Z.); bodex008@umn.edu (A.M.B.)
8 Department of Environmental Health Sciences, Robert Stempel College of Public Health and Social Work, Florida International University, Miami, FL 33199, USA
9 Department of Cell Biology & Pharmacology, Herbert Wertheim College of Medicine, Florida International University, Miami, FL 33199, USA
* Correspondence: hmansour@fiu.edu; Tel.: +1-(772)-345-4731

Citation: Eedara, B.B.; Manivannan, B.; Alabsi, W.; Sun, B.; Curiel-Lewandrowski, C.; Zhang, T.; Bode, A.M.; Mansour, H.M. Comprehensive Physicochemical Characterization, In Vitro Membrane Permeation, and In Vitro Human Skin Cell Culture of a Novel TOPK Inhibitor, HI-TOPK-032. *Int. J. Mol. Sci.* **2023**, *24*, 15515. https://doi.org/10.3390/ijms242115515

Academic Editors: Montserrat Fernández-Guarino, Asunción Ballester-Martinez and Andrés González-García

Received: 13 September 2023
Revised: 17 October 2023
Accepted: 19 October 2023
Published: 24 October 2023

Abstract: Nonmelanoma skin cancers (NMSC) are the most common skin cancers, and about 5.4 million people are diagnosed each year in the United States. A newly developed T-lymphokine-activated killer cell-originated protein kinase (TOPK) inhibitor, HI-TOPK-032, is effective in suppressing colon cancer cell growth, inducing the apoptosis of colon cancer cells and ultraviolet (UV) light-induced squamous cell carcinoma (SCC). This study aimed to investigate the physicochemical properties, permeation behavior, and cytotoxicity potential of HI-TOPK-032 prior to the development of a suitable topical formulation for targeted skin drug delivery. Techniques such as scanning electron microscopy (SEM), energy-dispersive X-ray (EDX) spectroscopy, differential scanning calorimetry (DSC), hot-stage microscopy (HSM), X-ray powder diffraction (XRPD), Karl Fisher (KF) coulometric titration, Raman spectrometry, confocal Raman microscopy (CRM), attenuated total reflectance-Fourier transform infrared spectroscopy (ATR-FTIR), and Fourier transform infrared microscopy were used to characterize HI-TOPK-032. The dose effect of HI-TOPK-032 on in vitro cell viability was evaluated using a 2D cell culture of the human skin keratinocyte cell line (HaCaT) and primary normal human epidermal keratinocytes (NHEKs). Transepithelial electrical resistance (TEER) at the air–liquid interface as a function of dose and time was measured on the HaCAT human skin cell line. The membrane permeation behavior of HI-TOPK-032 was tested using the Strat-M® synthetic biomimetic membrane with an in vitro Franz cell diffusion system. The physicochemical evaluation results confirmed the amorphous nature of the drug and the homogeneity of the sample with all characteristic chemical peaks. The in vitro cell viability assay results confirmed 100% cell viability up to 10 μM of HI-TOPK-032. Further, a rapid, specific, precise, and validated reverse phase-high performance liquid chromatography (RP-HPLC) method for the quantitative estimation of HI-TOPK-032 was developed. This is the first systematic and comprehensive characterization of HI-TOPK-032 and a report of these findings.

Keywords: NMSC; Strat-M; HaCaT cell line; NHEK cells; cell viability; TEER; air–liquid interface

1. Introduction

Skin cancer is the most common cancer in the United States (US) [1]. The American Academy of Dermatology estimates the diagnosis of about 9500 skin cancer cases in US every day [2]. Nonmelanoma skin cancers (NMSC), including basal cell carcinoma (BCC) and squamous cell carcinoma (SCC), are the most common skin cancers and are estimated to affect about 5.4 million people every year in the US [3]. Exposure to ultraviolet (UV) radiation from the sun is a major environmental carcinogen for approximately 98% of skin cancers.

TOPK (T-lymphokine-activated killer cell-originated protein kinase), a member of the mitogen-activated protein kinase (MAPK) protein family [4], is involved in many cellular functions, including tumor development, cell growth, apoptosis, and inflammation [5,6]. TOPK is highly expressed in many human cancers, such as leukemia, lymphoma, myeloma, breast cancer, and colorectal cancer [6–11]. Roh et al. [12] reported that acute UV irradiation increases the protein and phosphorylation levels of TOPK in human skin tissue. Thus, TOPK could be a promising molecular target for the prevention and control of UV-induced skin cancer [6].

At present, three TOPK-targeted and specific inhibitors have been developed as follows: HI-TOPK-032, OTS514/OTS964, and ADA-07 [13]. HI-TOPK-032 (N-(12-cyanoindolizino[2,3-b] quinoxalin-2-yl)-2-thiophenecarboxamide. Figure 1) directly inhibits TOPK activity in vitro and in vivo, and is effective in suppressing colon cancer cell growth and inducing the apoptosis of colon cancer cells [14]. Recently, Roh et al. [15] demonstrated that HI-TOPK-032 can suppress UV-induced SCC through the TOPK-c–Jun axis and its topical application can be used as a potential chemopreventive drug against SCC development.

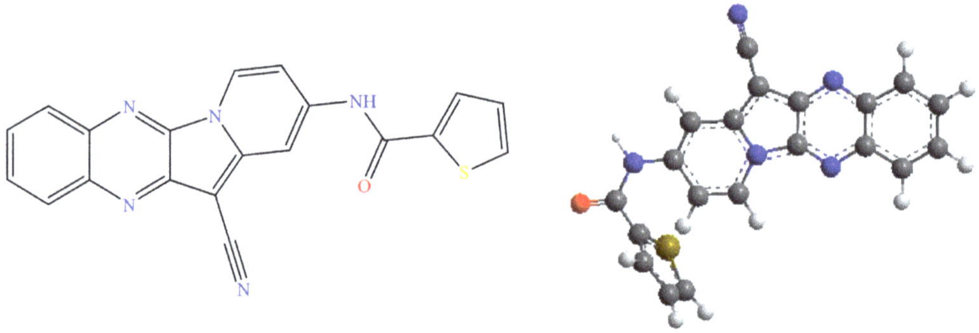

Figure 1. Chemical structures (drawn using Chem Draw® Ver. 21.0.0, CambridgeSoft, Cambridge, MA, USA) of HI-TOPK-032.

Prior to the development of various topical formulations of HI-TOPK-032, the comprehensive characterization of raw drugs to understand the physicochemical nature of the drug, permeation behavior, and cytotoxicity of this drug to human keratinocyte skin cells is necessary. The comprehensive physicochemical characterization of raw HI-TOPK-032 includes residual water content estimation using Karl Fisher coulometric titration (KFT), particle size and surface morphology using scanning electron microscopy (SEM), a solid-state nature using X-ray powder diffraction (XRPD) analysis, thermal behavior using differential scanning calorimetry, hot-stage microscopy, and molecular fingerprinting using Raman spectroscopy and attenuated total reflectance-Fourier transform infrared spectroscopy. The cytotoxicity potential of HI-TOPK-032 with increasing drug concentration (0.1 μM to 1000 μM) was evaluated using a 2D cell culture of the HaCaT human keratinocyte skin cell line. The permeation behavior of HI-TOPK-032 was determined using Strat-M® synthetic biomimetic membrane with a Franz cell diffusion system. Furthermore, a sensitive, reproducible, and reliable analytical method was required for the estimation of HI-TOPK-032 concentration. To the best of our knowledge, no chromatographic methods have been reported for the quantification of HI-TOPK-032. In this study, a rapid, specific, precise, and validated reverse phase-high performance liquid chromatographic (RP-HPLC) method for the quantitative estimation of HI-TOPK-032 is reported.

2. Results

2.1. Physicochemical Characterization

2.1.1. Scanning Electron Microscopy (SEM) and Energy-Dispersive X-ray (EDX) Spectroscopy

The SEM micrographs of HI-TOPK-032 (Figure 2A,B) showed irregular-shaped, aggregated particles with varying sizes and rough surfaces. The EDX spectrum (Figure 2C) of HI-TOPK-032 showed carbon (C), nitrogen (N), oxygen (O), and sulfur (S) elements along with platinum from the coating.

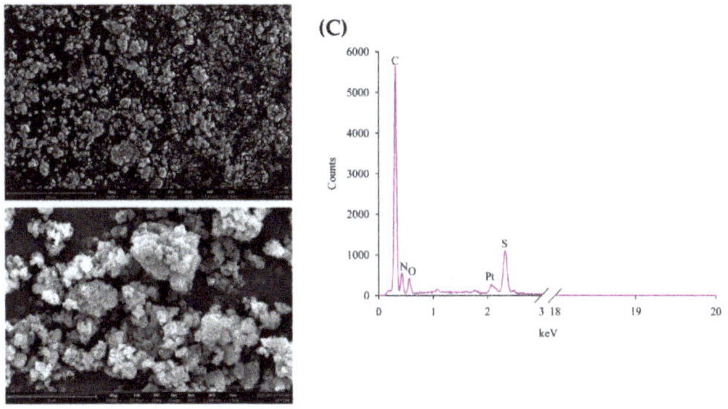

Figure 2. Representative scanning electron microscopic (SEM) images of raw HI-TOPK-032 at 2000× (**A**) and 20,000× (**B**) magnifications, and the energy-dispersive X-ray (EDX) spectrum (**C**) of raw HI-TOPK-032 showing characteristic elemental peaks.

2.1.2. Differential Scanning Calorimetry (DSC)

The raw HI-TOPK-032 DSC thermogram (Figure 3A) exhibited two endothermic peaks at ~145 °C and ~171 °C and a third exothermic peak at ~216 °C (Table 1). These observed peaks are a unique feature of raw HI-TOPK-032 red amorphous powder.

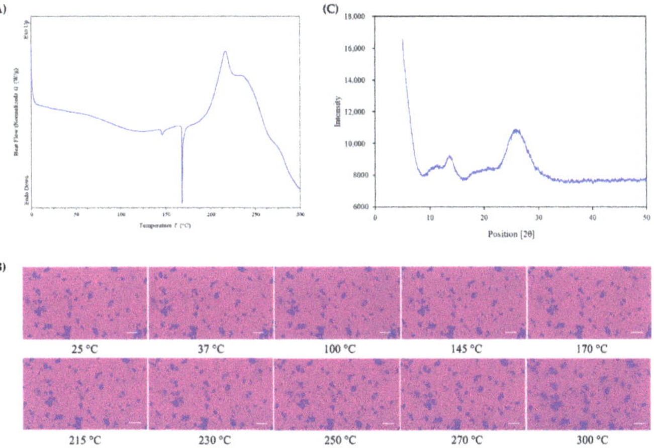

Figure 3. (**A**) Differential scanning calorimetry (DSC) thermogram of raw HI-TOPK-032 (n = 4); (**B**) Representative hot stage microscopy (HSM) images of raw HI-TOPK-032 (Scale bar = 50 µm, n = 3); (**C**) X-ray powder diffractograms (XRPD) of raw HI-TOPK-032 (n = 3).

Table 1. DSC thermal analysis data (n = 4, mean ± standard deviation).

Raw HI-TOPK-032				
Endotherm 1		Endotherm 2		Exotherm
T_{peak} (°C)	Enthalpy (J/g)	T_{peak} (°C)	Enthalpy (J/g)	T_{peak} (°C)
145.26 ± 3.4	0.3 ± 0.12	171.19 ± 3.41	1.26 ± 0.08	216.54 ± 0.95

2.1.3. Hot-Stage Microscopy (HSM)

As visualized by cross-polarized light microscopy, raw HI-TOPK-032 (Figure 3B) exhibited an absence of birefringence, indicating the amorphous nature of the drug. No visual changes or melting of the drug were observed upon heating up to 300 °C.

2.1.4. X-ray Powder Diffraction (XRPD)

The XRPD diffractogram of HI-TOPK-032 (Figure 3C) exhibited a typical halo with an absence of diffraction peaks, indicating the lack of long-range molecular order and the amorphous nature of the drug.

2.1.5. Karl Fisher (KF) Coulometric Titration

The residual water content of the raw HI-TOPK-032 was found to be 2.464 ± 0.235% (w/w) (n = 3, mean ± standard deviation). The low water content of the raw HI-TOPK-032 was consistent with the hydrophobic nature of the drug.

2.1.6. Raman Spectrometry and Confocal Raman Microscopy (CRM)

Characteristic peaks were identified using Raman spectrometry (Figure 4A) for raw HI-TOPK-032 and showed four prominent peaks (Figure 4B) representing 785.31 cm^{-1} (C-C functional group), 1638.61 cm^{-1} and 1677.49 cm^{-1} (>C=O mixed with NH deformation) and 2206.83 cm^{-1} (C≡C functional group). Raman microscopy mapping demonstrated the homogeneity of the sample (Figure 4C).

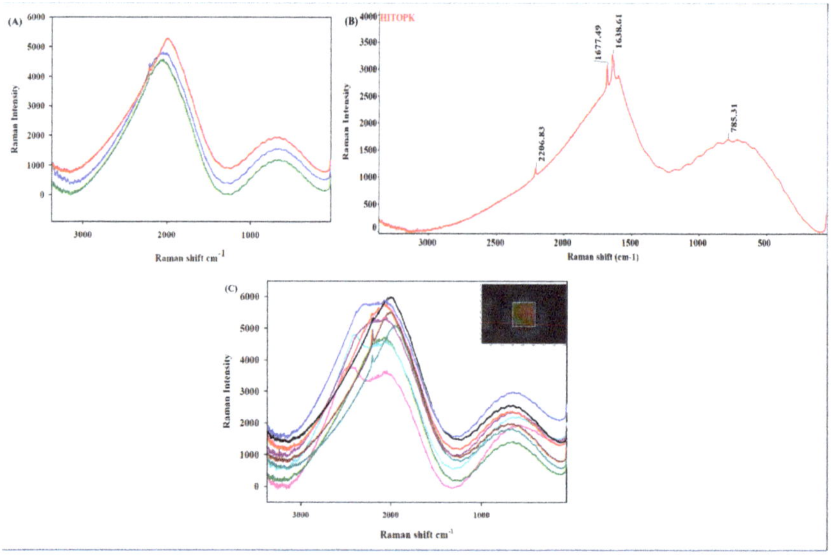

Figure 4. (**A**) Raman spectra (n = 3) of raw HI-TOPK-032 using 785 nm laser; (**B**) Representative HI-TOPK-032 Raman spectrum with peak values (n = 3); (**C**) Raman microscopy mapping of raw HI-TOPK-032 showing 9 spectra using 785 nm laser and Raman map (inset) with the area (white box) measured via the spectroscopic mapping method (n = 3).

2.1.7. Attenuated Total Reflectance-Fourier Transform Infrared Spectroscopy (ATR-FTIR) and Fourier Transform Infrared Microscopy

The ATR-FTIR spectrum (Figure 5A,B) of raw HI-TOPK-032 showed a prominent peak at 2203.82 cm^{-1} (C≡N functional group) with a consistent spectral pattern seen at the fingerprint region (<2000 cm^{-1}). The IR microscopy chemical map (Figure 5C) was consistent with the results obtained using FTIR spectrometry. Table 2 shows the important characteristic chemical peaks of HI-TOPK-032, which were identified via Raman spectrometry and FTIR spectrometry.

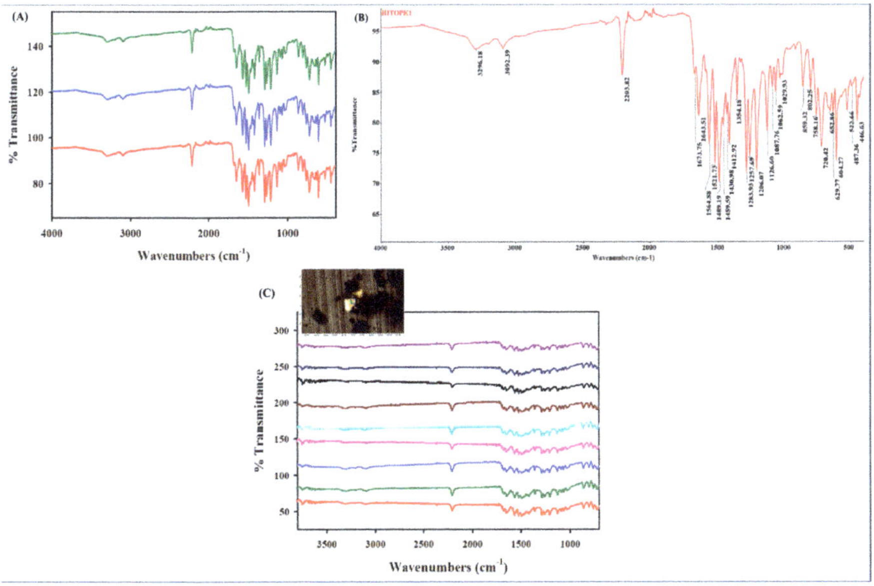

Figure 5. (**A**) ATR-FTIR spectrum of raw HI-TOPK-032 (n = 3; samples 1–3 represent spectra from three individual samples); (**B**) Representative HI-TOPK-032 FTIR spectrum with peak values (n = 3). (**C**) FTIR microscopy mapping of raw HI-TOPK-032 showing 9 spectra and an FTIR map (inset) with the approximate area (red box) measured by the spectroscopic mapping method (n = 3).

Table 2. Spectral peaks from Raman spectrometry and FTIR spectrometry of HI-TOPK-032 (n = 3).

Raman Spectrometry Peaks (cm^{-1})	FTIR Spectrometry Peak (cm^{-1})	
785.31	446.63	1257.69
1638.61	487.36	1283.93
1677.49	522.66	1354.18
2206.83	604.27	1412.92
	629.77	1430.98
	652.86	1459.59
	720.42	1489.19
	758.16	1521.73
	802.25	1564.88
	859.32	1643.51
	1029.93	1673.75
	1062.59	2203.82
	1087.76	3092.39
	1126.6	3296.18
	1206.07	

2.2. In Vitro 2D Cell Culture Dose–Response Assay with HaCaT and NHEK Cells

In vitro cell viability assays were conducted using HaCaT (Figure 6A) and NHEK cells (Figure 6B) with increasing HI-TOPK-032 concentrations and an exposure time of 48 h showed 100% viability at 0 μM (control), 0.1 μM, 1 μM, and 10 μM, and decreased viability with 100 μM (HaCaT- ≈27%; NHEK- ~39%) and 1000 μM (HaCaT- ≈8%; NHEK- ~6%) of the drug concentration, respectively.

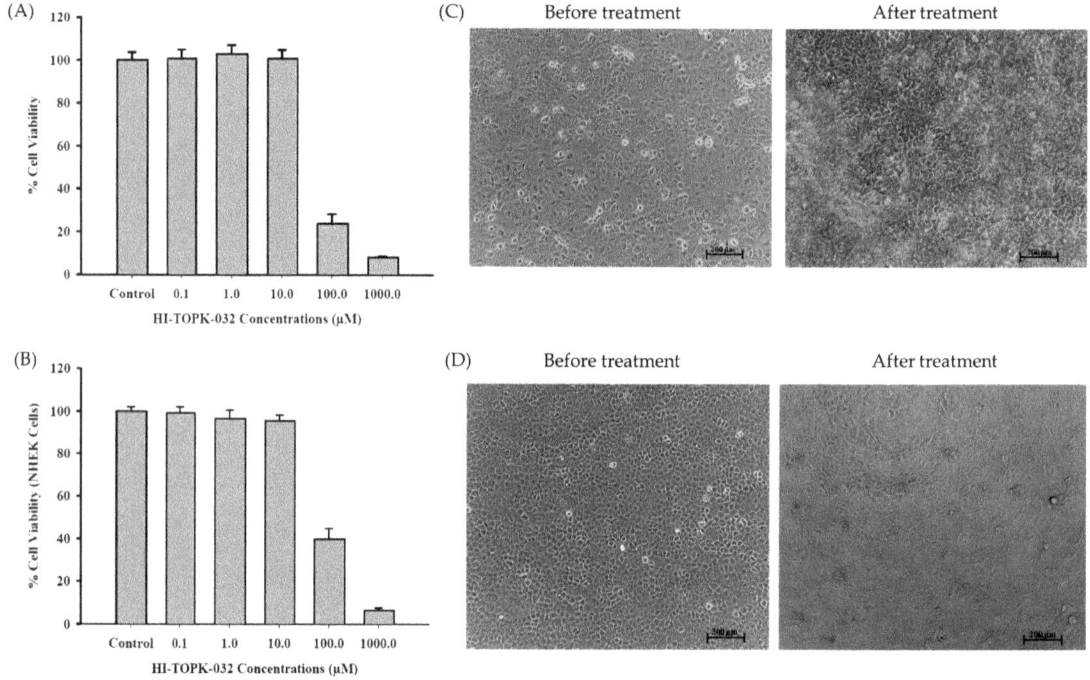

Figure 6. In vitro cell viability assay using (**A**) HaCaT cells (immortalized transformed human keratinocyte cell line) and (**B**) NHEK cells (normal human epidermal keratinocytes) and dose response with different concentrations of raw HI-TOPK-032 (n = 24 for each concentration). Representative images of the microscopic examination of HaCat (**C**) and NHEK (**D**) cell morphology before and after treatment with HI-TOPK-032.

HaCat cells were cultured (Figure 6C) in supplemented ADMEM (before treatment) and non-supplemented ADMEM (during HI-TOPK-032 treatments) with a simple microscopic observation showing a cuboidal and stratified shape with close packing from monolayer to multilayer at 48 h of exposure to the drug. Further visual inspection confirmed cell rounding, cytoplasmic vacuolation, and cell debris particles at concentrations of 100 μM and 1000 μM.

NHEK cells (Figure 6D) maintained in supplemented KGM (before treatment) and non-supplemented KGM (during HI-TOPK-032 treatments) upon microscopic observation showed a typical cobblestone-like morphology with proliferation to a multilayer morphology at 48 h of exposure time. Concentrations of 100 μM and 1000 μM showed observable cell rounding and floating cell debris using light microscopy.

2.3. In Vitro Transepithelial Electrical Resistance (TEER)

The in vitro TEER values recorded over a period of 7 days for the HaCaT immortalized and transformed keratinocyte cells, either naïve and treated with 100 μM of a raw HI-TOPK-032 concentration for 3 h, using ENDOHM-24G (Figure 7A) and ENOHM-6G (Figure 7B) chambers, indicating that treated cells (either HI-TOPK-032 or DMSO treated) recovered gradually over a period when compared to naïve cells.

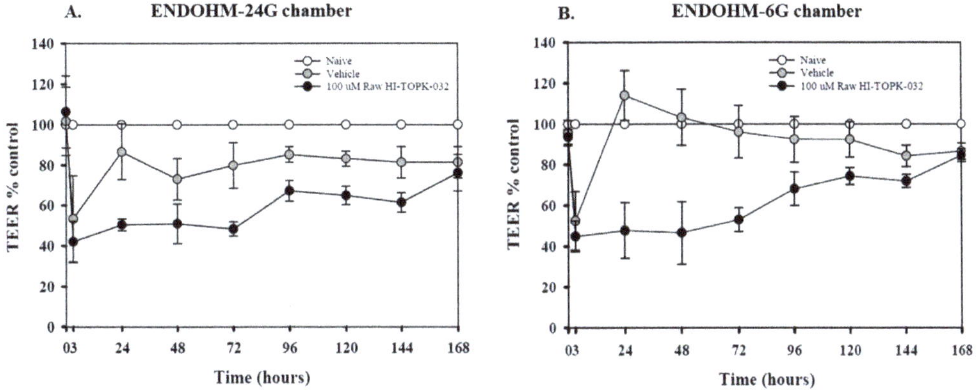

Figure 7. In vitro TEER values recorded using ENDOHM-24G (**A**) and ENDOHM-6G (**B**) chambers, of HaCaT cells at air–liquid interface (ALI) conditions exposed to 100 µM of a raw HI-TOPK-032 concentration for 3 h. TEER values were recorded before and after 3 h of HI-TOPK-032 exposure and subsequently at 24 h until 7 days. Data shown are the TEER values calculated as the percentage response of the control/naïve (non-treated) values using $n = 4$ replicates.

2.4. In Vitro Permeation of HI-TOPK-032 through Strat-M® Transdermal Diffusion Membrane

The in vitro permeation behavior of HI-TOPK-032 from a propylene glycol solution through the Strat-M transdermal diffusion membrane was evaluated using a Franz diffusion system. Figure 8 shows the increased permeation of HI-TOPK-032 over 6 h using the Strat-M membrane without any lag phase. At the end of 6 h, the permeation of HI-TOPK-032 was found to be 139.5 ± 12.4 µg/cm^2 with a steady state flux of 0.0241 ± 0.0023 µg/cm^2/h.

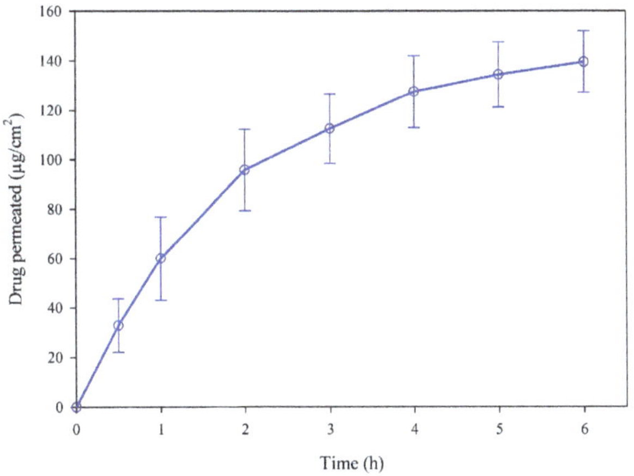

Figure 8. In vitro Franz-cell/Strat-M® permeation profile of HI-TOPK-032 ($n = 12$, mean ± standard deviation).

2.5. HPLC Method Development, Optimization, and Validation

Hi-TOPK-032 is hydrophobic and is almost insoluble in water and ethanol. It has a solubility of 4 mg/mL in DMSO. Thus, a primary stock solution of HI-TOPK-032 was prepared using DMSO. During analytical method development, the use of methanol or acetonitrile either alone with water or as a mobile phase resulted in an asymmetric peak with a >2 tailing factor. A combination of methanol and acetonitrile at 50:50 v/v with water produced a symmetric peak with a tailing factor of 1.3362. HI-TOPK-032 was eluted at a retention time of 4.373 min with a good peak shape and symmetry at a maximum wavelength of 205 nm, as depicted in Figure 9.

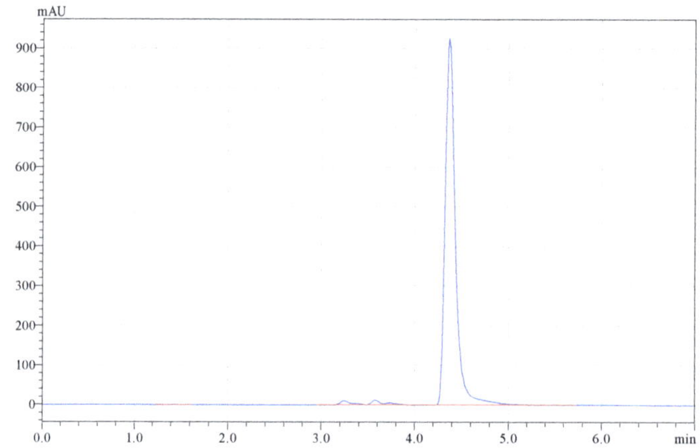

Figure 9. RP-HPLC chromatogram of HI-TOPK-032 (retention time = 4.3733 min) in a standard drug solution of 5 µg/mL.

2.5.1. System Suitability, Linearity and Sensitivity

The system's suitability parameters, such as peak retention time, area, height, the number of theoretical plates, and tailing factor, were determined by injecting six replicate injections of a standard HI-TOPK-032 solution of 5 µg/mL. The % CV of all the parameters was found to be within the acceptable limit of <2%, as shown in Table 3A. The developed analytical method was found to fulfill the requirements of system suitability.

Table 3. (A) System suitability parameters of the validated analytical method for HI-TOPK-032 (5 µg/mL). (B) Linearity and sensitivity results of HI-TOPK-032.

(A)					
	HI-TOPK-032 (5 µg/mL)				
	Retention Time (min)	**Peak Area**	**Peak Height (mAU)**	**Number of Theoretical Plates (USP)**	**Tailing Factor (10%)**
Mean	4.3733	6,892,319.33	927,983.83	7630.67	1.3362
S.D.	0.0005	9727.43	767.37	1.25	0.0004
%CV	0.0108	0.1411	0.0827	0.0163	0.0279

(B)	
	Mean ± S.D. (*n* = 6)
Slope	1,445,602 ± 7756
Intercept	114,432 ± 12,582
Correlation coefficient (r^2)	0.9993 ± 0.0002
LOD (µg/mL)	0.010
LOQ (µg/mL)	0.030

CV, coefficient of variation, LOD, limit of detection, LOQ, limit of quantification.

The standard calibration curves for HI-TOPK-032 were found to be linear in the concentration range of 0.5 to 8.0 μg/mL with a correlation coefficient (R^2) greater than 0.999 (Table 3B). Standard deviations of the slope and intercept for the calibration curves (n = 6) were 7756 and 12,582, respectively. The LOD and LOQ values were found to be 0.010 μg/mL and 0.030 μg/mL (Table 3B), respectively, indicating the high sensitivity of the developed analytical method.

2.5.2. Accuracy, Precision, and Recovery

The accuracy and precision values were calculated for the QC samples during intra- and inter-day runs, as shown in Table 4. The overall % recovery for the LQC, MQC, and HQC samples at intra- and inter-day runs was found in the range of 95–103%. The % of RSD and % of bias ranged between 0.05 and 2.90% and 1.02–4.88%, respectively, which were well within the acceptance criteria of <15%. These results indicate that the developed method represents the reliable analysis of HI-TOPK-032 in quality control laboratories.

Table 4. Intra- and inter-day accuracy and precision values at different concentration levels for the validated analytical method.

	Conc Level	Found Conc. (μg/mL)	% Recovery	% RSD	% Bias
Day 1	LQC (0.5 μg/mL)	0.511 ± 0.008	102.11 ± 1.61	1.58	−2.11
	MQC (5.0 μg/mL)	4.886 ± 0.002	97.72 ± 0.04	0.05	2.28
	HQC (8.0 μg/mL)	8.245 ± 0.027	103.06 ± 0.34	0.33	−3.06
Day 2	LQC (0.5 μg/mL)	0.482 ± 0.014	96.32 ± 2.79	2.90	3.68
	MQC (5.0 μg/mL)	5.171 ± 0.064	103.41 ± 1.28	1.24	−3.41
	HQC (8.0 μg/mL)	8.256 ± 0.097	103.20 ± 1.21	1.17	−3.20
Day 3	LQC (0.5 μg/mL)	0.476 ± 0.009	95.13 ± 1.79	1.88	4.88
	MQC (5.0 μg/mL)	4.949 ± 0.022	98.98 ± 0.44	0.45	1.02
	HQC (8.0 μg/mL)	7.676 ± 0.031	95.95 ± 0.38	0.40	4.05

2.5.3. Robustness, Carry-Over and Stability

To determine the robustness of the developed analytical method, the effect of the intended change in the mobile phase flow rate and oven temperature on peak retention time, peak area, the number of theoretical plates, tailing factor, and identified drug concentration were studied for the LQC, MQC, and HQC samples (Table 5). The slight variation (±5%) in the mobile phase flow rate and oven temperature showed a slight change in peak retention times (0.2 min with flow rate change and 0.01 min with oven temperature change) as expected. With the slight change in oven temperature and flow rate change, the tailing factor remained within acceptable limits (<2). The percentage of RSD values was found to be <2%. All the concentrations were identified with slight variation in the mobile phase flow rate, and over temperature were within the acceptable limits with a % bias <15%, indicating the robustness of the developed method.

No carry-over was found during the validation of the developed analytical method, indicating the suitability of the method for routine analysis.

The short-term stability of the drug solution under different storage conditions is shown in Table 6. The QC samples were stable when kept at bench top (~20 °C) in an auto-sampler (15 °C), refrigerator at 4 °C and freezer at −20 °C for 48 h. All the samples showed a percentage bias of <5% with the mean concentration after storage within the acceptable range of ±15% of the nominal concentration.

Table 5. Robustness of the validated analytical method.

Parameter	Conc. Level	Retention Time (min)		Peak Area		Number of Theoretical Plates (USP)		Tailing Factor (10%)		Found Conc. (μg/mL)		
		Mean ± S.D.	%RSD	Mean ± S.D.	%RSD	Mean ± S.D.	%RSD	Mean ± S.D.	%RSD	Mean ± S.D.	%RSD	%Bias
Change in mobile phase flow rate												
0.95 mL/min	LQC (0.5 μg/mL)	4.596 ± 0.002	0.052	831,928 ± 5673	0.682	8100.333 ± 48.016	0.593	1.313 ± 0.003	0.257	0.496 ± 0.004	0.791	−0.734
	MQC (5.0 μg/mL)	4.592 ± 0.002	0.053	8,067,694 ± 137,430	1.703	7792.778 ± 29.604	0.380	1.336 ± 0.002	0.1158	5.502 ± 0.095	1.728	10.034
	HQC (8.0 μg/mL)	4.592 ± 0.002	0.043	12,078,181 ± 96,746	0.801	7418.111 ± 46.620	0.628	1.344 ± 0.001	0.089	8.276 ± 0.067	0.809	3.450
1.00 mL/min	LQC (0.5 μg/mL)	4.373 ± 0.003	0.065	788,198 ± 5017	0.637	7819.111 ± 50.132	0.641	1.319 ± 0.004	0.334	0.466 ± 0.003	0.745	−6.784
	MQC (5.0 μg/mL)	4.369 ± 0.002	0.054	7,658,981 ± 131,529	1.717	7493.667 ± 67.180	0.896	1.342 ± 0.003	0.245	5.219 ± 0.091	1.743	4.379
	HQC (8.0 μg/mL)	4.369 ± 0.002	0.040	11,465,342 ± 108,979	0.951	7126.889 ± 53.813	0.755	1.353 ± 0.003	0.236	7.852 ± 0.075	0.960	−1.850
1.05 mL/min	LQC (0.5 μg/mL)	4.162 ± 0.003	0.063	756,240 ± 7580	1.002	7444.778 ± 41.593	0.559	1.327 ± 0.003	0.244	0.444 ± 0.005	1.181	−11.205
	MQC (5.0 μg/mL)	4.159 ± 0.003	0.061	7,307,762 ± 125,068	1.711	7227.000 ± 41.331	0.572	1.345 ± 0.003	0.216	4.976 ± 0.087	1.739	−0.480
	HQC (8.0 μg/mL)	4.159 ± 0.002	0.051	10,947,235 ± 92,631	0.846	6857.222 ± 56.790	0.828	1.352 ± 0.002	0.139	7.494 ± 0.064	0.855	−6.330
Change in oven temperature												
29 °C	LQC (0.5 μg/mL)	4.383 ± 0.003	0.070	792,882 ± 6295	0.794	7742.778 ± 47.316	0.611	1.319 ± 0.005	0.349	0.469 ± 0.004	0.928	−6.136
	MQC (5.0 μg/mL)	4.381 ± 0.002	0.054	7,674,089 ± 127,472	1.661	7469.333 ± 47.617	0.637	1.343 ± 0.003	0.201	5.229 ± 0.088	10.686	4.588
	HQC (8.0 μg/mL)	4.379 ± 0.002	0.043	11,492,951 ± 100,200	0.872	7102.222 ± 49.207	0.693	1.353 ± 0.002	0.181	7.871 ± 0.069	0.881	1.611
30 °C	LQC (0.5 μg/mL)	4.373 ± 0.003	0.065	788,198 ± 5017	0.637	7819.111 ± 50.132	0.641	1.319 ± 0.004	0.334	0.466 ± 0.003	0.745	−6.784
	MQC (5.0 μg/mL)	4.369 ± 0.002	0.054	7,658,981 ± 131,529	1.717	7493.667 ± 67.180	0.896	1.342 ± 0.003	0.245	5.219 ± 0.091	1.743	4.379
	HQC (8.0 μg/mL)	4.369 ± 0.002	0.040	11,465,342 ± 108,979	0.951	7126.889 ± 53.813	0.755	1.353 ± 0.003	0.236	7.852 ± 0.075	0.960	−1.850
31 °C	LQC (0.5 μg/mL)	4.360 ± 0.003	0.060	791,434 ± 8044	1.016	7789.333 ± 50.607	0.650	1.319 ± 0.004	0.331	0.468 ± 0.006	0.331	−6.336
	MQC (5.0 μg/mL)	4.357 ± 0.003	0.061	7,669,947 ± 126,954	1.655	7472.556 ± 65.934	0.882	1.342 ± 0.002	0.153	5.227 ± 0.088	1.680	4.531
	HQC (8.0 μg/mL)	4.356 ± 0.002	0.037	11,485,631 ± 95,252	0.829	7129.556 ± 44.199	0.620	1.351 ± 0.004	0.302	7.866 ± 0.066	0.838	−1.674

Table 6. Short-term stability of HI-TOPK-032 in quality control (QC) samples under different storage conditions (data are means, n = 3).

Condition		Conc Level	Found Conc. (µg/mL)	% Accuracy	% RSD	% Bias
Bench top	24 h	LQC (0.5 µg/mL)	0.496 ± 0.002	99.226 ± 0.438	0.442	0.774
		HQC (8.0 µg/mL)	8.286 ± 0.019	103.579 ± 0.243	0.235	−3.579
	48 h	LQC (0.5 µg/mL)	0.520 ± 0.001	103.903 ± 0.180	0.173	−3.903
		HQC (8.0 µg/mL)	7.812 ± 0.018	97.655 ± 0.227	0.233	2.345
Autosampler (15 °C)	24 h	LQC (0.5 µg/mL)	0.499 ± 0.002	99.705 ± 0.344	0.910	0.295
		HQC (8.0 µg/mL)	8.272 ± 0.075	103.397 ± 0.941	0.910	−3.397
	48 h	LQC (0.5 µg/mL)	0.517 ± 0.005	103.427 ± 0.960	0.928	−3.427
		HQC (8.0 µg/mL)	7.962 ± 0.023	99.521 ± 0.292	0.293	0.479
Refrigeration at 4 °C	24 h	LQC (0.5 µg/mL)	0.476 ± 0.004	95.190 ± 0.783	0.822	4.810
		HQC (8.0 µg/mL)	7.938 ± 0.218	99.228 ± 2.722	2.743	0.772
	48 h	LQC (0.5 µg/mL)	0.510 ± 0.004	101.980 ± 0.824	0.808	−1.980
		HQC (8.0 µg/mL)	7.745 ± 0.057	96.817 ± 0.708	0.732	3.183
Freezer at −20 °C	24 h	LQC (0.5 µg/mL)	0.491 ± 0.001	98.182 ± 0.122	0.124	1.818
		HQC (8.0 µg/mL)	8.151 ± 0.044	101.887 ± 0.548	0.538	−1.887
	48 h	LQC (0.5 µg/mL)	0.512 ± 0.009	102.401 ± 1.797	1.755	−2.401
		HQC (8.0 µg/mL)	7.883 ± 0.044	98.533 ± 0.547	0.555	1.467

3. Discussion

HI-TOPK-032 is a newly developed TOPK inhibitor, which is effective in suppressing colon cancer cell growth and inducing the apoptosis of colon cancer cells [14. Recently, HI-TOPK-032 has been shown to suppress UV-induced SCC [15]. A detailed physicochemical characterization and solid-state analysis of a new drug molecule is necessary to understand its properties prior to the development of a suitable formulation with optimum therapeutic efficacy. This manuscript reports for the first time a comprehensive physicochemical characterization of HI-TOPK-032, such as imaging via scanning electron microscopy with energy dispersive spectroscopy, X-ray powder diffraction analysis, thermal analysis, hot-stage microscopy, the residual water content estimation using KF titration, and molecular fingerprinting via spectroscopy. The X-ray diffractogram of HI-TOPK-032 indicates the amorphous nature of the drug in its supplied form without intense diffraction peaks. Further, the amorphous nature of HI-TOPK-032 was supported by the absence of crystalline birefringence in HSM. The DSC thermogram showed two solid phase transition peaks at ~145 °C and ~171 °C and an exothermic peak at ~216 °C indicative of a disorder-to-order solid-state first-order phase transition. The minimal residual water content of HI-TOPK-032 powder, which was confirmed from KFT, is consistent with the hydrophobic nature of the drug.

The cytotoxicity potential of HI-TOPK-032 was evaluated using a 2D human cell culture of HaCaT skin cells and NHEK cells. HaCaT cells are long-lived, immortalized human keratinocytes derived from adult trunk skin and have been widely used to study epidermal homeostasis and its pathophysiology [16]. HaCaT cells are a reproducible and reliable in vitro model for studies on epidermal architecture, inflammatory/repair responses, and skin metabolism [17–20]. Further, the p53 mutations of HaCaT cells are a distinctive feature of cutaneous SCC and are used as a model for analyzing skin cancer development. Primary keratinocytes, NHEK cells, which are isolated from an adult skin epidermis, have been widely used as a model for inflammatory skin diseases and skin responses to ultraviolet radiation or oxidative stress [17,21–23]. The in vitro cytotoxicity potential of HI-TOPK-032 (0–1000 µM) using human skin cells (2D cell culture) was successfully demonstrated, and the results show that the viability of HaCaT and NHEK cells remained high for up to 10 μM drug dose concentrations, which indicates that the drug may be safe to use at therapeutic doses. Both HaCaT and NHEK cell viability decreased significantly at a concentration > 100 μM for the drug dose concentration, indicating a dose-dependent effect on cell viability.

Strat-M® is a synthetic non-animal-based membrane model that mimics key structural and chemical features of human skin used for transdermal diffusion studies [24]. The tight top layer of the Strat-M membrane is coated with lipids simulating the lipid chemistry of the human stratum corneum (SC), and the lower porous layer simulates the epidermis and dermis layers of human skin [25]. The permeation behavior of HI-TOPK-032 from a propylene glycol solution using the Strat-M membrane was evaluated using the Franz cell diffusion system, and the results showed a linear increase without a lag phase. This demonstrates the necessity of suitable formulation development of HI-TOPK-032 for skin-targeted drug delivery with high drug retention for topical applications.

A simple, sensitive, isocratic reversed-phase HPLC method for the quantification of HI-TOPK-032 was developed and validated. This method was successfully used to evaluate the drug permeation behavior of HI-TOPK-032 through Strat-M® synthetic biomimetic membrane.

4. Materials and Methods

4.1. Materials

HI-TOPK-032 (N-(12-cyanoindolizino[2,3-b] quinoxalin-2-yl)-2-thiophenecarboxamide, $C_{20}H_{11}N_5OS$, molecular weight = 369.4 g/mol, red solid, >98% purity), as shown in Figure 1, was purchased from Bio-Techne Corporation (Minneapolis, MN, USA). Propylene glycol (PG, USP/FCC certified), HPLC-grade methanol, and acetonitrile were obtained from Fisher Scientific (Fair Lawn, NJ, USA). Dimethyl sulfoxide (DMSO, ≥99.5% (GC)), Tween® 80, and Hydranal®-Coulomat AD were obtained from Sigma-Aldrich (St. Louis, MO, USA). The Strat-M® membrane (47 mm), a synthetic, non-animal-based transdermal diffusion test model, was purchased from Millipore Sigma (Danvers, MA, USA).

Transformed keratinocytes from histologically normal human skin (HaCaT cells) were obtained from AddexBio® T0020001, San Diego, CA, USA. Advanced Dulbecco's Modified Eagle's Medium 1′ (ADMEM, Gibco®), Gibco® Collagen I, Rat Tail, Gibco® Fetal Bovine Serum (FBS), Gibco® Penicillin-Streptomycin (10,000 U/mL), Gibco® Amphotericin B (Fungizone), and 96-Well Black/Clear Bottom Plate and Falcon™ Tissue Culture T75 Flasks were obtained from Thermo Fisher Scientific™ (Thermo Fisher Scientific Inc., Miami, FL, USA). Resazurin sodium salt was purchased from Acros Organics (Thermo Fisher Scientific Inc., NJ, USA). In total, 12 mm of Snapwell® inserts (0.4 μm polyester membrane, 6-well plate) were obtained from Corning, Fisher Scientific, Suwanee, GA, USA). An ENDOHM-24G Chamber Cup (World Precision Instruments, Sarasota, FL, USA) was used to measure transepithelial electrical resistance (TEER).

Primary NHEKs (normal human epidermal keratinocytes) and the KGM™ Gold Keratinocyte Growth Medium BulletKit™ (Culture system containing KBM™ Gold™ Basal Medium and KGM™ Gold™ Single Quots™ supplements) were purchased from Lonza Walkersville Inc., MD, USA. Gibco® Collagen I (Rat Tail), 96-Well Black/Clear Bottom Plate, and Falcon™ Tissue Culture T75 Flasks were obtained from Thermo Fisher Scientific™ (Thermo Fisher Scientific Inc., Miami, FL, USA). Resazurin, sodium salt, was purchased from Acros Organics (Thermo Fisher Scientific Inc., NJ, USA) and Dimethyl Sulfoxide (DMSO) from Millipore-Sigma, St. Louis, MO, USA.

4.2. Physicochemical Characterization

4.2.1. Scanning Electron Microscopy (SEM) and Energy-Dispersive X-ray (EDX) Spectroscopy

The SEM and EDX data of raw HI-TOPK-032 were acquired with the Phenom ProX G6 (NanoScience Instruments, ThermoFisher Scientific, Phoenix, AZ, USA) following similar conditions reported previously [17,26]. The sample was mounted on an aluminum stub with a double-sided adhesive carbon tab (Ted Patella, Inc. Redding, CA, USA). The powder sample was coated with a platinum alloy (5 nm) using a Luxor platinum sputter coater (NanoScience Instruments, ThermoFisher Scientific, Phoenix, AZ, USA) under argon plasma (Airgas, Air Liquide, FL, USA). The SEM micrographs were captured using a Secondary Electron Detector (SED) at various magnifications at an accelerating voltage of 10 kV, a working distance of approximately 7 mm, and an intensity set on 'image' (Phenom ProX G6 software, NanoScience Instruments, Phoenix, AZ, USA)). The EDX spectrum of Hi-TOPK-032 powder was obtained at an accumulation voltage of 15 kV using a full Secondary Electron Detector at an 8000× *g* magnification.

4.2.2. Differential Scanning Calorimetry (DSC)

The thermal transitions of raw HI-TOPK-032 were determined using a Discovery Differential Scanning Calorimeter 250 with ultra-high purity (UHP) nitrogen gas (Airgas, Air Liquide, Palm Beach, FL, USA) with a flow rate of 50 mL/min and TRIOS v5.6.0.87 software for analysis (DSC250 with T-Zero® Technology (TA Instruments, New Castle, DE, USA). As described in previously published methods [27,28], briefly, 2–5 mg of the sample was packed into hermetic anodized aluminum T-Zero® DSC pan, and aluminum lids were hermetically sealed using a T-Zero® hermetic press (TA Instruments, New Castle, DE, USA). The reference pan was an empty, hermetically sealed T-Zero® aluminum pan. The raw HI-TOPK-032 samples were heated from 0 °C to 300 °C at a scanning rate of 5.00 °C/min. Experiments were performed in quadruplicate (n = 4).

4.2.3. Hot-Stage Microscopy (HSM)

Using similar conditions to those described previously, HSM of a raw HI-TOPK-032 powder sample was conducted. A microscopic glass slide containing a powder sample covered with a glass coverslip was placed on a Mettler FP82 hot stage (Columbus, OH, USA) attached to a Mettler FP 80 central processor heating unit and heated from 25.0 °C to 300.0 °C at a heating rate of 5.00 °C/min. Thermo-microscopic changes in the sample were observed under a cross-polarized light microscope (Leica DMLP, Wetzlar, Germany), and images were captured using a digital camera (Nikon Coolpix 8800, Nikon, Tokyo, Japan) under a 10× optical objective and 10× digital zoom.

4.2.4. X-ray Powder Diffraction (XRPD)

The crystallinity of raw HI-TOPK-032 powder was determined by X-ray powder diffraction (XRPD) analysis using similar conditions to those reported previously [17,26,28]. XRPD patterns of raw HI-TOPK-032 powder were recorded using a PANalytical X'pert diffractometer (PANalytical Inc., Westborough, MA, USA) equipped with a programmable incident beam slit and an X'celerator detector at room temperature. The powder sample was loaded onto a zero-background silicon sample holder as a thin layer and scanner over an angular range of 5.0 to 50.0° with a scanning rate of 2.00°/min using Ni-filtered Cu Kα (45 kV, 40 Ma, and λ = 1.5444 Å). All measurements were carried out in triplicate.

4.2.5. Karl Fisher (KF) Coulometric Titration

The residual water content of raw HI-TOPK-032 was analytically determined with Karl Fisher (KF) coulometric titration using similar conditions previously reported by the authors [29]. The measurements were carried out using a TitroLine® 7500 KF trace titrator (SI Analytics, Weilheim, Germany) coupled with a generator electrode TZ 1752 and a micro double platinum electrode KF 1150. Approximately 5 mg of the powder sample was added to the titration cell that contained the Hydranal™ Coulomat AD reagent (Honeywell Fluka™, Seelze, Germany). The residual water content of the sample was then accessed via endpoint titration. All samples were measured in triplicate.

4.2.6. Raman Spectrometry and Confocal Raman Microscopy (CRM)

Utilizing previously reported conditions [30–32], Raman acquisitions for molecular fingerprinting were obtained using a 785 nm laser of 30 mW in intensity in the DXR™ Raman system (Thermo Scientific™, Fitchburg, WI, USA) equipped with an Olympus BX41 confocal optical microscope with bright-field illumination (Olympus America, Inc., Chester Valley, PA, USA) and OMNIC™ for Dispersive Raman v9.12.1019 software. Briefly, each spectral point was acquired using 16 sample exposures each, with a detector exposure time of 4 s. A 50 μm confocal hole and 400 lines/mm grating were used. Spectra were baseline-corrected, and smoothing was performed prior to further analysis. All measurements were conducted in triplicate (n = 3).

Raman spectral maps were obtained using a 10× objective with 10 μm steps and 3 points each along the x and y axes to acquire 9 individual Raman acquisitions [33,34]. Each map point was acquired using 16 sample exposures with a 4 sec detector exposure time, 50 μm confocal hole, and 400 lines/mm grating. Baseline correction and smoothing were performed on the spectra prior to further analysis. These conditions have been described previously [35,36]. Mapping experiments were conducted in triplicate (n = 3).

4.2.7. Attenuated Total Reflectance-Fourier Transform Infrared Spectroscopy (ATR-FTIR) and Fourier Transform Infrared Microscopy

The ATR-FTIR spectroscopy was performed using the Nicolet™ iS50 FTIR spectrometer (Thermo Scientific™, USA) configured with a deuterated triglycine sulfate (DTGS) detector. Each spectrum was acquired with 32 scans at a spectral resolution of 8 cm^{-1} over the wavenumber range of 4000–400 cm^{-1}. The same experimental conditions were used to collect a background spectrum. Spectral data were obtained using the OMNIC v9.12.928 software. Baseline corrected and smoothed spectra were used for further analysis. The conditions used here have been reported previously [30,32,37].

FT-IR microscopy for chemical imaging and spectral mapping was performed using a Nicolet™ Continuum™ Infrared Microscope (Thermo Scientific™, USA) equipped with mercury–cadmium–telluride (MCT)/A detector, cooled by liquid nitrogen. Spectral maps were obtained with a 15× objective, step size 10 μm in the x and y direction, and the selected aperture was 100 × 100 μm. Nine individual acquisitions were acquired. Each spectrum was collected with 32 scans, an 8 cm^{-1} spectral resolution, and a wavelength number range of 4000–700 cm^{-1}. A background spectrum was collected under the same experimental conditions. Spectral data were acquired using the OMNIC v9.12.928 and the OMNIC Atlμs™ v9.12.990 software. Spectra were subjected to baseline correction and smoothening prior to further analysis.

4.3. *In Vitro 2D Cell Culture Dose–Response Assay with HaCaT Cells and NHEK Cells*

Following previously published growth conditions and methods [17,27,28,32,38], HaCaT cells (immortalized normal human keratinocyte cell line) were grown in collagen Type I-coated (concentration 5–10 μg/cm^2 in PBS) T-75 flasks using Advanced Dulbecco's Modified Eagle's Medium (ADMEM) 1× supplemented with 10% (v/v) FBS, 0.2% v/v Fungizone (0.5 μg/mL Amphotericin B, 0.41 μg/mL Sodium Deoxycholate), and 1% v/v Pen-Strep (100 Unit/mL Penicillin, 100 μg/mL Streptomycin) in a humidified incubator at 37 °C and a 5% CO_2 atmosphere. At 90% confluence, the HaCaT cells were seeded into a 96-well Black/Optical Bottom Plate at a density of 5000 cells/well in 100 μL of supplemented ADMEM, followed by incubation at 37 °C and 5% CO_2 for 48 h to allow the attachment of cells to the plate surface. After 48 h, cells were exposed to different HI-TOPK-032 concentrations. The HI-TOPK-032 solution was prepared by dissolving in 100% DMSO to produce an initial HI-TOPK-032 4 mg/mL concentration, which was diluted further with non-supplemented ADMEM. A 100 μL volume of the following drug concentrations was used: 0 μM (control), 0.1 μM, 1 μM, 10 μM, 100 μM, or 1000 μM was added to each well with 48 h exposure time and incubation at 37 °C and 5% CO_2. At the end of exposure time, the non-supplemented ADMEM with the drug was removed from each well and replaced with 100 μL of non-supplemented ADMEM containing 20 μL of 20 μM resazurin sodium salt dissolved in non-supplemented ADMEM followed by incubation for 4 h at 37 °C and 5% CO_2. At 4 h, the resorufin fluorescence intensity produced by viable cells was measured at 544 nm (excitation wavelength) and 590 nm (emission wavelength) using the BioTek Synergy H1 Microplate Reader equipped with Gen5 v2.09.2 software (BioTek Instruments Inc., Winooski, VT, USA). The relative % cell viability was calculated using Equation (1).

$$\text{Relative cell viability } (\%) = \frac{\text{Sample fluorescence intensity}}{\text{Control fluorescence intensity}} \times 100 \quad (1)$$

NHEKs were grown according to the manufacturer's instructions in a humidified incubator at 37 °C and 5% CO_2 in a collagen-coated T75 flask. After 90% confluence, 5000 cells/well were seeded in a 96-Well Black/Optical Bottom Plate in 100 μL of supplemented keratinocyte growth medium (KGM) and allowed 48 h for attachment to the plate surface in the humidified incubator at 37 °C and 5% CO_2. At 48 h, the cells were exposed to increasing concentrations of the raw HI-TOPK-032 drug. A 4 mg/mL raw HI-TOPK-032 stock was prepared in 100% DMSO and diluted further with non-supplemented KGM. The following drug concentrations: 0 μM (control), 0.1 μM, 1 μM, 10 μM, 100 μM, and 1000 μM were added to each well with 48 h exposure time in a humidified incubator at 37 °C and 5% CO_2 [17] as was conducted previously, to determine the dose-response of NHEKs (n = 24). After 48 h, the non-supplemented KGM with the drug was removed from each well and replaced by 100 μL non-supplemented KGM containing 20 μL of 20 μM resazurin sodium salt followed by 4 h humidified incubation at 37 °C and 5% CO_2. At 4 h, the resorufin fluorescence intensity produced by the viable cells was measured at 544 nm (excitation wavelength) and 590 nm (emission wavelength) using the BioTek Synergy H1 Microplate Reader with Gen5 v2.09.2 software (BioTek Instruments Inc., Winooski, VT, USA). The % relative cell viability was determined using Equation (1).

4.4. In Vitro Transepithelial Electrical Resistance (TEER) with Skin Epithelial Cells at Air-Liquid Interface (ALI)

TEER assesses the in vitro membrane barrier tightness and integrity of the cellular membrane by recording the blocked electrical signal through resistance measurements. TEER is an established marker of the tight junction function of cellular layers. HaCaT cells are nontumorigenic, immortalized keratinocytes from normal skin that exhibit normal morphogenesis. Using information from previously published methods [18,27,38], HaCaT cells were grown in supplemented Advanced Dulbecco's Modified Eagle's Medium (ADMEM), with 10% FBS, 1% Pen-Strep (100 U/mL penicillin, 100 μg/mL streptomycin), 0.2% Fungizone (0.5 μg/mL amphotericin B, 0.41 μg/mL sodium deoxycholate) and 1% GlutaMAX™ in a humidified incubator at 37 °C and 5% CO_2. After confluence, cells were seeded at ~400,000 cells per well in 12 mm Snapwell® inserts and ~50,000 cells per well in 6.5 mm Transwell® inserts (0.4 μm polyester membrane, 6-well plate and 24-well plate, Corning, Fisher Scientific, Suwanee, GA, USA) using supplemented ADMEM with appropriate volumes on the apical side and the basal side as per the manufacturer's guidelines. Supplemented ADMEM was changed every second day from the basal side. After a week, the cells appeared densely packed, forming a monolayer visible via light microscopy, and the transepithelial electrical resistance (TEER) values were measured using ENDOHM-24G and ENDOHM-6G Chamber Cups (World Precision Instruments, Sarasota, FL, USA). Under liquid-covered culture (LCC) conditions, when TEER values reached ~140 $\Omega \cdot cm^2$ for 12 mm inserts, and ~100 $\Omega \cdot cm^2$ for 6.5 mm inserts, media from the apical side were removed to facilitate air–liquid interface (ALI) conditions for 72 h. Under ALI conditions, TEER values were monitored when the value was stabilized at ~100 $\Omega \cdot cm^2$ for 12 mm (~70 $\Omega \cdot cm^2$ for 6.5 mm), the cells were exposed to 100 μM HI-TOPK-032 (4 mg/mL stock solution in DMSO) diluted using non-supplemented media. TEER values were recorded after 3 h of HI-TOPK-032 exposure with subsequent recordings every 24 h for up to 7 days using ENDOHM-24G and ENDOHM-6G Chamber Cups. TEER values for naïve- (non-treated) and vehicle (DMSO)- treated cells were also recorded simultaneously. TEER was recorded with 0.5 mL media added to each Snapwell® and Transwell® insert and immediately removed to return the cells to ALI conditions. SigmaPlot® v15 (SYSTAT Software, Inc., Palo Alto, CA, USA) was used to plot the TEER values between HI-TOPK-032-treated versus naïve (non-treated) HaCaT cells. All measurements were recorded from four separate cell inserts (n = 4 replicates). The plot represents data calculated as the percentage response of the control using Equation (2) [39]:

$$\text{TEER \% control} = \frac{\text{Sample TEER Value}}{\text{Control TEER Value}} \times 100\% \quad (2)$$

4.5. In Vitro Membrane Permeation of HI-TOPK-032

The in vitro permeation behavior of HI-TOPK-032 from a propylene glycol solution was determined using Franz diffusion cells (PermeGear, Inc., Hellertown, PA, USA), following similar conditions to those reported previously [17,28]. The Strat-M® membrane (Millipore Sigma, Danvers, MA, USA), a synthetic, non-animal-based transdermal diffusion test model membrane that is predictive of diffusion through human skin, was mounted between two O-rings with an orifice of 0.64 cm^2 and sandwiched between the donor and receptor chambers with a clamp. The receptor chamber was filled with 5 mL of freshly prepared phosphate-buffered saline (PBS, pH 7.4) containing Tween® 80 (5% w/v). Tween 80 was used as a solubilizer in the receptor medium to maintain sink conditions. The diffusion cells were maintained at 35 °C ± 0.05 °C using a precision reciprocal shaking bath model 25 (Thermo Fisher Scientific, Fair Lawn, NJ, USA) with 30 oscillations per minute. The HI-TOPK-032 solution was prepared by dissolving 1 mg of the drug in 0.4 mL of DMSO with the aid of sonication for 10 min followed by the addition of 0.6 mL propylene glycol. An aliquot of 200 µL of the drug solution was added to the donor compartment, and 200 µL samples were collected from the receptor chamber at 0.5, 1.0, 2.0, 3.0, 4.0, 5.0, and 6.0 h time intervals and replaced with an equal volume of the fresh medium. The samples were then analyzed using HPLC after appropriate dilution using methanol. The permeation experiments were conducted in triplicate. The cumulative amounts of drug permeated (µg/cm^2) were plotted as a function of time, and the flux at a steady state (J) was determined as the slope of linear regression analysis for the linear portion of the permeation curve [17,40].

4.6. High-Performance Liquid Chromatography (HPLC) Method Development, Optimization, and Validation

All HPLC runs were performed using a reverse-phase high-performance liquid chromatography (HPLC) LC 2050C 3D system (Shimadzu, Kyoto, Japan) equipped with the Luna® C_{18} silica column, 100 Å, 250 × 4.6 mm (Phenomenex, Torrance, CA, USA) maintained at 30 °C. This system was operated, and results were acquired and processed by LabSolutions software (Version 5.110) to control the instrument parameters.

Chromatographic analysis of HI-TOPK-032 was performed in the isocratic mode. The mobile phase consisted of 25:75 (% v/v) water and a mixture of methanol and acetonitrile (50:50 v/v), which was pumped at a flow rate of 1 mL/min. The sample injection volume was 10 µL, and the detection wavelength was 205 nm. The total run time was 7.5 min, and the total area of the peak was used for drug quantification. A mixture of methanol and acetonitrile (50:50 v/v) was used as a diluent.

4.6.1. Preparation of Calibration Standard and Quality Control (QC) Samples

A stock solution of HI-TOPK-032 was prepared by dissolving 1 mg of the accurately weighed drug in 0.4 mL of DMSO with the aid of sonication for 10 min, followed by dilution to 1 mL using a mixture of methanol/ acetonitrile (50:50 v/v) as a diluent. Standard solutions of HI-TOPK-032 with drug concentrations in the range of 5–80 µg/mL were prepared through the dilution of the stock solution with a diluent. An aliquot of 100 µL of the standard solution was transferred into microcentrifuge tubes (1.6 mL) and diluted to a final volume of 1 mL with the diluent to prepare calibration standards with drug concentrations of 0.5, 1, 2, 4, 6, and 8 μg/mL. Three QC samples were at concentrations of 0.5, 5, and 8 μg/mL representing the low, medium, and high concentrations, respectively.

4.6.2. Assay Validation

Assay validation was carried out according to the International Conference on Harmonization (ICH) guidelines [41].

4.6.3. System Suitability, Linearity and Sensitivity

The system's suitability was evaluated using six replicate injections of standard solution at 5 μg/mL of HI-TOPK-032. The percentage coefficient of variation (%CV) for the peak retention time, peak area, peak height, the number of theoretical plates, and tailing factor was determined with an acceptance criterion of ±2%.

The linearity was determined by the construction of calibration curves using the calibration standards in triplicate. Linearity was evaluated by linear regression analysis and calculated by the least square regression method.

The sensitivity of the developed analytical method was determined by estimating the limit of detection (LOD) and limit of quantification (LOQ) from the signal-to-noise ratio. The LOD indicates the lowest concentration level, resulting in a peak area of three times the baseline noise. The LOQ indicates the lowest concentration level that provides a peak area with a signal-to-noise ratio higher than 10, with precision (% CV) and accuracy (% bias) within ± 10%. LOD and LOQ were calculated using Equations (3) and (4):

$$LOD = \frac{3.3\sigma}{S} \tag{3}$$

$$LOQ = \frac{10\sigma}{S} \tag{4}$$

where σ is the standard deviation of the peak response at the lowest concentration of a regression line and S is the slope of the calibration curve.

4.6.4. Accuracy, Precision and Recovery

Intra-day and inter-day precision (as relative standard deviation, RSD), accuracy (as concentration bias (%)), and recovery (%) were determined using an assay of 6 replicates of QC samples on 3 different days. The RSDs for intra-day precision were calculated using the mean values of 6 replicates at each concentration for a single day, and inter-day RSDs were calculated from the mean value of 18 determinations on 3 different days. The bias (%) was calculated as 100 × (nominal concentration − measured concentration)/nominal concentration). Recovery was determined through a comparison of the measured concentration to the nominal concentration (0.5, 5, and 10 μg/mL of QC samples).

4.6.5. Robustness, Carry-Over and Stability

The robustness of the developed analytical method was evaluated by injecting QC samples with a deliberate variation of ±5% units of the mobile phase flow rate (1 mL/min) and the column temperature (30 °C). The effect of variation on the peak areas, retention times, found drug concentrations, the number of theoretical plates, and tailing factor were evaluated.

Carry-over was determined through the injection of a diluent directly following a high QC sample run.

The short-term stability of the drug solution was tested by an analysis of triplicate low and high QC samples during storage for 24 h and 48 h under the following conditions: on the bench at an ambient temperature (~20 °C); in autosampler vials at 15 °C; in a refrigerator at 4 °C; in a freezer at −20 °C.

4.7. Statistical Analysis

Data (mean ± standard deviation (SD)) were subjected to one-way analysis of variance (ANOVA) and Student–Newman–Keuls post hoc testing using Sigma Plot® version 15.0 (Systat Software Inc., San Jose, CA, USA). A probability level of 5% ($p \leq 0.05$) was considered statistically significant.

5. Conclusions

In conclusion, this systematic and comprehensive study reports a complete physicochemical characterization of a new TOPK inhibitor, HI-TOPK-032, for the first time. The physicochemical evaluation results confirmed the amorphous nature of the drug and the homogeneity of the sample with all characteristic chemical peaks. The in vitro cell viability assay results confirmed 100% cell viability for up to 10 µM of HI-TOPK-032, demonstrating biocompatibility as a function of drug dose. An isocratic reversed-phase HPLC assay with a photodiode array detector for the quantification of HI-TOPK-032 was developed and validated. This method is simple, accurate, and precise without the use of an internal standard. This method was used to evaluate the drug permeation behavior of HI-TOPK-032 using the Strat-M® synthetic biomimetic membrane.

Author Contributions: Conceptualization, C.C.-L., A.M.B. and H.M.M.; methodology, B.B.E., B.M., W.A., B.S., C.C.-L., T.Z., A.M.B. and H.M.M.; formal analysis, B.B.E., B.M., W.A., B.S., C.C.-L., A.M.B. and H.M.M.; resources, C.C.-L., A.M.B. and H.M.M.; writing—original draft preparation, B.B.E., B.M., W.A., B.S. and H.M.M.; writing—review and editing, B.B.E., B.M., W.A., B.S., C.C.-L., T.Z., A.M.B. and H.M.M.; project administration, C.C.-L., A.M.B. and H.M.M.; funding acquisition, C.C.-L., A.M.B. and H.M.M.; supervision, C.C.-L., A.M.B. and H.M.M. All authors have read and agreed to the published version of the manuscript.

Funding: This work was supported by a federal grant award NIH NCI P01CA229112.

Institutional Review Board Statement: Not applicable.

Informed Consent Statement: Not applicable.

Data Availability Statement: The data presented in this study are available on request from the corresponding author.

Acknowledgments: The authors thank the X-ray Diffraction Facility of the Department of Chemistry and Biochemistry at The University of Arizona. The authors sincerely thank Andrei Astachkine for the core facility access and assistance.

Conflicts of Interest: The authors declare no conflict of interest.

References

1. Guy, G.P., Jr.; Machlin, S.R.; Ekwueme, D.U.; Yabroff, K.R. Prevalence and costs of skin cancer treatment in the U.S., 2002–2006 and 2007–2011. *Am. J. Prev. Med.* **2015**, *48*, 183–187. [CrossRef] [PubMed]
2. Skin Cancer: American Academy of Dermatology. Updated 22 April 2022. Available online: https://www.aad.org/media/stats-skin-cancer (accessed on 1 June 2023).
3. Basal and Squamous Cell Skin Cancer: American Cancer Society. Updated 12 January 2023. Available online: https://www.cancer.org/cancer/basal-and-squamous-cell-skin-cancer/about/key-statistics.html (accessed on 1 June 2023).
4. Abe, Y.; Matsumoto, S.; Kito, K.; Ueda, N. Cloning and Expression of a Novel MAPKK-like Protein Kinase, Lymphokine-activated Killer T-cell-originated Protein Kinase, Specifically Expressed in the Testis and Activated Lymphoid Cells. *J. Biol. Chem.* **2000**, *275*, 21525–21531. [CrossRef] [PubMed]
5. Hu, Q.-F.; Gao, T.-T.; Shi, Y.-J.; Lei, Q.; Liu, Z.-H.; Feng, Q.; Chen, Z.-J.; Yu, L.-T. Design, synthesis and biological evaluation of novel 1-phenyl phenanthridin-6(5H)-one derivatives as anti-tumor agents targeting TOPK. *Eur. J. Med. Chem.* **2019**, *162*, 407–422. [CrossRef]
6. Zykova, T.A.; Zhu, F.; Vakorina, T.I.; Zhang, J.; Higgins, L.A.; Urusova, D.V.; Bode, A.M.; Dong, Z. T-LAK Cell-originated Protein Kinase (TOPK) Phosphorylation of Prx1 at Ser-32 Prevents UVB-induced Apoptosis in RPMI7951 Melanoma Cells through the Regulation of Prx1 Peroxidase Activity*[S]. *J. Biol. Chem.* **2010**, *285*, 29138–29146. [CrossRef]
7. Nandi, A.; Tidwell, M.; Karp, J.; Rapoport, A.P. Protein expression of PDZ-binding kinase is up-regulated in hematologic malignancies and strongly down-regulated during terminal differentiation of HL-60 leukemic cells. *Blood Cells Mol. Dis.* **2004**, *32*, 240–245. [CrossRef] [PubMed]

8. Simons-Evelyn, M.; Bailey-Dell, K.; Toretsky, J.A.; Ross, D.D.; Fenton, R.; Kalvakolanu, D.; Rapoport, A.P. PBK/TOPK Is a Novel Mitotic Kinase Which Is Upregulated in Burkitt's Lymphoma and Other Highly Proliferative Malignant Cells. *Blood Cells Mol. Dis.* **2001**, *27*, 825–829. [CrossRef]
9. Côté, S.; Simard, C.; Lemieux, R. Regulation of growth-related genes by interleukin-6 in murine myeloma cells. *Cytokine* **2002**, *20*, 113–120. [CrossRef]
10. Park, J.H.; Lin, M.L.; Nishidate, T.; Nakamura, Y.; Katagiri, T. PDZ-binding kinase/T-LAK cell-originated protein kinase, a putative cancer/testis antigen with an oncogenic activity in breast cancer. *Cancer Res.* **2006**, *66*, 9186–9195. [CrossRef]
11. Zhu, F.; Zykova, T.A.; Kang, B.S.; Wang, Z.; Ebeling, M.C.; Abe, Y.; Ma, W.; Bode, A.M.; Dong, Z. Bidirectional Signals Transduced by TOPK-ERK Interaction Increase Tumorigenesis of HCT116 Colorectal Cancer Cells. *Gastroenterology* **2007**, *133*, 219–231. [CrossRef]
12. Roh, E.; Lee, M.H.; Zykova, T.A.; Zhu, F.; Nadas, J.; Kim, H.G.; Bae, K.B.; Li, Y.; Cho, Y.Y.; Curiel-Lewandrowski, C.; et al. Targeting PRPK and TOPK for skin cancer prevention and therapy. *Oncogene* **2018**, *37*, 5633–5647. [CrossRef]
13. Herbert, K.J.; Ashton, T.M.; Prevo, R.; Pirovano, G.; Higgins, G.S. T-LAK cell-originated protein kinase (TOPK): An emerging target for cancer-specific therapeutics. *Cell Death Dis.* **2018**, *9*, 1089. [CrossRef] [PubMed]
14. Kim, D.J.; Li, Y.; Reddy, K.; Lee, M.-H.; Kim, M.O.; Cho, Y.-Y.; Lee, S.-Y.; Kim, J.-E.; Bode, A.M.; Dong, Z. Novel TOPK Inhibitor HI-TOPK-032 Effectively Suppresses Colon Cancer Growth. *Cancer Res.* **2012**, *72*, 3060–3068. [CrossRef]
15. Roh, E.; Han, Y.; Reddy, K.; Zykova, T.A.; Lee, M.H.; Yao, K.; Bai, R.; Curiel-Lewandrowski, C.; Dong, Z. Suppression of the solar ultraviolet-induced skin carcinogenesis by TOPK inhibitor HI-TOPK-032. *Oncogene* **2020**, *39*, 4170–4182. [CrossRef] [PubMed]
16. Seo, M.D.; Kang, T.J.; Lee, C.H.; Lee, A.Y.; Noh, M. HaCaT Keratinocytes and Primary Epidermal Keratinocytes Have Different Transcriptional Profiles of Cornified Envelope-Associated Genes to T Helper Cell Cytokines. *Biomol. Ther.* **2012**, *20*, 171–176. [CrossRef]
17. Ruiz, V.H.; Encinas-Basurto, D.; Sun, B.; Eedara, B.B.; Dickinson, S.E.; Wondrak, G.T.; Chow, H.-H.S.; Curiel-Lewandrowski, C.; Mansour, H.M. Design, Physicochemical Characterization, and In Vitro Permeation of Innovative Resatorvid Topical Formulations for Targeted Skin Drug Delivery. *Pharmaceutics* **2022**, *14*, 700. [CrossRef]
18. Colombo, I.; Sangiovanni, E.; Maggio, R.; Mattozzi, C.; Zava, S.; Corbett, Y.; Fumagalli, M.; Carlino, C.; Corsetto, P.A.; Scaccabarozzi, D.; et al. HaCaT cells as a reliable in vitro differentiation model to dissect the inflammatory/repair response of human keratinocytes. *Mediat. Inflamm.* **2017**, *2017*, 7435621. [CrossRef] [PubMed]
19. Schürer, N.; Köhne, A.; Schliep, V.; Barlag, K.; Goerz, G. Lipid composition and synthesis of HaCaT cells, an immortalized human keratinocyte line, in comparison with normal human adult keratinocytes. *Exp. Dermatol.* **1993**, *2*, 179–185. [CrossRef]
20. Zhang, N.; Liang, H.; Farese, R.V.; Li, J.; Musi, N.; Hussey, S.E. Pharmacological TLR4 inhibition protects against acute and chronic fat-induced insulin resistance in rats. *PLoS ONE* **2015**, *10*, e0132575. [CrossRef]
21. Dazard, J.-E.; Gal, H.; Amariglio, N.; Rechavi, G.; Domany, E.; Givol, D. Genome-wide comparison of human keratinocyte and squamous cell carcinoma responses to UVB irradiation: Implications for skin and epithelial cancer. *Oncogene* **2003**, *22*, 2993–3006. [CrossRef]
22. Liu, L.; Xie, H.; Chen, X.; Shi, W.; Xiao, X.; Lei, D.; Li, J. Differential response of normal human epidermal keratinocytes and HaCaT cells to hydrogen peroxide-induced oxidative stress. *Clin. Exp. Dermatol.* **2012**, *37*, 772–780. [CrossRef]
23. Meephansan, J.; Tsuda, H.; Komine, M.; Tominaga, S.-i.; Ohtsuki, M. Regulation of IL-33 expression by IFN-γ and tumor necrosis factor-α in normal human epidermal keratinocytes. *J. Investig. Dermatol.* **2012**, *132*, 2593–2600. [CrossRef] [PubMed]
24. Arce, F.J.; Asano, N.; See, G.L.; Itakura, S.; Todo, H.; Sugibayashi, K. Usefulness of Artificial Membrane, Strat-M®, in the Assessment of Drug Permeation from Complex Vehicles in Finite Dose Conditions. *Pharmaceutics* **2020**, *12*, 173. [CrossRef] [PubMed]
25. Haq, A.; Goodyear, B.; Ameen, D.; Joshi, V.; Michniak-Kohn, B. Strat-M® synthetic membrane: Permeability comparison to human cadaver skin. *Int. J. Pharm.* **2018**, *547*, 432–437. [CrossRef]
26. Muralidharan, P.; Hayes, D.; Fineman, J.R.; Black, S.M.; Mansour, H.M. Advanced Microparticulate/Nanoparticulate Respirable Dry Powders of a Selective RhoA/Rho Kinase (Rock) Inhibitor for Targeted Pulmonary Inhalation Aerosol Delivery. *Pharmaceutics* **2021**, *13*, 2188. [CrossRef] [PubMed]
27. Acosta, M.F.; Muralidharan, P.; Grijalva, C.L.; Abrahamson, M.D.; Hayes, D., Jr.; Fineman, J.R.; Black, S.M.; Mansour, H.M. Advanced therapeutic inhalation aerosols of a Nrf2 activator and RhoA/Rho kinase (ROCK) inhibitor for targeted pulmonary drug delivery in pulmonary hypertension: Design, characterization, aerosolization, in vitro 2D/3D human lung cell cultures, and in vivo efficacy. *Ther. Adv. Respir. Dis.* **2021**, *15*, 25.
28. Ruiz, V.H.; Encinas-Basurto, D.; Sun, B.; Eedara, B.B.; Roh, E.; Alarcon, N.O.; Curiel-Lewandrowski, C.; Bode, A.M.; Mansour, H.M. Innovative Rocuronium Bromide Topical Formulation for Targeted Skin Drug Delivery: Design, Comprehensive Characterization, In Vitro 2D/3D Human Cell Culture and Permeation. *Int. J. Mol. Sci.* **2023**, *24*, 8776. [CrossRef] [PubMed]
29. Gomez, A.I.; Acosta, M.F.; Muralidharan, P.; Yuan, J.X.J.; Black, S.M.; Hayes, D.; Mansour, H.M. Advanced spray dried proliposomes of amphotericin B lung surfactant-mimic phospholipid microparticles/nanoparticles as dry powder inhalers for targeted pulmonary drug delivery. *Pulm. Pharmacol. Ther.* **2020**, *64*, 101975. [CrossRef] [PubMed]
30. Muralidharan, P.; Hayes, D., Jr.; Black, S.M.; Mansour, H.M. Microparticulate/Nanoparticulate Powders of a Novel Nrf2 Activator and an Aerosol Performance Enhancer for Pulmonary Delivery Targeting the Lung Nrf2/Keap-1 Pathway. *Mol. Syst. Des. Eng.* **2016**, *1*, 48–65. [CrossRef]

31. Li, X.; Vogt, F.G.; Hayes, D., Jr.; Mansour, H.M. Design, characterization, and aerosol dispersion performance modeling of advanced spray-dried microparticulate/nanoparticulate mannitol powders for targeted pulmonary delivery as dry powder inhalers. *J. Aerosol Med. Pulm. Drug Deliv.* **2014**, *27*, 81–93. [CrossRef]
32. Acosta, M.F.; Abrahamson, M.D.; Encinas-Basurto, D.; Fineman, J.R.; Black, S.M.; Mansour, H.M. Inhalable nanoparticles/microparticles of an AMPK and Nrf2 activator for targeted pulmonary drug delivery as dry powder inhalers. *AAPS J.* **2020**, *23*, 2. [CrossRef]
33. Rzhevskii, A. Basic aspects of experimental design in raman microscopy. *Spectroscopy* **2016**, *31*, 40–45.
34. Mansour, H.M.; Hickey, A.J. Raman characterization and chemical imaging of biocolloidal self-assemblies, drug delivery systems, and pulmonary inhalation aerosols: A review. *AAPS PharmSciTech* **2007**, *8*, E99. [CrossRef] [PubMed]
35. Meenach, S.A.; Vogt, F.G.; Anderson, K.W.; Hilt, J.Z.; McGarry, R.C.; Mansour, H.M. Design, physicochemical characterization, and optimization of organic solution advanced spray-dried inhalable dipalmitoylphosphatidylcholine (DPPC) and dipalmitoylphosphatidylethanolamine poly(ethylene glycol) (DPPE-PEG) microparticles and nanoparticles for targeted respiratory nanomedicine delivery as dry powder inhalation aerosols. *Int. J. Nanomed.* **2013**, *8*, 275–293. [CrossRef]
36. Park, C.-W.; Rhee, Y.-S.; Vogt, F.G.; Hayes, D.; Zwischenberger, J.B.; DeLuca, P.P.; Mansour, H.M. Advances in microscopy and complementary imaging techniques to assess the fate of drugs ex vivo in respiratory drug delivery: An invited paper. *Adv. Drug Deliv. Rev.* **2012**, *64*, 344–356. [CrossRef] [PubMed]
37. Meenach, S.A.; Anderson, K.W.; Zach Hilt, J.; McGarry, R.C.; Mansour, H.M. Characterization and aerosol dispersion performance of advanced spray-dried chemotherapeutic PEGylated phospholipid particles for dry powder inhalation delivery in lung cancer. *Eur. J. Pharm. Sci.* **2013**, *49*, 699–711. [CrossRef]
38. Muralidharan, P.; Acosta, M.F.; Gomez, A.I.; Grijalva, C.; Tang, H.; Yuan, J.X.; Mansour, H.M. Design and Comprehensive Characterization of Tetramethylpyrazine (TMP) for Targeted Lung Delivery as Inhalation Aerosols in Pulmonary Hypertension (PH): In Vitro Human Lung Cell Culture and In Vivo Efficacy. *Antioxidants* **2021**, *10*, 427. [CrossRef]
39. Meenach, S.A.; Anderson, K.W.; Hilt, J.Z.; McGarry, R.C.; Mansour, H.M. High-performing dry powder inhalers of paclitaxel DPPC/DPPG lung surfactant-mimic multifunctional particles in lung cancer: Physicochemical characterization, in vitro aerosol dispersion, and cellular studies. *AAPS PharmSciTech* **2014**, *15*, 1574–1587. [CrossRef]
40. Park, C.-W.; Mansour, H.M.; Oh, T.-O.; Kim, J.-Y.; Ha, J.-M.; Lee, B.-J.; Chi, S.-C.; Rhee, Y.-S.; Park, E.-S. Phase behavior of itraconazole–phenol mixtures and its pharmaceutical applications. *Int. J. Pharm.* **2012**, *436*, 652–658. [CrossRef]
41. Q2(R1) Validation of Analytical Procedures: Text and Methodology Guidance for Industry. 2005. Available online: https://www.fda.gov/regulatory-information/search-fda-guidance-documents/q2r1-validation-analytical-procedures-text-and-methodology-guidance-industry (accessed on 1 June 2023).

International Journal of
Molecular Sciences

MDPI

Article

Value of the Lymphocyte Transformation Test for the Diagnosis of Drug-Induced Hypersensitivity Reactions in Hospitalized Patients with Severe COVID-19

Carlos Fernández-Lozano [1,†], Emilio Solano Solares [2,†], Isabel Elías-Sáenz [2], Isabel Pérez-Allegue [2], Monserrat Fernández-Guarino [3], Diego Fernández-Nieto [3], Laura Díaz Montalvo [2], David González-de-Olano [2], Ana de Andrés [4], Javier Martínez-Botas [1,*] and Belén de la Hoz Caballer [2,*]

1 Biochemistry-Research Department, Hospital Universitario Ramón y Cajal, Instituto Ramón y Cajal de Investigación Sanitaria, Carretera de Colmenar Km 9, 28034 Madrid, Spain; carlitos4mb@hotmail.com
2 Allergy Service, Hospital Universitario Ramón y Cajal, Instituto Ramón y Cajal de Investigación Sanitaria, Carretera de Colmenar Km 9, 28034 Madrid, Spain; emilio.solano.solares@gmail.com (E.S.S.); isaes014@gmail.com (I.E.-S.); ipallegue@gmail.com (I.P.-A.); lauragdm97@gmail.com (L.D.M.); dgolano@yahoo.es (D.G.-d.-O.)
3 Dermatology Service, Hospital Universitario Ramón y Cajal, Instituto Ramón y Cajal de Investigación Sanitaria, Carretera de Colmenar Km 9, 28034 Madrid, Spain; montsefdez@msn.com (M.F.-G.); fnietodiego@gmail.com (D.F.-N.)
4 Immunology Service, Hospital Universitario Ramón y Cajal, Instituto Ramón y Cajal de Investigación Sanitaria, Carretera de Colmenar Km 9, 28034 Madrid, Spain; aandresm@salud.madrid.org
* Correspondence: javier.botas@hrc.es (J.M.-B.); belen.hoz@salud.madrid.org (B.d.l.H.C.); Tel.: +34-91336-8466 (J.M.B.); +34-91336-8341 (B.d.l.H.C.)
† These authors contributed equally to this work.

Abstract: In the first wave of COVID-19, up to 20% of patients had skin lesions with variable characteristics. There is no clear evidence of the involvement of the SARS-CoV-2 virus in all cases; some of these lesions may be secondary to drug hypersensitivity. To analyze the possible cause of the skin lesions, we performed a complete allergology study on 11 patients. One year after recovery from COVID-19, we performed a lymphocyte transformation test (LTT) and Th1/Th2 cytokine secretion assays for PBMCs. We included five nonallergic patients treated with the same drugs without lesions. Except for one patient who had an immediate reaction to azithromycin, all patients had a positive LTT result for at least one of the drugs tested (azithromycin, clavulanic acid, hydroxychloroquine, lopinavir, and ritonavir). None of the nonallergic patients had a positive LTT result. We found mixed Th1/Th2 cytokine secretion (IL-4, IL-5, IL-13, and IFN-γ) in patients with skin lesions corresponding to mixed drug hypersensitivity type IVa and IVb. In all cases, we identified a candidate drug as the culprit for skin lesions during SARS-CoV-2 infection, although only three patients had a positive drug challenge. Therefore, it would be reasonable to recommend avoiding the drug in question in all cases.

Keywords: delayed drug hypersensitivity; skin reaction; SARS-CoV-2; LTT; interleukins

Citation: Fernández-Lozano, C.; Solano Solares, E.; Elías-Sáenz, I.; Pérez-Allegue, I.; Fernández-Guarino, M.; Fernández-Nieto, D.; Díaz Montalvo, L.; González-de-Olano, D.; de Andrés, A.; Martínez-Botas, J.; et al. Value of the Lymphocyte Transformation Test for the Diagnosis of Drug-Induced Hypersensitivity Reactions in Hospitalized Patients with Severe COVID-19. *Int. J. Mol. Sci.* **2023**, *24*, 11543. https://doi.org/10.3390/ijms241411543

Academic Editor: Motonari Kondo

Received: 28 June 2023
Revised: 12 July 2023
Accepted: 14 July 2023
Published: 17 July 2023

1. Introduction

SARS-CoV-2 is a respiratory virus that can affect multiple organs, causing a wide range of symptoms in some patients [1]. Cutaneous involvement, in which many types of skin lesions are identified [2], was described in the first published papers on SARS-CoV-2. COVID-19 skin reactions were found to be generally higher in Western Europe than in Asia, with 6.6% reported in Europe compared with 0.2% in Asia [3]. Initially, an Italian group described six types of skin lesions: maculopapular rashes, urticarial rashes, vesicular rashes, erythema multiforme, cutaneous vasculitis, and chilblain-like lesions [4]. These lesions were considered secondary to the infection, but hypersensitivity to the treatments received could not be ruled out with absolute certainty [5]. The lesions described in patients with SARS-CoV-2 infection were very heterogeneous and had a similar pattern to those observed in delayed drug hypersensitivity reactions (e.g., maculopapular exanthema (MPE) and fixed drug eruption (FDE)), drug-induced liver injury (DILI), and severe cutaneous adverse reactions (SCARs) (e.g., Stevens–Johnson syndrome (SJS), toxic epidermal necrolysis (TEN), drug reactions with eosinophilia and systemic symptoms (DRESSs), and acute generalized exanthematous pustulosis (AGEP)) [6–9]. The most common drugs prescribed for COVID-19 treatment were hydroxychloroquine (18.5%), azithromycin (11.1%), lopinavir (7.4%), ritonavir (7.4%), and paracetamol (9.2%) [3].

Late skin reactions to drugs belong to a mechanism of type IV hypersensitivity mediated by T cells. Advances in our knowledge of the cells and cytokines involved in these types of reactions have allowed them to be classified into four types (IVa-IVd) [10]. Type IVa corresponds to T-helper type 1 (Th1) cytokine-driven responses associated with high IFN-γ/TNF-α secretion. Type IVb corresponds to T-helper type 2 (Th2) cytokine-driven reactions with the increased secretion of IL-4, IL-5, and IL-13. Type IVc corresponds to the cytotoxic reactions mediated by cytotoxic CD8 T cells and seems to be the primary mechanism of bullous skin reactions, such as SJS and TEN. Type IVd represents the T-cell-induced sterile neutrophilic inflammatory response, e.g., AGEP [11].

Diagnostic tests for delayed drug hypersensitivity are scarce. In vivo tests like epicutaneous patches are the most readily available. These patches must be prepared with the suspected drug involved in the reactions (based on a very detailed allergy clinical history) with an appropriate concentration and vehicle in order to yield accurate results. A positive result confirms the involvement of the drug, but the predictive value of a negative test is unknown. Therefore, a drug challenge is still considered the gold standard for diagnosing a drug allergy. In most delayed reactions, this option is not possible due to the patient's risk of reaction and the lack of standardization of the challenged drugs, as a complete single dose of a drug may rule out an immediate IgE-mediated reaction but not a delayed reaction that may occur after consecutive doses in a longer treatment.

In recent years, the lymphocyte transformation test (LTT) has been used to diagnose delayed drug-induced hypersensitivity reactions by detecting the proliferation of drug-specific memory T cells [12]. In addition, previous studies have shown that the measurements of cytokine secretion in PBMCs may be useful in diagnosing drug hypersensitivity [11,13,14].

Our group conducted a prospective, observational, and descriptive study to determine whether drug hypersensitivity was the real cause of skin lesions. The results have been reported previously [15]. The aim of the present study was to confirm the mechanism of hypersensitivity and the drugs involved in the skin lesions observed in patients with SARS-CoV-2 infection by means of an immunological study.

2. Results

2.1. Design and Setting

Patients were selected from our previous study, which was a prospective, observational, and descriptive study for which its main objective was to determine whether drug hypersensitivity could have been a cause of skin lesions in patients admitted to our hospital with SARS-CoV-2 infection between March and May 2020 [15]. Of the 72 patients included in this study, 37 were classified as having a possible drug-caused lesion according to the Spanish Pharmacovigilance System (ASPS) [16]. Of these, only 16 agreed to continue in the study. In all cases, a complete allergological study was performed via skin tests, epi-patches, and oral challenges against the drugs used during the period of infection and skin lesions [15]. In the present study, 11 of these 16 patients agreed to finish the "in vitro" study (Figure 1). We also included five nonallergic patients (NAPs) who were exposed to these drugs but did not develop lesions. The main treatments used were dolquine (hydroxychloroquine (HCQ)); azithromycin (AZT); kaletra (lopinavir/ritonavir (LOP/RIT)); and/or beta-lactam antibiotics, such as amoxicillin/clavulanic acid (AMOX/CLA) or ceftriaxone (Table 1).

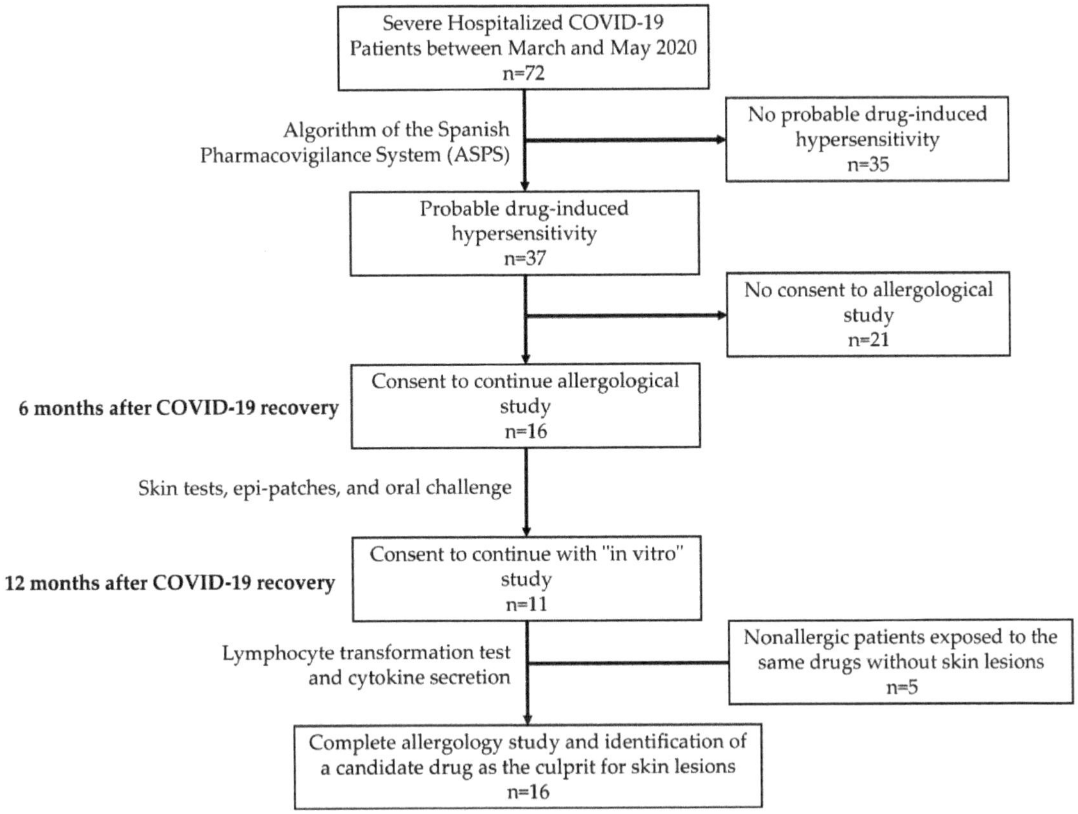

Figure 1. Study design.

The patients included in this study presented three types of cutaneous lesions: maculopapular exanthema (MPE), urticarial exanthema (UEX), and vesicular exanthema (VEX). Accordingly, patients were classified as generalized exanthema (n = 10) or cutaneous vasculitis (n = 1) (Table 1). In all cases, the time from the start of treatment to the onset of lesions was between 1 and 15 days, with a mean of 7.5 days. Consistently with the general characteristics of the most severe COVID-19 patients, 75% of the patients were male and had a median age of 62 years (IQR 71-58.75).

Epicutaneous patch tests were performed 4–6 months after hospital discharge, with a negative result for the eleven patients. In the case of beta-lactam antibiotics, the skin prick test with late-reaction lecture ware was also performed, and all results were negative. Afterward, a drug provocation test (DPT) was performed with the implicated drugs on alternative days. DPTs were performed in 9 out of the 11 patients. Two patients had no exposure to a DPT; one had no exposure because of the severity of his initial lesions due to cutaneous vasculitis, and the other refused the DPT. The DPT results were positive in three patients: two for AZT (late maculopapular exanthema and vesicular exanthema) and one for AMOX/CLA (macular exanthema). It is important to mention that patient P2 presented an immediate reaction to 12.5 mg of AZT. In all three cases, the cutaneous lesions were consistent with the initial ones during COVID-19 treatment (Table 1).

Table 1. Clinical characteristics of the patients and allergological study.

Patient	Age (Years)/Sex	COVID-19 Treatments	Reaction	Epicutaneous Patch Test		Oral Challenges		LTT	
				Positive	Negative	Positive	Negative	Positive	Negative
P1	60/F	AZT, DOL	MPE [(1)]		AZT, DOL		AZT, DOL	HCQ	AZT, AMOX, CLA, LOP, RIT
P2	61/M	AZT, KAL, DOL, CEL	UEX [(1)]		AZT, DOL, KAL, CEL	AZT [§]	DOL, KAL		HCQ, AZT, AMOX, LOP, RIT
P3	53/M	AZT, KAL, DOL, CEL, AMOX/CLA	MPE [(1)]		DOL, KAL, CEL, AMOX	AMOX/CLA	KAL, AZT, HCQ	CLA	HCQ, AZT, AMOX, LOP, RIT
P4	63/F	AZT, KAL, DOL, CEL	MPE [(1)], VEX [(2)]		AZT, DOL, KAL		AZT, HCQ, KAL	LOP, RIT	HCQ, AZT, AMOX
P5	66/M	AZT, KAL, DOL, CEL	MPE [(1)], VEX [(2)]		AZT, DOL, KAL, CEL	AZT	KAL, CEL	AZT, HCQ	AMOX, LOP, RIT
P6	61/F	AZT, DOL	MPE [(1)] VEX [(2)]		AZT, DOL		DOL, AZT	AZT, LOP, RIT	HCQ, AMOX
P7	77/F	KAL, DOL, CEL	MPE [(1)]			*	*	LOP, RIT	HCQ, AZT, AMOX
P8	84/M	AZT, KAL, DOL, CEL	MPE [(1)], VEX [(2)]		AZT, DOL, KAL, CEL		AZT, DOL, KAL, CEL	LOP, RIT	HCQ, AZT, AMOX
P9	76/M	AZT, DOL	VEX [(2)]		AZT, DOL		AZT, DOL	HCQ, RIT	AZT, AMOX, LOP
P10	74/M	AZT, DOL, CEL	CVAS [(3)], CLL [(4)]		AZT, DOL, CEL	*	*	AZT, RIT	AZT, AMOX, LOP
P11	64/M	AZT, KAL, DOL	MPE [(1)]		AZT, KAL, DOL		AZT, KAL, DOL	LOP, RIT	HCQ, AZT, AMOX
NAP1	58/M	AZT, KAL, DOL							HCQ, AZT, AMOX, LOP, RIT
NAP2	52/M	AZT, KAL, DOL, CEL							HCQ, AZT, AMOX, LOP, RIT
NAP3	59/M	AZT, KAL, DOL, CEL							HCQ, AZT, AMOX, LOP, RIT
NAP4	49/M	AZT, DOL							HCQ, AZT, AMOX, LOP, RIT
NAP5	70/M	AZT, KAL, DOL, CEL							HCQ, AZT, AMOX, LOP, RIT

[(1)] Generalized exanthema: MPE—maculopapular exanthem or UEX—urticarial exanthem; [(2)] VEX—vesicular exanthem; [(3)] CVAS—cutaneous vasculitis; [(4)] CLL—chilblain-like lesion. Abbreviations: AZT—azitromicin; AMOX—amoxicillin; CLA—clavulanic acid; DOL—dolquine; HCQ—hydroxychloroquine; KAL—kaletra; LOP—lopinavir; RIT—ritonavir; CEL—ceftriaxona. [§] Immediate reaction with 12.5 mg. * Oral challenge not possible because of generalized severe reaction.

2.2. Lymphocyte Transformation Test (LTT)

In order to identify the possible culprit drugs causing skin lesions in these patients, we performed an LTT one year after recovery from COVID-19. An LTT was also performed in five nonallergic patients. The study was conducted one year after recovery from COVID-19. In all cases, the LTT was performed using three doses of AZT, AMOX, CLA, HCQ, LOP, and RIT (Table 2). Ceftriaxone was excluded from the LTT study due to the limited sample size and the results of the allergology study. The test was considered positive with a stimulation index ≥ 3. Except for patient 2, who had an immediate reaction to AZT, all patients had a positive LTT result for at least one of the drugs tested. Three patients tested positive for AZT (P5, P6, and P10). Of these, patient 5 also had a positive DPT. One patient tested positive for CLA with a positive DPT (P3). Three patients tested positive for HCQ (P1, P5, and P9). Four patients tested positive for LOP (P4, P6, P7, and P8). Seven patients tested positive for RIT (P4, P6, P7, P8, P9, P10, and P11). None of the patients responded to AMOX. Two patients responded to only one drug, and eight responded to two drugs. None of the nonallergic patients had a positive LTT result for any of the drugs tested. All results are shown in Table 2.

2.3. Cytokine Secretion

Next, we analyzed the cytokine secretion of PBMCs in response to all relevant drugs four days after drug stimulation. In patients with cutaneous lesions, cytokine release was measured in all conditions with a positive LTT result and at least one negative drug. In the case of patient 2, who had an immediate reaction to AZT, cytokine secretion was analyzed at all concentrations of this drug (0.1, 1, and 10 μg/μL) and at 5 μg/μL of RIT. In the group of nonallergic patients without cutaneous lesions, cytokine secretion was analyzed at a representative concentration for each drug except for AZT, which did not give any positive LTT results. In the group of patients with cutaneous lesions, the LTT-positive drugs strongly induced the secretion of IL-4, IL-5, and IL-13 (Figure 2 and Supplementary Table S1) in most patients. The levels of these cytokines in the nonallergic patient's group were consistently low, and no increase was observed with any of the selected drugs. Although there was an apparent increase in IFN-γ with the LTT-positive drugs, an increase in IFN-γ was also observed in three nonallergic patients, which occurred with all tested drugs. It is interesting to note that patient 2, who had an immediate response to AZM and a negative LTT result, had very low levels of these cytokines. The response of the other cytokines studied, IL-1β, Il-6, TNF-α, and IL-10, was inconsistent, as they increased with some treatments but not others. These cytokines were also increased by some non-proliferation-stimulating drugs and in control patients.

Table 2. Lymphocyte transformation test (LTT) results.

Patient	(Dynabeads™ CD3/CD28)	Azitromicin			Amoxicillin			Clavulanic Acid			Hidroxiloroquine			Lopinavir			Ritonavir		
		0.1 µg/µL	**1 µg/µL**	**10 µg/µL**	**100 µg/µL**	**200 µg/µL**	**500 µg/µL**	**1 µg/µL**	**10 µg/µL**	**100 µg/µL**	**1 µg/µL**	**10 µg/µL**	**100 µg/µL**	**0.2 µg/mL**	**1 µg/mL**	**5 µg/mL**	**0.2 µg/µL**	**1 µg/µL**	**5 µg/µL**
P1	10.2	0.8	1.5	1.5	1.4	1.4	1.2	1.4	1.6	1.6	1.4	**3.2**	0.3	1.7	2.1	2.2	1.4	1.2	1.2
P2	12.2	0.5	1.0	0.5	0.9	1.4	1.5	1.2	1.2	1.4	1.2	1.8	1.9	1.1	0.8	0.9	1.3	1.0	0.8
P3	15.0	1.3	1.5	1.9	1.7	1.7	1.4	1.9	**3.2**	**3.4**	1.4	1.8	0.3	2.0	1.8	0.9	2.0	1.8	1.8
P4	5.8	0.8	0.7	0.9	0.7	2.1	0.7	0.7	0.7	0.8	0.6	1.1	0.1	**3.9**	0.6	0.9	**3.5**	0.3	0.5
P5	9.0	1.7	1.4	**3.1**	1.6	1.4	2.8	1.9	1.7	1.6	**3.4**	0.8	0.7	1.3	1.0	0.8	1.1	1.2	0.6
P6	11.6	**3.0**	1.7	1.0	1.9	1.6	1.9	2.4	2.5	2.3	1.3	1.8	1.6	1.9	**3.0**	2.8	2.9	**3.2**	2.6
P7	9.4	1.4	0.9	1.4	1.8	1.1	1.5	1.8	1.5	1.4	1.7	2.0	1.8	1.9	2.3	**3.4**	2.3	1.0	**3.2**
P8	7.4	1.9	1.7	1.6	1.9	1.8	1.9	1.9	1.5	1.6	1.6	1.9	1.9	1.1	3.3	1.6	1.8	1.5	**3.2**
P9	6.7	1.5	1.3	1.2	1.3	1.2	1.2	1.4	1.3	1.2	1.6	**3.2**	1.5	1.2	2.7	1.8	1.6	**3.0**	**3.4**
P10	8.2	1.1	1.8	**3.1**	0.7	0.9	1.2	1.0	1.3	1.1	0.9	0.8	1.0	2.4	1.5	1.3	2.6	**3.1**	2.1
P11	8.4	1.6	1.4	1.2	1.4	1.2	1.2	1.5	1.8	1.4	1.5	1.3	1.3	1.7	2.1	**3.2**	1.9	2.7	**3.3**
NAP1	6.3	1.4	1.1	1.0	1.1	0.9	0.9	0.9	1.0	0.9	0.4	1.4	0.9	1.1	1.2	1.2	0.9	1.2	0.9
NAP2	5.5	1.9	1.0	1.5	1.3	0.9	0.7	1.6	1.0	0.8	0.4	1.7	0.9	1.8	1.4	1.2	1.8	1.5	1.2
NAP3	5.2	1.5	1.1	1.7	1.9	2.0	1.5	1.9	1.2	1.3	1.8	0.8	1.6	1.0	0.6	0.8	0.9	0.8	0.7
NAP4	9.9	1.8	1.6	2.0	2.0	1.9	1.8	1.9	1.4	1.8	1.9	1.3	1.1	1.5	2.0	1.8	1.9	1.9	1.8
NAP5	7.8	1.4	1.2	0.9	0.8	0.8	0.7	0.9	0.9	0.7	0.3	0.2	1.1	1.9	0.9	0.7	0.9	0.8	0.6

As the standard criteria, an SI ≥ 3 in at least one concentration was considered positive (bold and highlighted in grey).

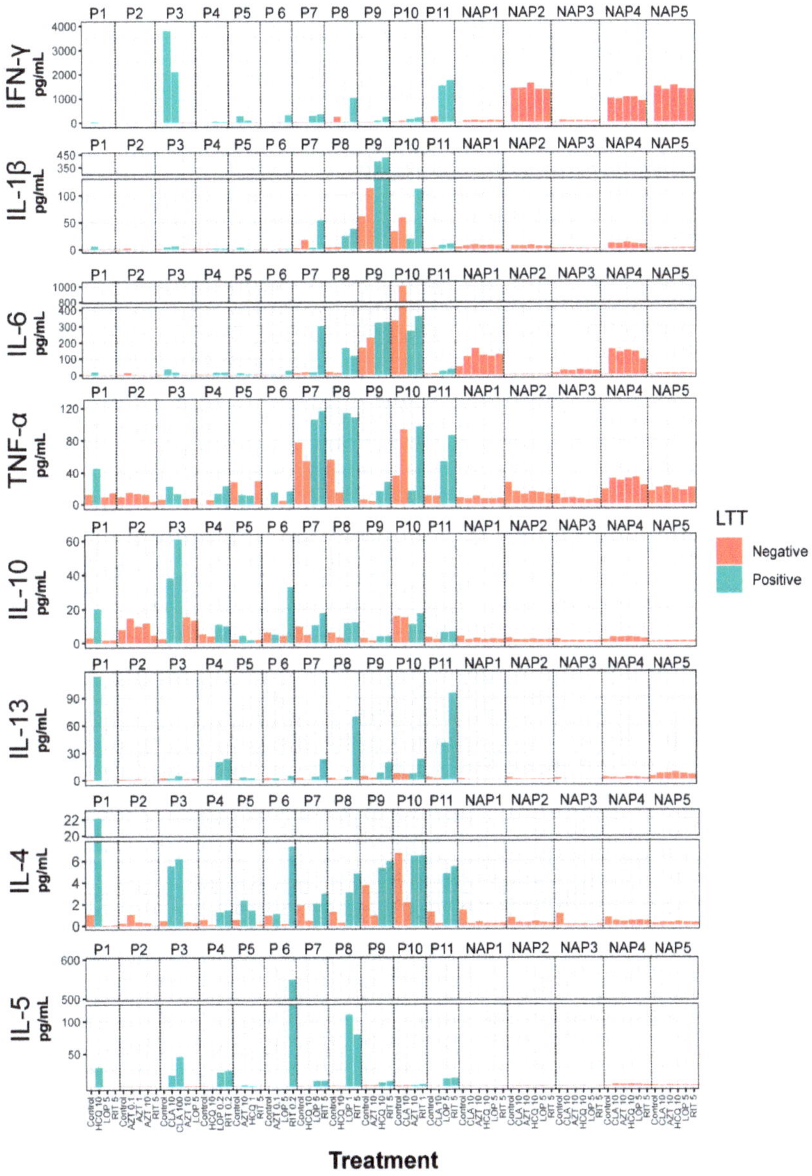

Figure 2. Cytokine secretion of PBMCs in response to all relevant drugs. The red bars correspond to the condition where the LTT result was negative, and the blue bars correspond to the condition where the LTT result was positive.

3. Discussion

During the first wave of the COVID-19 pandemic, up to 20% of patients had skin lesions of different characteristics [4,17,18]. The skin lesions associated with COVID-19 were classified into six categories: maculopapular exanthems, urticarial exanthems, vesicular exanthems, erythema multiforme, cutaneous vasculitis, and chilblain-like lesions [4]. Due to the heterogeneity of the treatments, it has not been possible to clearly establish whether or not some of the skin lesions that were presented in patients during the first wave of COVID-19 could be secondary to drug hypersensitivity. In the present study, we analyzed the possible cause of skin lesions during SARS-CoV-2 infection in 11 patients. Using lymphocyte proliferation and cytokine secretion assays, we identified a drug candidate as the culprit despite only three patients having positive drug provocation test results.

The fact that skin manifestations were greatly reduced in subsequent waves when COVID-19 treatments were changed supports the view that the skin manifestations observed in the first wave were mainly due to hypersensitivity reactions to the drugs used at that time [19] or to the combination of both the drugs used and the viral strain in the subsequent waves of COVID-19. Such interactions between drugs and viral infections have been widely reported for the viruses of the Herpesviridae family and less commonly for other viruses such as influenza, chikungunya, or HIV [7].

An LTT is recommended for the diagnosis of drug hypersensitivity reactions (DHRs) in which the distal effector phase is mediated by T cells [12]. After the PBMC culture, the activation of the lipocytes begins within minutes due to a specific drug antigen presented by major histocompatibility complex (MHC) class I or II antigen-presenting cells (APCs). Following T-cell receptor (TCR) activation, Ca^{2+} increases, and a signaling cascade activates early antigen recognition genes. Over the next few hours, the expression of genes encoding several cytokines (IL-2, 3, 4, 5, and 6; IFN-γ; and TGF-β) and early activation markers increases. One to two days after T-cell activation, IL-2 induces the proliferation of activated T-cells; consequently, DNA synthesis starts. Approximately three to five days after activation, T cells enter the functional differentiation phase and produce different cytokine patterns: Th1, Th2, or Th3. Th1 is mainly associated with the production of IL-2, IFN-γ, and TNF-α; Th2 is associated with the production of IL-4, IL-5, and IL-13; Th3 is associated with the production of IL-17A and IL-17F. The type of specific T cell produced depends on the sensitization phase, and these cytokine patterns determine the effector functions of T lymphocytes [11]. Several studies have shown that cytokine secretion in the supernatant of drug-stimulated PBMCs may also be useful in the diagnosis of drug hypersensitivity [13,14]. The production of Th1 cytokines, mainly IL-2, IFN-γ, and TNF-α, in PBMCs has been associated with DHR in several studies [11]. High IFN-γ production by drug-stimulated PBMCs has been observed during the acute allergic phase in SCARs such as SJS, TEN, DRESS, or AGEP [20]. IL-5 increases in patients with drug-induced MPE and DRESS [21,22], and it has been proposed as a useful in vitro method for detecting drug sensitization. Furthermore, the combination of IL-5 measures and the LTT may better indicate drug sensitization than the LTT alone [23]. Other studies have shown a mixed Th1/Th2 cytokine pattern with the production of IL-5, IL-4, and IL-13 in addition to IFN-γ. Indeed, high levels of IL-5 and IFN-γ secretion by CD4 cells are associated with maculopapular exanthema [10] and have been proposed as promising in vitro indicators of drug hypersensitivity [11,24]. Lochmatter et al. [13] extensively studied the secretion of 17 cytokines and chemokines in PBMCs from patients with well-documented drug allergies. They found that the measurement of IL-5 combined with IFN-γ, IL-13, or IL-2 is the more sensitive marker for detecting T-cell sensitization to drugs.

Consistently with this, we found mixed Th1/Th2 cytokine secretion (IL-4, IL-5, IL-13, and IFN-γ) in patients with skin lesions. Therefore, this allows us to classify these patients as having mixed type IVa and IVb drug hypersensitivity reactions, corresponding to T-helper type 1 (Th1) cytokine-driven responses that are associated with high levels of IFN-γ secretion and Th2 cytokine-driven responses that are associated with high levels of IL-4, IL-5, and IL-13 secretion.

It is important to note that we found elevated levels of IFN-γ in some patients without skin lesions, a phenomenon that has been described previously [25,26].

Among the eleven patients studied, an immediate clinical response was observed in only one case, which was confirmed by a positive oral challenge and a negative LTT result for AZT. In the remaining cases, a specific immune response to some of the drugs that the patients had received during treatment could be established, which was not found in patients with SARS-CoV-2 infection but in those without skin lesions. Interestingly, only two patients had a positive oral challenge: one relative to AZT and one relative to CLA. The discordant results between the oral challenge and LTT could be due to two situations. Firstly, the drugs were not given for a sufficient time or at a sufficient dose during the oral challenge. This may be because the drugs used are so toxic that they cannot be given for long periods without clinical necessity [11]. Alternatively, this may be because the patient was no longer in an inflammatory state that was present during the viral infection. the study was carried out 6 months later; therefore, the patient did not have the cofactor necessary to trigger the cutaneous symptoms again. The 12-month period was chosen for the in vitro study because this is the recommended latency period for LTT studies in severe late drug reactions such as DRESS or exanthema multiforme.

On the other hand, it is important to emphasize the importance of performing the LTT at least 2 months after the resolution of the infection [13,27], with the recommendation being between 6 and 12 months [28]; otherwise, the risk of false-positive results increases, as described previously. Indeed, a case of COVID-19-related cutaneous manifestations has been described in which the proliferation assay was performed 21 days after infection and reported sensitization to all drugs tested [29]. This may be a sign of hyperreactivity caused by a viral infection and, consequently, may be a false-positive LTT result.

Therefore, considering that all patients with late reactions presented skin lesions and had a positive LTT result with a mixed Th1/Th2 cytokine release, it would be reasonable to recommend avoiding the drug in question in all cases. If drug administration is necessary, an exhaustive study under allergological supervision with appropriate dosage and administration time should be carried out. These results highlight the need for a multidisciplinary approach to the management of adverse drug reactions [5].

4. Materials and Methods

4.1. Lymphocyte Transformation Test (LTT)

The LTT was performed according to Giraldo-Tugores et al. with minor modifications [30]. PBMCs were freshly isolated from heparinized venous blood samples (30 mL) using Ficoll (LymphoPrep™) gradient centrifugation. The cells were resuspended in AIM-V medium (Gibco, Thermo Fisher Scientific Inc., Waltham, MA, USA) (2×10^6 cell/mL) and cultured in 96-well U-bottomed plates (200 µL/well) containing the following stimuli: Dynabeads Human T-Activator CD3/CD28 (1 µL/well) (Gibco) as the positive control; AIM-V or DMSO medium as the negative control (unstimulated condition); and azitromicin (0.1 µg/µL, 1 µg/µL, and 10 µg/µL), amoxicilin (100 µg/µL, 200 µg/µL, and 500 µg/µL), clavulanate (1 µg/µL, 10 µg/µL, and 100 µg/µL), hydroxychloroquine (1 µg/µL, 10 µg/µL, and 100 µg/µL), lopinavir (0.02 µg/µL, 0.1 µg/µL, 0.5 µg/µL, and 2.5 µg/µL), and ritonavir (0.04 µg/µL, 0.2 µg/µL, 1 µg/µL, and 5 µg/µL). Cultures were performed in triplicate and incubated for 4 days in a humidified incubator (37 °C and 5% CO_2). On day 4, the culture plates were centrifuged, and 100 µL aliquots of the culture supernatant were transferred to another 96-well plate and stored at −40 °C for cytokine analysis. Then, 100 µL of fresh AIM-V medium containing 10 µCi of ^{3}H-thymidine (PerkinElmer, Waltham, MA, USA) was added to the cells and gently resuspended on the cell pellet. On day 6, the cultures were transferred to a Multiscreen®-HV 96-Well Filter Plate (Merck Millipore, Burlington, MA, USA), and cells were harvested using a MultiScreen®Vacuum Manifold (Millipore). Each 96-well filter was punched into a scintillation vial, and radioactivity incorporated into the DNA was measured using a liquid scintillation counter (PerkinElmer). The proliferative response was expressed as a stimulation index (SI), which was calculated using the ratio of disintegrations per minute (dpm) of the drug-stimulated T cells and the mean of dpm of the unstimulated T cells. As part of the standard criteria, an SI > 3 in at least one concentration was considered positive.

4.2. Secreted Cytokine Measurement

Four-day cell-culture supernatants were centrifuged and stored at −40 °C. Th1 (IFN-γ, IL-1β, and TNF-α) and Th2 (IL-5, IL-4, IL-6, IL-10, and IL-13) cytokines were measured using the MILLIPLEX® MAP Human High Sensitivity T Cell Magnetic Beads panel (Merck Millipore) according to the manufacturer's instructions and were acquired on the Luminex Magpix System (Luminex, Austin, TX, USA).

5. Conclusions

Using lymphocyte proliferation and cytokine secretion assays, we identified a drug candidate as the culprit of skin lesions during SARS-CoV-2 infection despite only three patients having positive drug provocation test results. Therefore, considering that all patients with late reactions had presented skin lesions and had a positive LTT result with an increase in cytokine secretion, it would be reasonable to recommend avoiding the drug in question in all cases.

Supplementary Materials: The supporting information can be downloaded at: https://www.mdpi.com/article/10.3390/ijms241411543/s1.

Author Contributions: Conceptualization, M.F.-G., J.M.-B. and B.d.l.H.C.; sample collection and data acquisition, C.F.-L., E.S.S., I.E.-S., I.P.-A. and D.F.-N.; data analysis, C.F.-L., E.S.S., D.F.-N., A.d.A., J.M.-B. and B.d.l.H.C.; writing—original draft preparation, E.S.S., J.M.-B. and B.d.l.H.C.; writing—review and editing, C.F.-L., I.E.-S., I.P.-A., L.D.M., A.d.A., D.F.-N., D.G.-d.-O. and M.F.-G.; visualization, C.F.-L., E.S.S., J.M.-B. and B.d.l.H.C.; supervision, M.F.-G., J.M.-B. and B.d.l.H.C.; funding acquisition, M.F.-G., J.M.-B. and B.d.l.H.C. All authors have read and agreed to the published version of the manuscript.

Funding: This research was funded by FONDO SUPERA COVID-19, grant identification "Cutinmfarm"; by the SANTADER FOUNDATION; and in association with the Instituto Ramón y Cajal de Investigación Sanitaria (IRYCIS) and Alcala University (AU) of Madrid (Spain).

Institutional Review Board Statement: The study was conducted in accordance with the Declaration of Helsinki and approved by the Institutional Review Board (or Ethics Committee) of the HOSPITAL UNIERSITARIO RAMÓN Y CAJAL (protocol code 197/20, 22 June 2020).

Informed Consent Statement: Informed consent was obtained from all subjects involved in the study.

Data Availability Statement: Not applicable.

Acknowledgments: J.M.-B. is a researcher at FIBio-HRC and is supported by the Consejería de Sanidad (Comunidad Autónoma de Madrid).

Conflicts of Interest: The authors declare no conflict of interest.

References

1. Riggioni, C.; Comberiati, P.; Giovannini, M.; Agache, I.; Akdis, M.; Alves-Correia, M.; Anto, J.M.; Arcolaci, A.; Azkur, A.K.; Azkur, D.; et al. A compendium answering 150 questions on COVID-19 and SARS-CoV-2. *Allergy* **2020**, *75*, 2503–2541. [CrossRef] [PubMed]
2. Galvan Casas, C.; Catala, A.; Carretero Hernandez, G.; Rodriguez-Jimenez, P.; Fernandez-Nieto, D.; Rodriguez-Villa Lario, A.; Navarro Fernandez, I.; Ruiz-Villaverde, R.; Falkenhain-Lopez, D.; Llamas Velasco, M.; et al. Classification of the cutaneous manifestations of COVID-19: A rapid prospective nationwide consensus study in Spain with 375 cases. *Br. J. Dermatol.* **2020**, *183*, 71–77. [CrossRef] [PubMed]
3. Sameni, F.; Hajikhani, B.; Yaslianifard, S.; Goudarzi, M.; Owlia, P.; Nasiri, M.J.; Shokouhi, S.; Bakhtiyari, M.; Dadashi, M. COVID-19 and Skin Manifestations: An Overview of Case Reports/Case Series and Meta-Analysis of Prevalence Studies. *Front. Med.* **2020**, *7*, 573188. [CrossRef]
4. Recalcati, S.; Gianotti, R.; Fantini, F. COVID-19: The experience from Italy. *Clin. Dermatol.* **2021**, *39*, 12–22. [CrossRef]
5. Cabrera-Hernandez, R.; Solano-Solares, E.; Chica-Guzman, V.; Fernandez-Guarino, M.; Fernandez-Nieto, D.; Ortega-Quijano, D.; de-Andres-Martin, A.; Moreno, C.; Carretero-Barrio, I.; Garcia-Abellas, P.; et al. SARS-CoV-2, skin lesions and the need of a multidisciplinary approach. *J. Eur. Acad. Dermatol. Venereol.* **2020**, *34*, e659–e662. [CrossRef]

6. Mitamura, Y.; Schulz, D.; Oro, S.; Li, N.; Kolm, I.; Lang, C.; Ziadlou, R.; Tan, G.; Bodenmiller, B.; Steiger, P.; et al. Cutaneous and systemic hyperinflammation drives maculopapular drug exanthema in severely ill COVID-19 patients. *Allergy* **2022**, *77*, 595–608. [CrossRef] [PubMed]
7. Ramirez, G.A.; Ripa, M.; Burastero, S.; Benanti, G.; Bagnasco, D.; Nannipieri, S.; Monardo, R.; Ponta, G.; Asperti, C.; Cilona, M.B.; et al. Drug Reaction with Eosinophilia and Systemic Symptoms (DRESS): Focus on the Pathophysiological and Diagnostic Role of Viruses. *Microorganisms* **2023**, *11*, 346. [CrossRef]
8. Karimi, A.; Pourbakhtiaran, E.; Fallahi, M.; Karbasian, F.; Armin, S.; Babaie, D. Is It Stevens-Johnson Syndrome or MIS-C with Mucocutaneous Involvement? *Case Rep. Pediatr.* **2021**, *2021*, 1812545. [CrossRef]
9. Lootah, S.; Alshammari, E.; Alqanatish, J. Complete Remission in a Child with Multisystem Inflammatory Syndrome and Stevens-Johnson Syndrome Treated with Infliximab. *Cureus* **2023**, *15*, e37076. [CrossRef]
10. Pichler, W.J. Delayed drug hypersensitivity reactions. *Ann. Intern. Med.* **2003**, *139*, 683–693. [CrossRef]
11. Porebski, G.; Gschwend-Zawodniak, A.; Pichler, W.J. In vitro diagnosis of T cell-mediated drug allergy. *Clin. Exp. Allergy* **2011**, *41*, 461–470. [CrossRef] [PubMed]
12. Sachs, B.; Fatangare, A.; Sickmann, A.; Glassner, A. Lymphocyte transformation test: History and current approaches. *J. Immunol. Methods* **2021**, *493*, 113036. [CrossRef] [PubMed]
13. Lochmatter, P.; Beeler, A.; Kawabata, T.T.; Gerber, B.O.; Pichler, W.J. Drug-specific in vitro release of IL-2, IL-5, IL-13 and IFN-γ in patients with delayed-type drug hypersensitivity. *Allergy* **2009**, *64*, 1269–1278. [CrossRef] [PubMed]
14. Srinoulprasert, Y. Lymphocyte transformation test and cytokine detection assays: Determination of read out parameters for delayed-type drug hypersensitivity reactions. *J. Immunol. Methods* **2021**, *496*, 113098. [CrossRef]
15. Solano-Solares, E.; Chica-Guzman, V.; Perez-Allegue, I.; Cabrera-Hernandez, R.; Fernandez-Guarino, M.; Fernandez-Nieto, D.; Moreno-Garcia-Del-Real, C.; de-Andres-Martin, A.; Garcia-Bermejo, L.; Gonzalez-de-Olano, D.; et al. Role of Drug Hypersensitivity in the Cutaneous Manifestations of SARS-CoV-2 Infection. *J. Investig. Allergol. Clin. Immunol.* **2022**, *32*, 218–220. [CrossRef] [PubMed]
16. Cabanas, R.; Ramirez, E.; Sendagorta, E.; Alamar, R.; Barranco, R.; Blanca-Lopez, N.; Dona, I.; Fernandez, J.; Garcia-Nunez, I.; Garcia-Samaniego, J.; et al. Spanish Guidelines for Diagnosis, Management, Treatment, and Prevention of DRESS Syndrome. *J. Investig. Allergol. Clin. Immunol.* **2020**, *30*, 229–253. [CrossRef]
17. Mendez Maestro, I.; Pena Merino, L.; Udondo Gonzalez Del Tanago, B.; Aramburu Gonzalez, A.; Orbea Sopena, A.; Sanchez De Vicente, J.; Raton Nieto, J.A.; Acebo Marinas, E.; Gardeazabal Garcia, J. Skin manifestations in patients hospitalized with confirmed COVID-19 disease: A cross-sectional study in a tertiary hospital. *Int. J. Dermatol.* **2020**, *59*, 1353–1357. [CrossRef]
18. Nakashima, C.; Kato, M.; Otsuka, A. Cutaneous manifestations of COVID-19 and COVID-19 vaccination. *J. Dermatol.* **2023**, *50*, 280–289. [CrossRef]
19. Fernandez-Nieto, D.; Ortega-Quijano, D.; Suarez-Valle, A.; Jimenez-Cauhe, J.; Jaen-Olasolo, P.; Fernandez-Guarino, M. Lack of skin manifestations in COVID-19 hospitalized patients during the second epidemic wave in Spain: A possible association with a novel SARS-CoV-2 variant—A cross-sectional study. *J. Eur. Acad. Dermatol. Venereol.* **2021**, *35*, e183–e185. [CrossRef]
20. Suthumchai, N.; Srinoulprasert, Y.; Thantiworasit, P.; Rerknimitr, P.; Tuchinda, P.; Chularojanamontri, L.; Rerkpattanapipat, T.; Chanprapaph, K.; Disphanurat, W.; Chakkavittumrong, P.; et al. The measurement of drug-induced interferon γ-releasing cells and lymphocyte proliferation in severe cutaneous adverse reactions. *J. Eur. Acad. Dermatol. Venereol.* **2018**, *32*, 992–998. [CrossRef]
21. Yawalkar, N.; Shrikhande, M.; Hari, Y.; Nievergelt, H.; Braathen, L.R.; Pichler, W.J. Evidence for a role for IL-5 and eotaxin in activating and recruiting eosinophils in drug-induced cutaneous eruptions. *J. Allergy Clin. Immunol.* **2000**, *106*, 1171–1176. [CrossRef] [PubMed]
22. Sachs, B.; Erdmann, S.; Malte Baron, J.; Neis, M.; al Masaoudi, T.; Merk, H.F. Determination of interleukin-5 secretion from drug-specific activated ex vivo peripheral blood mononuclear cells as a test system for the in vitro detection of drug sensitization. *Clin. Exp. Allergy* **2002**, *32*, 736–744. [CrossRef]
23. Merk, H.F. Diagnosis of drug hypersensitivity: Lymphocyte transformation test and cytokines. *Toxicology* **2005**, *209*, 217–220. [CrossRef]
24. Glassner, A.; Wurpts, G.; Roseler, S.; Yazdi, A.S.; Sachs, B. In vitro detection of T cell sensitization by interferon-γ secretion in immediate-type drug allergy. *Clin. Exp. Allergy* **2023**, *53*, 222–225. [CrossRef] [PubMed]
25. Halevy, S.; Cohen, A.; Livni, E. Acute generalized exanthematous pustulosis associated with polysensitivity to paracetamol and bromhexine: The diagnostic role of in vitro interferon-γ release test. *Clin. Exp. Dermatol.* **2000**, *25*, 652–654. [CrossRef] [PubMed]
26. Gaspard, I.; Guinnepain, M.T.; Laurent, J.; Bachot, N.; Kerdine, S.; Bertoglio, J.; Pallardy, M.; Lebrec, H. Il-4 and IFN-γ mRNA induction in human peripheral lymphocytes specific for β-lactam antibiotics in immediate or delayed hypersensitivity reactions. *J. Clin. Immunol.* **2000**, *20*, 107–116. [CrossRef]
27. Cabanas, R.; Calderon, O.; Ramirez, E.; Fiandor, A.; Caballero, T.; Heredia, R.; Herranz, P.; Madero, R.; Quirce, S.; Bellon, T. Sensitivity and specificity of the lymphocyte transformation test in drug reaction with eosinophilia and systemic symptoms causality assessment. *Clin. Exp. Allergy* **2018**, *48*, 325–333. [CrossRef]
28. Glassner, A.; Dubrall, D.; Weinhold, L.; Schmid, M.; Sachs, B. Lymphocyte transformation test for drug allergy detection: When does it work? *Ann. Allergy Asthma Immunol.* **2022**, *129*, 497–506.e3. [CrossRef]

Table 1. Skin cancer treatment modalities [15–18].

Surgery	– Mohs micrographic surgery (gold-standard treatment); – Conventional excision;
Physical therapies	– Electrodessication/curettage; – Electrochemotherapy; – Radiotherapy; – Ablative CO_2 laser;
Topical therapies	– Imiquimod; – 5-fluorouracil; – Photodynamic therapy; – Tirbanibulin;
Intralesional therapies	– IFN-α; – Methotrexate; – 5-fluorouracil; – Bleomycin; – Papillomavirus vaccine;
Systemic therapies	– Immune checkpoint inhibitors (PD-1/PD-L1); – Hedgehog pathway inhibitors (vismodegib, sonidegib); – BRAF/MEK inhibitors; – Chemotherapy; – Others.

Topical therapies are reserved as intentional healing therapies for low-risk tumours (i.e., small and superficial), although they can also be employed as palliative strategies in patients with a high morbidity index or in cases where surgical resection is not feasible or is contraindicated [11,16].

Among topical therapies, immune response modifiers (IRM) stand out for their direct and indirect stimulation of antitumor innate and adaptative immune responses, tissue-sparing and function-preserving properties [1,5,14,19]. Imiquimod (IM) is the most used topically applied IRM and was first approved by the Food and Drug Administration (FDA) in 1997 for the treatment of adult external genital and perianal warts [1,4,20]. Indications for head and scalp non-hypertrophic actinic keratoses (AK) and non-head and neck superficial basal cell carcinoma (sBCC) were added in 2004 [1,11,13,21]. Since then, it has been employed off-label for different infectious and neoplastic superficial skin disorders, such as Bowen's disease (BD), nodular basal cell carcinoma (nBCC), SCC, lentigo maligna (LM), melanoma metastases, cutaneous T-cell lymphomas and pyogenic granuloma [1,2,21–23]. However, the scientific evidence supporting its use in these latter conditions is anecdotical and relies mostly on case series and open-label trials, with varying and inconsistent treatment regimens [24].

Despite its frequent use by dermatologists, the physiologic pathways involved in the therapeutic action of IM remained elusive in the first years after its approval. This "enigma" has been partially resolved due to the publication of several articles reporting the effects of IM on skin cancer cells [10,23,25–27]. For these reasons, the aim of this review is to better define the molecular mechanisms of action of IM and its indications in cutaneous neoplastic disorders.

2. Chemical Structure and Pharmacokinetics

The chemical structure of IM is 1-(2-methylpropyl)-1H-imadazo[4,5-c]quinolin-4-amine (imidazoquinoline) [1,14,28]. This small molecule (240.3 Da) and nucleoside analogue was initially discovered in a programme to develop inhibitors of herpes simplex virus replication [6,10,14,28–30].

IM is commercially available as an oil-in-water-based 3.75–5% varnishing cream in sachets [11,31]. Manufacturers recommend its application at bedtime [28]. No more than one sachet should be applied to a contiguous area during each application [11,31]. While treating periocular tumours, it is suggested to apply the product with a swab onto the lesion to avoid contact with the cornea or conjunctiva [20]. Occlusion should be avoided since it does not increase efficacy and causes more severe local reactions [1,14,32]. Despite IM lacking the potential for inducing phototoxic and photoallergic reactions, the exposure to UV radiation should be minimized because of an increased sunburn susceptibility secondary to the vehicle [11,14]. Consequently, the site of treatment should be cleaned with soap and water 8 h afterwards [11,31]. Patients need to wash their hands before and after its use [11,31].

Therapeutic regimens are individualized according to clinical and/or histological diagnosis, the severity of the condition and expected tolerance and compliance by the patient [14]. The frequency of use is highly variable and may be daily with rest periods, 2–3 times/week [14]. etc. The duration of the treatment commonly ranges from 6 to 16 weeks [1].

Despite minimal systemic absorption, with a median bioavailability from 1% (one-two sachets, five times/week) to 3% (six sachets, five times/week), IM is still classified as a pregnancy category C drug [14]. Thus, contraception is encouraged for women of childbearing age while on treatment [11]. In relation to other special populations, it is unknown whether IM is excreted in the milk [1]. In contrast, its safety in paediatric subjects aged 2–12 years has been assessed in double-blind RCTs [14].

3. Mechanisms of Action

UV-induced skin carcinogenesis mostly relies on two mechanisms:

- DNA damage. Chronic UV exposure leads to the accumulation of DNA mutations that surpass the physiological repair mechanisms [4,22]. Whereas UVA (320–400 nm) causes indirect genetic damage through photooxidative stress, UVB (290–320 nm) directly induces the formation of thymidine dimers and C-T/CC-TT conversions [33].
- Impaired T-cell immune surveillance, either locally through the reduction in and inactivation of Langerhans cells (LC), or systemically by skewing the differentiation of T helper cells to an immunosuppressive phenotype [29,34].

Immunosurveillance is vital for the survival of malignant cells [28]. Tumours develop different mechanisms to escape recognition by immune cells, such as the following:

- Reduced expression of major histocompatibility complex (MHC) I, preventing antigen presentation [4].
- Generation of an immunosuppressive tumoral microenvironment through the liberation of pro-tumoral cytokines (i.e., IL-10 and TFG-β) and the recruitment of $CD4^+CD25^+FoxP3^+$ regulatory T cells, myeloid-derived suppressor cells, N2-polarized neutrophils, tumour-associated macrophages and tolerogenic dendritic cells (DC) [4,34,35].
- Resistance to apoptosis [4].

For these reasons, therapeutic agents, such as IM, that simultaneously bypass tumoral resistance to apoptosis and stimulate immune recognition have a considerable clinical benefit in the management of cutaneous malignancies [28].

Depending on the molecular target, the effects of IM can be divided into TLR7-dependent and TLR7-independent.

3.1. TLR7-Dependent Effects

TLR7 plays an important role in recognizing pathogen-associated molecular patterns (PAMPs) [14,35]. This membrane receptor is mostly found in macrophages, monocytes, DCs and LCs, although it can be also expressed by other immune cell types [5].

IM mainly binds TLR7, although it can also serve as a TLR8 analogue in high concentrations [28,35]. TLR7-IM binding triggers a MyD88-dependent signalling cascade, recruiting protein kinases and ultimately stimulating the NF-κβ transcription factor, enhancing the transcription of numerous pro-inflammatory genes [1,14,19,28].

The effects of IM are thus pleiotropic, strongly activating the innate immune system while providing a link to the adaptative immunity [1,14]:

- The innate immune system is the first line of defence against non-specific infectious pathogens and different physical or chemical insults [1]. Several cell types (neutrophils, eosinophils, natural killer (NK) cells, basophils and mast cells) participate through phagocytosis, chemokine synthesis and inflammatory mediators [1].
- Epidermal and dermal plasmacytoid dendritic cells (pDC) are the primary skin cell population responsive to IM since they are stimulated in vitro using lower doses than other cell types [14]. IM specifically induces their functional maturation and migration to regional lymph nodes, which is essential for triggering a profound tumour-directed T cell response [14,28,34].
- After pDC, macrophages are one of the cell lines more sensitive to this IRM [14]. IM not only stimulates the survival of macrophages through the upregulation of potent apoptosis inhibitors, such as Fas-associated death domain-like IL-1β-converting enzyme inhibitory protein (FLICE), but also strongly activates their function through the upregulation of macrophage inflammatory proteins (MIP)-1α, MIP-1β, IL-1α, nitric oxide synthase (NOS) and CD40 [14].
- IM has been demonstrated to stimulate the synthesis of IFN-α, IFN-γ, TNF-α, IL-1a, IL-2, IL-6, IL-8, IL-10, IL-12, G-CSF and GM-CSF via macrophages and DC [1,5,14,19,28]. These molecules (specially IFN-γ, IL-12 and TNF-α), together with LC, skew naïf T cell differentiation towards a Th_1 phenotype, fostering a potent and antigen-specific adaptative immune response against tumour-associated antigens (TAA) [1,5,14,19,28].
- Interferons play an essential role in the antitumoral effects of IM [4,19]. IFN-α2a and IFN-α2b inhibit the growth of malignant cells and increase the expression of IL-12βR in CD4+ T cells [4,19]. The activation of this receptor leads to an additional synthesis of IFN-γ by naïve T cells [19]. Berman et al. [26] showed that after IFN-α treatment, BCC cells expressed FasR. FasR-FasL binding can occur after BCC cell– and/or BCC cell–T-cell interaction and activates the apoptotic extrinsic pathway [26]. Even a suicidal activation of FasR by BCC cells co-expressing FasR and FasL may happen [26].
- IM also upregulates vital cytokines (i.e., CCL5, CXCL9, CXCL10) for homing T cells [25]. After 3–6 days of treatment application, a brisk lichenoid and peritumoral inflammatory infiltrate consisting mainly of CD45RO+ T lymphocytes, DC and macrophages develops [2,14,24,29]. Afterwards, the peritumoral and intratumoral macrophage count increases [14].
- IM also enhances the antigen's further presentation process to T cells through the upregulation of costimulatory membrane receptors in antigen-presenting cells (APC), such as CD40, CD80, CD86 and ICAM1, and the expression of MHC I and MHC II [1,14]. Increased expression of MHC-I has also been confirmed in BCC cells [4].
- NK cells can also respond to IM [14,28,34]. For instance, it induces the expression of 2′5′-oligoadenylate synthetase and NOS [14,28,34].
- Additional mechanisms through which IM can hamper tumour growth and dissemination have been described [14,34,36]. It has shown clear antiangiogenic mechanisms by increasing the synthesis of anti-angiogenic molecules (IL-10, IL-12, tissue inhibitor of matrix metalloproteinase (TIMP), thrombospondin 1 and 2 (TSP-1/TSP-2)) and simultaneously downregulating the expression of pro-angiogenic factors (basic fibroblast growth factor (bFGF), matrix metalloproteinase-9 (MMP-9), vascular endothelial growth factor (VEGF), angiogenin and IL-8) [14,34,36]. This could be useful in neoplasms with a considerable formation of vessels, such as pyogenic granuloma, Kaposi's sarcoma, infantile haemangioma and angiosarcoma [34].
- After exposure to IM, the levels of MMP inhibitors (TIMP-1 and TIMP-2) are increased 14- and 5-fold, respectively, [34]. The cleavage of collagen IV by MMP is essential for local malignant invasion and systemic dissemination [34].
- Interestingly, IM inhibits IL-13 signalling, which is over-stimulated in most malignant neoplasms [5,25,28].

These immune effects correlate with the clinical findings observed in the RCTs and case series [32,37–41]. Whereas the initial intense inflammatory response within the first days of treatment depends on the activation of the innate immune system, the continuing improvement after treatment discontinuation (i.e., AK) might be secondary to the reversal of local immunosuppression of chronically sun-damaged areas, thus leading to a persistent and protective antitumoral skin Th_1-skewed immunity ("vaccination effect") [1,14,28].

3.2. TLR7-Independent Effects

It was initially though that the mechanism of action of IM relied only on the stimulation of the immune system [1]. This assertion was called into question when various authors reported the clearance of cutaneous lesions after treatment without clinically evident inflammatory signs [14]. Biopsies taken from BCC and AK after the discontinuation of IM confirmed the preservation of non-neoplastic cells [26]. Had its mechanism of action been entirely dependent on immunomodulation, the surrounding normal cells would have been damaged by the inflammatory infiltrate [29].

Since then, several works have been published that confirm that IRM displays direct antineoplastic activity:

- Impaired viability of neoplastic cells [29]. Schön et al. [29] detected a mean reduction in cell count of 40–70% after SCC and HaCaT lines were cultured with IM 50 μg/mL. The proapoptotic effect was dose-dependent [29].
- Disruption of the electron transport chain through the inhibition of the mitochondrial complex and cytosolic NQO2, facilitating electron leakage and robust production and accumulation of ROS [23]. The mitochondrial membrane collapse leads to ATP depletion, mitophagy and, ultimately, cell death [23].
- Mitochondrial fragmentation through dynamin-related GTPases, such as MFN1/2, OPA1 and DRP1, facilitating mitophagy [23].
- Activation of inflammasome, leading to increased synthesis of IL-1β and IL-18 [14,23].
- Inhibition of adenosine intracellular receptors in clinical dosing settings, showing the highest affinity for A_1 and A_{2A} subtypes [28]. This blocks an immunosuppressive feedback which strongly activates proinflammatory pathways [14,28].

These phenomena are more dominant in skin cancer cells than in normal keratinocytes [23]. Among these effects, the induction of autophagy is considered one of the most relevant mechanisms of action of IM [35]. Autophagy is a cellular response to bioenergetic stress that permits cell survival via a dual mechanism [10,27,35]:

- Engulfment of large cytoplasmic portions containing damaged organelles and long-lived macromolecules within double-membrane autophagosomes, subsequently fusing with lysosomes [10,27,35]. This leads to considerable internal remodelling and helps in maintaining the proper quality of the mitochondrial population [35].
- Generation of glycolytic substrates for ATP synthesis [10].

Autophagy is regulated by a family of highly preserved genes known as the ATG family and can be activated via the following processes [23,27]:

- ER-stress/PERK/PKR axis through ROS-dependent manner [23].
- Release of cathepsins B (CTB) and D (CTD) into the cytosol [27]. Massive ROS production induces lysosomal membrane peroxidation, affecting its integrity and increasing its permeability [27]. The release of cathepsins lowers the cytosolic pH and activates additional hydrolases, leading to the indiscriminate digestion of cellular components and, ultimately, to autophagic apoptosis [23,27]. If severe, it could result in uncontrolled cell necrosis [27].

Autophagy plays a dual role in cancer cells depending on the cell type and therapeutic mechanism of the drug [23]. For instance, IM-induced autophagy in APC accelerates the elimination of intracellular antigens and fosters the innate immune response [29,35].

Apart from these, IM shows noteworthy proapoptotic effects in clinical dosing settings, even in the absence of immune cells, overcoming the resistance of neoplastic cells to death signals [28]:

Extrinsic pathway (death-receptor induced apoptosis) [27]:

- The longevity of BCC cells is due, at least in part, to the absence of CD95 [26]. On the other hand, these cells strongly and diffusely express CD95 ligand (FasL), which is involved in the apoptosis of infiltrating antitumoral T cells, allowing the BCC to escape the host's immune surveillance [26].
- IM stimulates the expression of membrane-bound death receptors in sBCC cells, such as CD95 and CD95L (FasR, Fas-APO1 receptor system) [14,28,29]. CD4+ cells can trigger the apoptosis of malignant cells through CD95-CD95 ligand binding [4]. When this occurs, a signalling cascade ensues, which ultimately results in DNA fragmentation, cell–membrane blebbing and the expression of phagocytosis signalling molecules on the cell surface (Figure 1) [26]. These effects have been confirmed in vivo by Berman et al. [26], who excised 10 non-head primary BCC immediately after treatment with either IM 5% or placebo, applied five times/week for two weeks. The histological clearance rate was 80% in IM-treated BCC (vs. 0% in the placebo group) [26]. The expression of CD95 in BCC cells was 75% in IM-treated patients (vs. 0% in the placebo group) [26].
- Nevertheless, the expression and activation of CD95 and TRAIL receptors R1-R4 in SCC cell lines do not significantly change after exposure to IM [29].

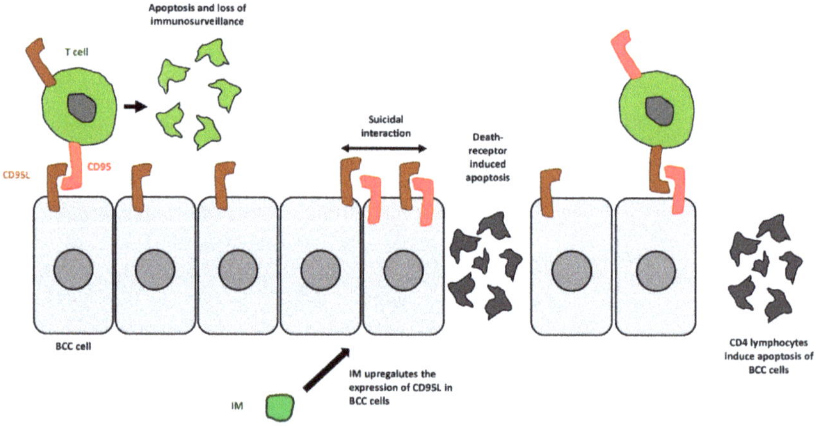

Figure 1. Extrinsic pathway of apoptosis induced by imiquimod (IM). Under normal conditions, basal cell carcinoma cells (BCC) lack CD95, which allows them to elude immunosurveillance. IM upregulates the expression of CD95 and CD95L in BCC cells, triggering the extrinsic pathway of apoptosis through BCC cell–BCC cell and BCC cell–CD4$^+$ T cell contact.

Intrinsic pathway (chemically induced apoptosis) [29]:

- It is the main apoptotic mechanism in SCC and melanoma cells, although it has been observed in BCC as well [10,27]. As a death-receptor-independent apoptosis pathway, its role in IM-induced apoptosis is critical since its inhibition in vitro with Z-IETD-FMK leads to increased cell viability [27].
- This pathway is mainly triggered by the bcl-2-dependent release of mitochondrial cytochrome C into the cytosol [14]. Then, cytochrome C binds APAF-1 and pro-caspase-9, building apoptosomes, which further activate caspase-9 and caspase-3 [28,29]. This has been confirmed in BCC cell lines [28,29]. Caspases are essential in IM-induced apoptosis, since the in vitro use of pan-caspase inhibitors completely abrogates it [28,29].

- The translocation of cytochrome c depends on the ratio between antiapoptotic (bcl-2, mcl-1, bcl-x_L) and proapoptotic (bax, bak, bid) mitochondrial membrane-bound proteins [28,29]. IM dramatically and rapidly inhibits the translation of bcl-2, mcl-1, bcl-x_L and other antiapoptotic proteins in BCC cells (Figure 2) [10,14,28]. It has been shown that IM blocks the initiation and elongation phases of mcl-1 translation by decreasing the levels of phosphorylated 4E-BP1 and stimulating the phosphorylation of eEf2 [10].
- CTSB and CTSD, whose release into the cytosol is induced by IM, activate the proapoptotic protein Bid [27]. This increases the permeability of the mitochondrial outer membrane, causing cytosolic translocation of cytochrome c, inhibition of mitochondrial complex I and a decrease in mitochondrial membrane potential [27].
- CTSD indirectly activates effector caspases (caspase-3 and caspase-7), which, in turn, target proteins involved in the apoptotic response [27,29]. Importantly, the activation of caspase-3 has been confirmed in SCC cell lines after treatment with IM, increasing the pro-caspase-3/caspase-3 ratio to 10:1 compared with that of vehicle-treated cultures [27,29].
- Downregulation of antiapoptotic genes (hurpin and HAX-1) in AK cells [28].
- Oncogenic signalling modulation:
- Downregulation of several MAPK-related genes (MAP2K4, MAPK1, MAPK11 and MAP3K5) in BSM [25].
- Inhibition of Hedgehog signalling through adenosine receptor/protein kinase A-mediated GLI phosphorylation [34].

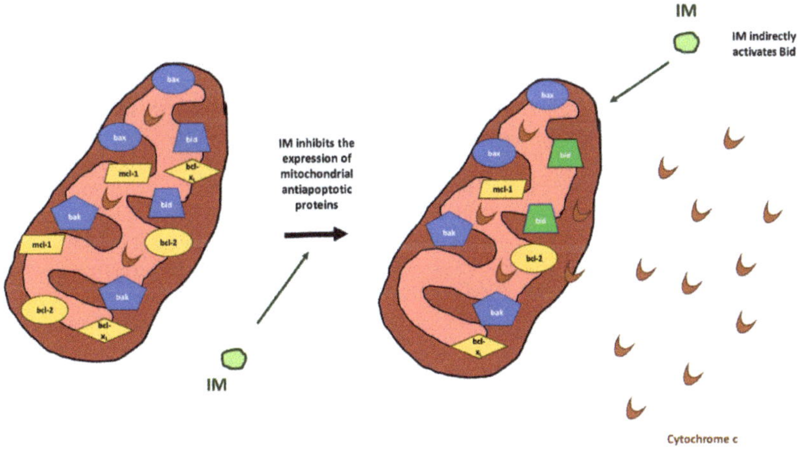

Figure 2. Intrinsic pathway of apoptosis induced by imiquimod (IM). IM induces a disbalance between mitochondrial proapoptotic (blue: bax, bak, bid) and antiapoptotic (yellow: bcl-2, bcl-x_L, mcl-1), favouring the translocation of cytochrome c into the cytosol. This leads to the activation of caspases and, ultimately, cell death.

In conclusion, IM fosters a potent tumour-directed response through the activation of simultaneous and synergistic antineoplastic pathways [14].

4. Clinical Indications

4.1. Actinic Keratoses

AK are intraepithelial dysplasias that involve the basal cell layer and can additionally extend to the overlying strata [33]. They consist of proliferating atypical keratinocytes with large nucleus/cytoplasm ratios, hyperchromatic nuclei, marked nuclear and cell pleomorphism, disordered terminal differentiation and a loss of polarity [33].

They are the most frequent carcinoma diagnosed in situ in humans [24,33]. AK arise in chronically light-exposed areas (face, back of the hands, and scalp in bald individuals) and are thus associated with cumulative lifetime sun exposure (i.e., outdoor work) [8,14,33,42]. Their incidence has continue to increased over the past few decades [33]. The prevalence of AK in the United Kingdom is estimated to be 34% in males and 18% in females older than 70 years of age [33]. Immunosuppressed hosts have a 250-fold risk of developing AK, with at least 40% of affected individuals progressing to invasive squamous cell carcinoma [33]. Given its high prevalence, AK pose a considerable burden for healthcare systems [43]. Their diagnosis and treatment cost in the United States surpasses USD 1 billion dollars annually [43].

Clinically, AK are defined as multiple red-to-brown dry and rough macules or papules, ranging from a few millimetres up to 2 cm [33]. Sometimes, they are covered by an overlying hyperkeratotic scale [33].

AK are the best clinical indicator for the development of future cutaneous malignant neoplasms, especially SCC [42]. They are indeed regarded as the initial stage of a biological continuum that ranges from AK to BD and SCC [5]. These entities share mutations (p53, expression of telomerases) and chromosomic aberrations [33].

Nevertheless, the clinical behaviour of AK is unpredictable [43]. Whereas some lesions tend towards spontaneous regression (approximately 25% per annuum) or persistence without further changes, others convert to truly invasive carcinomas [43]. The annual progression rate to SCC has been recently estimated to range from 0% to 0.5% per lesion-year [43]. The risk seems to be lower in individuals with no history of previous NMSC [44]. Overall, the clinical factors for predicting the subsequent progression of AK are unfortunately not well-defined [5,44]. Given this uncertainty, every patient suffering from AK should be offered prompt and appropriate management [33,44]. AK are often managed in the clinical setting as chronic disorders, requiring different and even the repetition of distinct treatment modalities over the course of time [44,45].

IM is approved as a field cancerization treatment for the management of scalp and facial non-hypertrophic AK located in a contiguous area measuring 25 cm^2 or less [1,31]. Formulations of 2.5%, 3.75% and 5% are approved by the FDA [6]. Less concentrated formulations display similar efficacy with higher tolerability [6].

It must be applied once to three times per week for one to four months [11,14,18,31]. Additional doses could be prescribed to patients with an incomplete clinical response [11]. The duration and frequency are usually individualized according to the number of lesions and the severity of the disease, although treatment should not be extended for missed doses [1,14].

Short-term complete clearance at 3–6 months varies between 17.4–39%, with a mean reduction in lesion counts ranging from 55 to 86.6% [11,37,40,42,46–51]. At least 59% of patients experience a reduction in AK lesions by more than 75% [1]. The preventive potential effect against new clinically evident AK declines after the discontinuation of the treatment, practically disappearing 9 months afterwards, with a relapse rate of 17.4–39% and a lesion count near 50% of the baseline numbers [42,45].

Similarly to 5-fluorouracil (5-FU), IM may unmask subclinical preneoplastic changes during the first weeks of treatment in up to a half of patients, which is not associated with a worse final clinical outcome [1,22,45].

Nonetheless, IM is not the most efficacious treatment for preventing the progression of AK into SCC [44]. In a single-blind multicentre RCT in the Netherlands, the risk of developing SCC in the following four years after different field cancerization-directed treatments was assessed [44]. Immunocompetent patients older than 18 years of age with Fitzpatrick's phototypes I-IV and at least five AK lesions at the initial visit within a treatment area of 25–100 cm^2 were included [44]. A total of 156 patients were treated with IM 5%, three times/week, for 4 weeks [44]. The risk of developing SCC was 5.8% in patients treated with IM, which was higher than that in patients initially treated with 5-FU [44].

On the other hand, since there is a wide array of field cancerization-directed treatments with distinct and specific mechanisms of action, the combination of IM with other therapeutic options (photodynamic therapy (PDT), 5-FU, tirbanibulin, diclofenac) may display synergistic effects that could ultimately lead to improved clinical and histological outcomes [39,52,53]:

- IM + PDT. According to the available literature data, there are only two prospective trials where these two strategies were simultaneously or sequentially employed in the management of AK [52,53].
    - Sequential regimen. Pre-treatment with PDT may have several advantages: it reduces the lesion count, possibly increasing the tolerability of IM; and generates a residual inflammatory response that may bolster IM-induced stimulation of the immune system, thus increasing its efficacy [53]. Shaffelburg [53] performed a double-blind, vehicle-controlled, split-face clinical trial of 25 patients with at least 10 facial AK. They were first treated with PDT (20% 5-ALA, blue light, two monthly sessions), followed, one month later, by the application of IM 5% cream (two times/week, 16 weeks) only to a single half of the face [53]. The median AK lesion reduction at month 12 was higher in the sequential treatment group (86.7% vs. 73.1%, $p = 0.0023$) [53]. The adverse reactions reported were not severe [53].
    - Simultaneous regimen. Tanaka et al. [52] conducted a single-centre clinical trial where 18 patients with AK on the face, head and scalp where randomly allocated to receive 5% IM cream (three times/week for one month), PDT (20% 5-ALA PDT, red light, 50 J/cm^2, once/week for three weeks) or a simultaneous combination of both treatments (5-ALA PDT, 50 J/cm^2, every Monday for three weeks + IM 5% cream, every Wednesday and Friday for one month) [52]. The patients were clinically assessed one month after treatment discontinuation [52]. The clinical clearance rate was higher with IM+PDT (100% vs. 66.7% (IM) vs. 47.1% (PDT), $p < 0.05$) [52]. Adverse events were mild to moderate, and no statistically significant differences were found between the three groups, either in their incidence or in their severity [52].
- IM + 5-FU.
- To the best of our knowledge, the benefits of this specific combination in the management of AK have only been assessed in one single-centre open-label study [39]. A total of 64 patients with extensive AK on the face, scalp, upper limbs, or legs were concomitantly treated with three courses of 5-FU 5% cream (once daily in the morning, for seven days) and IM 5% cream (once daily in the night, for six days), with a hiatus of three to four weeks between each cycle [39]. A total of 25% of participants withdrew from the study, although the authors reported that only two patients (3.13%) abandoned the study because of side effects [39]. Interestingly, adverse reactions were rarer and milder in the second and third cycles, which could be secondary to a reduction in lesion count [39]. Treatment breaks were deemed essential to improve the tolerability of the combination and secure a proper compliance [39]. The authors claimed this technique was beneficial since the total duration of the regimen was still shorter than those commonly used in monotherapies [39]. Nevertheless, the lack of clinical variables (objective lesion count), comparison groups and histological assessment clearly affects the validity of their observations [39].
- Interestingly, Nahm et al. [54] recently published the results of a single-centre retrospective review of 327 patients with AK on the face or ears who employed a combination of IM 5% cream, 5-FU 2% solution and tretinoin 0.1% cream [54]. The participants applied the mix up to 30 times within a 76-day period at their discretion, at a maximum frequency of five times/week for six weeks [54]. They were instructed to individualize the frequency for mitigating excessive irritation [54]. One year after the discontinuation of the treatment, the risk of in-field (OR = 0.06, 95% CI [0.02, 0.15]) and out-field NMSC (OR = 0.25, 95% CI [0.14, 0.42]) was dramatically inferior to that in the year

before field-treatment [54]. The participants required fewer sessions of cryotherapy for managing AK (2.3 vs. 1.5, $p < 0.001$) [54]. Notwithstanding these excellent results, there were several biases: a retrospective nature, limited post-treatment follow-up and an undetermined AK count [54]. Future prospective studies and RCT are warranted to confirm and better understand these findings.

- There are no RCT that evaluate the efficacy of combination treatments of IM with tirbanibulin or diclofenac.

Moreover, the effectiveness and tolerability of the combination of IM with lesion-directed treatments has also been studied, especially with cryotherapy [55]. In a multicentre vehicle-controlled double-blind RCT, 247 patients with at least 10 typical facial AK were randomly treated with IM 3.75% cream (once daily for two weeks on the treatment, two weeks off the treatment, and once daily for two weeks on the treatment (two–two–two regimen)) or placebo [55]. At the first visit, a minimum of five AK were treated with cryosurgery in every participant of both groups according to the investigator's usual clinical practice [55]. There was a greater median percent reduction in lesion count at week 26 for the cryosurgery/IM group (86.5% vs. 50%, $p < 0.0001$) [55]. However, a considerable limitation of this study was the absence of a comparison between cryotherapy+IM and IM in monotherapy [55].

4.2. Bowen's Disease

BD is an intraepithelial dysplasia where the stratum basale is preserved, leading to a "horizon" appearance under a microscope [14]. It clinically manifests as enlarging erythematous, desquamative and often well-defined plaques [14].

The surgical treatment of BD is challenging due to its common location in difficult-to-treat areas (i.e., shins), extension and multifocal nature [14]. Thus, IM could serve as an adequate medical treatment [11]. Nevertheless, the scientific evidence is low and mainly consists of case reports [1,2,5,11,14,31]. Different regimens have been used (once daily, three times and five times per week for 3–20 weeks). The overall clearance rate ranges between 57 and 80% [1,2,5,11,14,31]. Thickness lesion and hyperkeratosis are associated with a poorer response [11].

4.3. Basal Cell Carcinoma

BCC is the most common human malignant neoplasm and the tumour with the highest mutational burden [6,14]. In total, 4.3 million cases of BCC are annually diagnosed in the U.S [6]. Its age-standardized incidence rate in Australia was set at 770 per 100,000 person years [6]. BCC incidence increases annually by 2–10%, especially in young women [3,9,34]. Intermittent and high UV exposure during recreational activities (i.e., sunburns during childhood and adolescence) is deemed to be the most important factor in the carcinogenesis of BCC [8]. They are most commonly located in the head and neck (70%) of middle-aged/elderly light-skin individuals [3,6,30]

Although its growth rate is usually slow, its clinical behaviour remains unpredictable [3,56]. If left untreated or inappropriately managed, BCC may cause considerable morbidity through the local invasion and destruction of surrounding tissues [3,6]. Nevertheless, it seldom metastasizes (0.0028–0.55%) [3,6,30].

Several histological subtypes have been described, with the most important being the following: superficial (sBCC, 20%, the commonest subtype in Australia), nodular (nBCC, 50–79%), infiltrative, morpheaform (5–10%), cystic, metatypical and basosquamous [3,6,8,30,57]. The histological classification is a key factor in deciding which is the most appropriate treatment for the patient since the cure and relapse rates differ between variants [6]. Consequently, depending on the clinical and histological patterns, BCC can be divided into two main risk categories (Table 2) [3].

Table 2. Differences between high-risk and low-risk basal cell carcinoma [3,15].

	Low Risk	High Risk
Histological subtype	– Superficial – Macronodular	– Morpheaform – Infiltrative – Micronodular
Perineural/perivascular infiltration	No	Yes
Size	<5 cm	>5 cm
Location	Remaining	– Centrofacial – Periocular – Ears
Other	Primary naïve tumour without associated high-risk factors	– Relapsing – Immunosuppression

As a non-surgical therapy, IM is reserved for the management of low-risk BCC where the control of histological margins is less important [3]. The application of the product should encompass a margin of 1–3 cm perilesional normal-appearing skin [24].

Most RCTs excluded sBCC and nBCC in immunosuppressed hosts, tumours with a surface area larger than 2 cm^2, BCC located in certain areas (anogenital region, hands, feet, within 1 cm of the hairline, eyes, nose, mouth or ears) and previously treated cases [1,3,57].

sBCC:

- IM is the most efficacious FDA-approved treatment for sBCC and is the preferred modality in low-risk areas [2,6]. sBCC is more responsive to IM than nBCC [1,5,6,14]. Only the 5% formulation is licensed [6].
- Different regimens have been employed: twice daily, once daily, and every other day for 6–16 weeks [15,58]. IM presents a clear dose–frequency relationship in the management of BCC [1,5,32,59]. Histological clearance at week 12 was complete if the patients were treated twice daily [14]. When the frequency was reduced, the rate progressively decreased to 82% (five times/week) and 52% (three times/week) [6,14]. A once-daily dosing, five days/week, for six weeks is the regimen approved by the FDA since it achieves a good complete clearance rate (81–90%) with an adequate safety profile [1,6,14,60].
- Overall clinical and histological clearance rates at 3–12 months range from 60% to 80% in well-defined RCTs [15]. The cure rates with varying treatment regimens, from twice daily to twice weekly, and with follow-ups between 12 weeks and 5 years range from 43% to 94% [12].

nBCC:

- IM is used off-label in the management of nBCC [6]. The preferred regimen (five times/ week for 12 weeks) shows a clearance rate of 50–65% [2,3,12,32]. Therefore, the overall efficacy of IM in nBCC is poor, with at least a third of the patients presenting residual disease after treatment discontinuation [11,61].
- Given these results, it has been hypothesized that pre-treatment with cryotherapy could enhance tumour immunogenicity and even provide a clinical benefit in BCC refractory to IM in monotherapy [62]. Messeguer et al. [62] selected 23 BCC (sBCC = 11, nBCC = 12), 1 to 2 cm in size, resistant to IM 5% cream in monotherapy, administered five times/week for six weeks [62]. Cryotherapy was applied one month after the completion of the initial therapy [62]. Beginning the same day, the participants applied a second cycle of IM 5% cream with the same dosing regimen [62]. The complete clearance rate at one month was 83%, which was still lower in nBCC (67% vs. 91%) [62]. Only one relapse was detected in the follow-up period (at least one year) [62]. Four tumours still required an additional cycle of cryoimmunotherapy [62]. However,

these results have several limitations: the study was open-label and lacked a control group, the follow-up period was limited, and a complete cure was not confirmed via biopsy [62].

- Additionally, IM can be employed as an adjunctive therapy to Mohs' surgery, electrodessication and curettage [8,14,63]. For instance, in an open-label uncontrolled single-site study, 14 patients with high-risk BCC (>2 cm) unfit for surgery, chemotherapy and radiotherapy were sequentially treated with initial vaporization with aCO_2 laser in ablative mode (initial parameters: 600 μs pulse duration, 45 mJ energy, repeat time 10 ms, stack level 2), followed by cycle therapies of diclofenac sodium 3% gel (once daily for five days) plus IM 5% cream (once daily for two days), up to a maximum of 24 weeks [64]. Nine patients relapsed during the treatment period [64]. Despite these interesting approaches, surgical excision remains the gold-standard treatment [15]. For instance, Sinx et al. [65] directed a multicentre noninferiority clinical trial where 145 immunocompetent patients with histologically proven primary nBCC of 4 to 20 mm, with or without a superficial component, were randomly assigned to be treated with surgical excision with a 3 mm safety margin, or curettage followed by treatment with 5% IM (five times per week, six weeks) [65]. The patients underwent clinical and dermoscopic assessment one year after the discontinuation of the treatment [65]. If treatment failure was suspected, a punch biopsy was carried out to confirm tumoral relapse [65]. One year after treatment, the relapse rate was superior in the group of curettage+IM (13.7% vs. 0%, $p = 0.0004$) [65]. Nonetheless, it should be highlighted that approximately a quarter of the patients (23.7%) treated with curettage+IM did not fully comply with the regimen [65]. No differences were detected as regards severe pain (13.5% vs. 27%, $p = 0.208$) [65]. However, the investigator-reported cosmetic outcome was superior [65].

4.4. Lentigo Maligna

Lentigo maligna is an in situ phase of melanoma which arises in chronically sun-damaged skin areas [14]. Since malignant cells are restricted to the epidermis, its metastasizing potential is limited [6,66]. It accounts for approximately 80% of all melanoma in situ (MIS) [66].

Its incidence is higher in elderly individuals, and it is most frequently located on the face [66]. A total of 53,120 new cases of MIS were reported in 2009 [66].

Although surgical excision is still considered the gold-standard treatment, its commonly large size at diagnosis and the patients' comorbidities make non-invasive treatment modalities good alternatives for the management of this condition [66]. Since melanoma is one of the most immunogenic malignancies, IM could theoretically serve as an appropriate antineoplastic treatment [67]. IM is in fact reserved as a third-line treatment for cases in which surgical excision or radiotherapy are not feasible, such as in elderly and/or fragile patients [6,14,17,66]. The clearance rates reported with IM have ranged from 66% to 100% [66]. The guidelines do not specify the optimal dosing, schedule or length of treatment [6,11,66]. However, reviews that assessed the outcomes of non-surgical therapies for LM recommended at least 60 applications, six to seven times/week [68,69]. Large controlled RCTs with long follow-up periods are nevertheless needed to define the best dosing regimen [6]. On the other hand, as the effects of IM are non-ablative, a hypothetical risk of local recurrence and progression to invasive melanoma exists [14]. These doubts are mainly raised by the difficulty in objectively assessing histological clearance after treatment [66].

Additionally, IM can be used as an adjuvant treatment to other therapeutic approaches, such as surgery or radiotherapy [6,11,35]. In this sense, Cho et al. [35] studied the synergistic effect of IM in radiotherapy-treated murine melanoma cell lines B16F1 and B16F10. After incubation for 24 h, an increase in autophagy-associated proteins was detected [35].

4.5. Melanoma Skin Metastases

The management of metastatic melanoma is extremely complex [1]. Patients commonly require the combination of different treatments to better control the burden of the disease [14]. It has not been demonstrated whether the treatment of melanoma cutaneous and subcutaneous metastases has an impact on overall survival [1].

Although it can eradicate accessible dermal metastases, IM does not treat subcutaneous metastases and does not prevent lymphatic and systemic metastatic spreading [5,14,36]. Good clearance rates have been reported in refractory cases where IM was combined with isolated limb perfusion, intralesional IL-2, Bacillus Calmette–Guérin (BCG) vaccine, 5-fluorouracil or curettage [6,14,70–74].

RCTs are needed to better define the efficacy, dosing, schedule, and length of the treatment. The dosing schedule varies as follows: twice daily, once daily, five days/week (the most frequent) and once daily three times/week, for 8–72 weeks [6,14,70–74]. A complete clinical and histological regression was observed in approximately 82.3% of patients [36]. Clinical benefits may be detected after only 2 months of therapy [36].

4.6. Breast Cancer Skin Metastases

Breast cancer is the second most common malignancy to metastasize to the skin after melanoma [25]. BSM management is often challenging [25]. Although surgical resection and radiotherapy are the preferred treatments, BSM tend to relapse, leading to chest wall ulceration, pain and bleeding, which causes a great impact on the patient's physical and emotional well-being [25,75].

The scientific evidence regarding the use of IM in this condition relies solely on single case reports [75]. For instance, Henriques et al. [75] successfully treated a 26-year-old woman with a triple-negative invasive ductal carcinoma with skin metastases in her left lower neck and left supraclavicular region and upper back [75]. They were refractory to systemic chemotherapy, trastuzumab, lapatinib and locoregional radiotherapy [75]. A regimen of IM 5% three times/week for four months was prescribed. The lesions partially regressed and the pain intensity was decreased [75].

4.7. Extramammary Paget's Disease (EMPD)

EMPD is a rare skin malignancy that frequently arises in apocrine gland-rich anatomical regions, such as the anogenital area [5,76]. Its clinical course is often unpredictable, ranging from an indolent entity to an invasive neoplasm with locoregional and systemic dissemination [5]. The incidence is higher in patients aged 60 to 80 years [76]. It often presents as a genital plaque [76]. A better prognosis is expected if neoplastic cells are restricted to the epidermis [76]. Dermally invasive EMPD is associated with a risk of locoregional and systemic dissemination [76].

Due to its multifocal nature, aggressive surgical interventions have a high local recurrence risk [5]. For this reason, non-aggressive topical treatments such as IM are preferred, especially during the initial stages [5].

Data regarding the efficacy of IM are mostly based on case reports and series [5,76]. Sawada et al. [77] conducted a single-site nonrandomized prospective study where nine patients with in situ EMPD were enrolled. IM 5% cream was used three times per week for 6–16 weeks [77]. The product was applied in the lesions with a 1–2 cm circumferential margin [77]. The participants were assessed one month after the discontinuation of the treatment [77]. A complete clearance (clinical and histological) was achieved in five patients (56%) [77]. Nevertheless, the recurrence rate was high since three patients relapsed in the follow-up period (up to 46 months) [77]. No patient abandoned the study due to side effects [77]. Additionally, Cowan et al. [78] performed a nonrandomized prospective pilot trial study in eight patients with recurrent primary EMPD of the vulva. All of them had previously undergone partial or total vulvectomy [78]. IM 5% cream was used three times per week for 12 weeks. A complete clinical and histological response was observed in six patients (75%) by the follow-up appointment [78]. No participants progressed to invasive cancer while receiving active therapy [78]. Overall, the treatment was well-tolerated [78].

In conclusion, different treatment modalities have been used (daily to three times/week for 6–16 weeks) [5,76–78]. A regimen of 3–4 times/week for 6 months is the most recommended option [5,76–78].

4.8. Mycosis Fungoides

Primary cutaneous lymphomas (PCL) comprise a wide range of rare non-Hodgkin malignant monoclonal proliferations arising from skin-resident lymphocytes [79]. Cutaneous T-cell lymphomas represent the largest group of PCL (75%) [5], with mycosis fungoides (MF) being the most common form [5,79]. This disease is generally associated with an indolent clinical course [41].

IM could serve as a promising skin-directed drug for the management of cutaneous T-cell lymphomas at initial stages or even of plaques refractory to conventional treatments, such as psoralen+UVA or retinoids [5,80]. To the best of our knowledge, there are only two prospective studies that have evaluated the efficacy and safety of IM 5% cream in MF [41,81].

Deeths et al. [81] assessed the effectiveness of IM in six patients diagnosed with stable MF (stages IA-IIB). IM 5% cream was applied to a maximum of five lesions, three times per week for three months [81]. Three participants concomitantly received systemic therapy (photochemotherapy (n = 2) and systemic retinoids (n = 1)) [81]. All patients except one experienced some degree of clinical improvement [81]. The lesions were completely cleared in three participants, which was confirmed in the follow-up biopsy one month after the discontinuation of the treatment [81].

In a double-blind placebo-controlled RCT conducted by Chong et al. [41], four male patients with stage IB MF (T2N0M0) were treated with IM 5% cream once daily for 16 weeks [41]. The target area measured approximately 20 cm^2. Simultaneously, a distant control area was chosen [41]. At week 32, the lesions treated with IM showed a mean decrease in surface area of 8.9% (vs. 39.9%) [41]. The treatment was well-tolerated [41].

Subsequently, several case reports have been published that indicated a possible benefit of IM in the management of MF [80]. Most patients had limited skin involvement, with solitary patches or plaques not ideally suited for systemic treatments [41,80,82,83]. Different regimens were employed: once daily, every other day, and five times weekly [41,80,82,83]. The treatment's duration ranged from two weeks to six months [41,80,82,83]. The follow-up periods ranged from six to ten months [41,80,82,83]. However, future RCT with larger samples and longer follow-up periods are warranted to confirm these findings.

5. Adverse Reactions

IM has an overall good safety profile [5]. Most adverse reactions are mild to moderate, are easily manageable and do not require the discontinuation of the treatment, which only occurs in 2–3% of the cases [1,8]. Up to a third of patients might need pharmacological therapy to mitigate the side effects [45].

Nearly every single patient develops a local reaction consisting of a variable degree of erythema, and scaling in the treatment area [1]. In severe cases, they can be accompanied by erosions, ulceration, crusting and pain [1]. Irritation may even extend to the surrounding areas [11]. Interestingly, these inflammatory side effects occur only in previously damaged or pathological cutaneous tissue [1]. When IM is applied to healthy skin, it has been found to be no more irritating than a moisturizing lotion [1].

Since these adverse reactions are dose- and time-dependent, balancing its efficacy and tolerance is critical for assuring an adequate compliance on the patient's part [15,20]. If significant inflammation develops, the frequency of application can be reduced, which is needed in approximately 16% of the cases [11].

It is controversial whether the severity of the side effects is associated with a better clinical and histological response [15,34]. Several risk factors for intense local reactions have been described, such as low Fitzpatrick's phototypes (I-II), severe actinic damage and being of the female sex [1].

Apart from the classical side effects, other rarer complications have been identified [1,5,14], as follows:

- Scarring and hypopigmentation have been reported in isolated cases, especially in high-frequency regimens [5]. Nevertheless, the evidence on this topic is contradictory since patients treated with IM in AK studies showed an improvement in scarring and pigmentary scores after the treatment [1].
- Cytokine-release syndrome has seldom been noted and has been attributed to a larger synthesis and systemic release of IFN and other inflammatory mediators [1]. Its severity correlates with the size of the treated area and the degree of the local reaction induced [1].
- Contact sensitization and the exacerbation of pre-existing eczematous conditions [14].
- Hypertrophic lupus erythematosus-like reaction [21], which might be caused by the activation of plasmacytoid dendritic cells through TLR binding [21].
- Other autoimmune disorders, such as *pemphigus foliaceus*, psoriasis, autoimmune spondyloarthropathy and vitiligo [11,14].
- Angioedema [11,14].
- *Erythema multiforme* [11,14].
- Eruptive epidermoid cysts [11,14].
- Schönlein–Henoch purpura [11,14].
- Chronic neuropathic pain [11,14].

After its approval, there was a safety concern regarding the use of IM in transplanted hosts [84]. Due to an increase in IFN levels, it was hypothesized that the exposure to IM could lead to an increased risk of allograft rejection [84]. In double-blind, single-centre placebo RCT, 21 immunosuppressed renal transplant recipients were treated with IM 5% three times/week for 16 weeks for AK and viral warts [84]. None of the patients treated with IM had a deleterious effect on their renal allograft in the 1-year follow-up [84]. Nevertheless, a reduced efficacy was observed when compared to that of studies concerning immunocompetent hosts [84]. Higher-frequency regimens and combinations with other therapies should be taken into consideration in the clinical setting.

6. Conclusions

IM is a topically self-applied IRM that strongly activates the innate immune system and fosters a tumour-targeted T-cell response. Its mechanism of action is nonetheless pleiotropic since it displays direct antineoplastic effects through the stimulation of apoptosis, autophagy and mitochondrial disfunction. IM could represent a solid alternative to surgical resection in certain cases of skin cancer. Due to its non-aggressive nature, it preserves the cosmesis and functionality of critical areas better. Its side effects are often mild, predictable, and easily manageable. Although several case series and observational studies underline its efficacy in off-label indications, such as LM or nBCC, more RCTs are needed to confirm these findings and better define the optimal regimens.

Author Contributions: Conception, E.G.-M.; acquisition, analysis or interpretation of data, E.G.-M. and S.B.-A.; data curation, E.G.-M.; writing—original draft preparation, E.G.-M.; writing—review and editing, E.G.-M., E.B.-R., B.d.N.-R., C.A.-L., L.A.-M.d.S. and S.B.-A. All authors have read and agreed to the published version of the manuscript.

Funding: This research has been funded by a Spanish grant from Instituto de Salud Carlos III MINECO and Peder Funds (PI21/00315) and by Fundación para la Investigación Biomédica del Hospital Universitario Ramón y Cajal (2020/0142).

Institutional Review Board Statement: Not applicable.

Informed Consent Statement: Not applicable.

Data Availability Statement: All the data are presented in this study.

Conflicts of Interest: The authors declare no conflict of interest.

Abbreviations

5-FU	5-fluorouracil
AK	actinic keratosis
APC	antigen-presenting cells
BCC	basal cell carcinoma
BCG	Bacillus Calmette–Guérin
BD	Bowen's disease
BSM	breast skin metastases
bFGF	basic fibroblast growth factor
CTB	cathepsin B
CTD	cathepsin D
EMPD	extramammary Paget's disease
DC	dendritic cells
FDA	Food and Drug Administration
FLICE	Fas-associated death domain-like IL-1β-converting enzyme inhibitory protein
G-CSF	granulocyte colony stimulating factor
GM-CSF	granulocyte and monocyte stimulating factor
HPV	human papillomavirus
IM	imiquimod
IRM	immune response modifiers
LC	Langerhans cells
LM	lentigo maligna
MF	mycosis fungoides
MHC	major histocompatibility complex
MIP	macrophage inflammatory proteins
MIS	melanoma in situ
MMP-9	matrix metalloproteinase-9
NK cells	natural killer cells
NMSC	nonmelanoma skin cancer
NOS	nitric oxide synthase
nBCC	nodular basal cell carcinoma
pDC	plasmacytoid dendritic cells
PCL	primary cutaneous lymphoma
PDT	photodynamic therapy
PTCH	protein patched homolog
RCT	randomized clinical trial
sBCC	superficial basal cell carcinoma
PAMP	pathogen-associated molecular pattern
PCL	primary cutaneous lymphoma
SCC	squamous cell carcinoma
TAAs	tumour-associated antigens
TIMP	tissue inhibitor of matrix metalloproteinase
TLR	Toll-like receptor
TRAIL	TNF-related apoptosis-inducing ligand
TSP-1	thrombospondin-1
UV	ultraviolet
VEGF	vascular endothelial growth factor

References

1. Burns, C.A.; Brown, M.D. Imiquimod for the Treatment of Skin Cancer. *Dermatol. Clin.* **2005**, *23*, 151–164. [CrossRef] [PubMed]
2. Collins, A.; Savas, J.; Doerfler, L. Nonsurgical Treatments for Nonmelanoma Skin Cancer. *Dermatol. Clin.* **2019**, *37*, 435–441. [CrossRef] [PubMed]
3. Thomson, J.; Hogan, S.; Leonardi-Bee, J.; Williams, H.C.; Bath-Hextall, F.J. Interventions for Basal Cell Carcinoma of the Skin. *Cochrane Database Syst. Rev.* **2020**, *11*, CD003412. [CrossRef] [PubMed]
4. Ghafouri-Fard, S.; Ghafouri-Fard, S. Immunotherapy in Nonmelanoma Skin Cancer. *Immunotherapy* **2012**, *4*, 499–510. [CrossRef]
5. Urosevic, M.; Dummer, R. Role of Imiquimod in Skin Cancer Treatment. *Am. J. Clin. Dermatol.* **2004**, *5*, 453–458. [CrossRef]

6. Cullen, J.K.; Simmons, J.L.; Parsons, P.G.; Boyle, G.M. Topical Treatments for Skin Cancer. *Adv. Drug Deliv. Rev.* **2020**, *153*, 54–64. [CrossRef]
7. Nahm, W.J.; Shen, J.; Zito, P.M.; Gonzalez, A.M.; Nagrani, N.; Moore, K.; Badiavas, E.V.; Kirsner, R.S.; Nichols, A.J. A Non-Surgical and Cost-Effective Treatment Approach Employing Topical Imiquimod, 5-Fluorouracil, and Tretinoin for Primary Non-Melanoma Skin Cancers. *J. Drugs Dermatol. JDD* **2021**, *20*, 260–267. [CrossRef]
8. Čeović, R.; Petković, M.; Mokos, Z.B.; Kostović, K. Nonsurgical Treatment of Nonmelanoma Skin Cancer in the Mature Patient. *Clin. Dermatol.* **2018**, *36*, 177–187. [CrossRef]
9. Banzhaf, C.A.; Themstrup, L.; Ring, H.C.; Mogensen, M.; Jemec, G.B.E. Optical Coherence Tomography Imaging of Non-Melanoma Skin Cancer Undergoing Imiquimod Therapy. *Skin Res. Technol. Off. J. Int. Soc. Bioeng. Skin ISBS Int. Soc. Digit. Imaging Skin ISDIS Int. Soc. Skin Imaging ISSI* **2014**, *20*, 170–176. [CrossRef]
10. Huang, S.-W.; Chang, C.-C.; Lin, C.-C.; Tsai, J.-J.; Chen, Y.-J.; Wu, C.-Y.; Liu, K.-T.; Shieh, J.-J. Mcl-1 Determines the Imiquimod-Induced Apoptosis but Not Imiquimod-Induced Autophagy in Skin Cancer Cells. *J. Dermatol. Sci.* **2012**, *65*, 170–178. [CrossRef]
11. Micali, G.; Lacarrubba, F.; Dinotta, F.; Massimino, D.; Nasca, M.R. Treating Skin Cancer with Topical Cream. *Expert Opin. Pharmacother.* **2010**, *11*, 1515–1527. [CrossRef]
12. Bahner, J.D.; Bordeaux, J.S. Non-Melanoma Skin Cancers: Photodynamic Therapy, Cryotherapy, 5-Fluorouracil, Imiquimod, Diclofenac, or What? Facts and Controversies. *Clin. Dermatol.* **2013**, *31*, 792–798. [CrossRef] [PubMed]
13. Ruiz, E.S.; Cohen, J.L.; Friedman, A. Before or after: Is There a Connection between the Use of Adjunctive Nonmelanoma Skin Cancer Treatments and Subsequent Invasive Tumors? *J. Drugs Dermatol. JDD* **2015**, *14*, 450–452.
14. Papadavid, E.; Stratigos, A.J.; Falagas, M.E. Imiquimod: An Immune Response Modifier in the Treatment of Precancerous Skin Lesions and Skin Cancer. *Expert Opin. Pharmacother.* **2007**, *8*, 1743–1755. [CrossRef] [PubMed]
15. Work Group; Invited Reviewers; Kim, J.Y.S.; Kozlow, J.H.; Mittal, B.; Moyer, J.; Olencki, T.; Rodgers, P. Guidelines of Care for the Management of Basal Cell Carcinoma. *J. Am. Acad. Dermatol.* **2018**, *78*, 540–559. [CrossRef]
16. Peris, K.; Fargnoli, M.C.; Garbe, C.; Kaufmann, R.; Bastholt, L.; Seguin, N.B.; Bataille, V.; Marmol, V.D.; Dummer, R.; Harwood, C.A.; et al. Diagnosis and Treatment of Basal Cell Carcinoma: European Consensus-Based Interdisciplinary Guidelines. *Eur. J. Cancer Oxf. Engl. 1990* **2019**, *118*, 10–34. [CrossRef] [PubMed]
17. Robinson, M.; Primiero, C.; Guitera, P.; Hong, A.; Scolyer, R.A.; Stretch, J.R.; Strutton, G.; Thompson, J.F.; Soyer, H.P. Evidence-Based Clinical Practice Guidelines for the Management of Patients with Lentigo Maligna. *Dermatol. Basel Switz.* **2020**, *236*, 111–116. [CrossRef] [PubMed]
18. Eisen, D.B.; Asgari, M.M.; Bennett, D.D.; Connolly, S.M.; Dellavalle, R.P.; Freeman, E.E.; Goldenberg, G.; Leffell, D.J.; Peschin, S.; Sligh, J.E.; et al. Guidelines of Care for the Management of Actinic Keratosis. *J. Am. Acad. Dermatol.* **2021**, *85*, e209–e233. [CrossRef]
19. Woodmansee, C.; Pillow, J.; Skinner, R.B. The Role of Topical Immune Response Modifiers in Skin Cancer. *Drugs* **2006**, *66*, 1657–1664. [CrossRef]
20. Avallone, G.; Merli, M.; Dell'Aquila, C.; Quaglino, P.; Ribero, S.; Zalaudek, I.; Conforti, C. Imiquimod-Side Effects in the Treatment of Periocular Skin Cancers: A Review of the Literature. *Dermatol. Ther.* **2022**, *35*, e15326. [CrossRef]
21. Safadi, M.G.; Hassan, S.; Patel, V.; Viglione, M.; Zahner, S.L. Imiquimod-Induced Hypertrophic Lupus Erythematosus-like Reaction. *Dermatol. Online J.* **2022**, *28*, 12. [CrossRef]
22. Kopera, D. Earliest Stage Treatment of Actinic Keratosis with Imiquimod 3.75% Cream: Two Case Reports-Perspective for Non Melanoma Skin Cancer Prevention. *Dermatol. Ther.* **2020**, *33*, e13517. [CrossRef]
23. Chuang, K.-C.; Chang, C.-R.; Chang, S.-H.; Huang, S.-W.; Chuang, S.-M.; Li, Z.-Y.; Wang, S.-T.; Kao, J.-K.; Chen, Y.-J.; Shieh, J.-J. Imiquimod-Induced ROS Production Disrupts the Balance of Mitochondrial Dynamics and Increases Mitophagy in Skin Cancer Cells. *J. Dermatol. Sci.* **2020**, *98*, 152–162. [CrossRef]
24. Uhoda, I.; Quatresooz, P.; Piérard-Franchimont, C.; Piérard, G.E. Nudging Epidermal Field Cancerogenesis by Imiquimod. *Dermatol. Basel Switz.* **2003**, *206*, 357–360. [CrossRef] [PubMed]
25. Rozenblit, M.; Hendrickx, W.; Heguy, A.; Chiriboga, L.; Loomis, C.; Ray, K.; Darvishian, F.; Egeblad, M.; Demaria, S.; Marincola, F.M.; et al. Transcriptomic Profiles Conducive to Immune-Mediated Tumor Rejection in Human Breast Cancer Skin Metastases Treated with Imiquimod. *Sci. Rep.* **2019**, *9*, 8572. [CrossRef] [PubMed]
26. Berman, B.; Sullivan, T.; De Araujo, T.; Nadji, M. Expression of Fas-Receptor on Basal Cell Carcinomas after Treatment with Imiquimod 5% Cream or Vehicle. *Br. J. Dermatol.* **2003**, *149* (Suppl. S66), 59–61. [CrossRef] [PubMed]
27. Chang, S.-H.; Lin, P.-Y.; Wu, T.-K.; Hsu, C.-S.; Huang, S.-W.; Li, Z.-Y.; Liu, K.-T.; Kao, J.-K.; Chen, Y.-J.; Wong, T.-W.; et al. Imiquimod-Induced ROS Production Causes Lysosomal Membrane Permeabilization and Activates Caspase-8-Mediated Apoptosis in Skin Cancer Cells. *J. Dermatol. Sci.* **2022**, *107*, 142–150. [CrossRef]
28. Schön, M.P.; Schön, M. The Small-Molecule Immune Response Modifier Imiquimod--Its Mode of Action and Clinical Use in the Treatment of Skin Cancer. *Expert Opin. Ther. Targets* **2006**, *10*, 69–76. [CrossRef] [PubMed]
29. Schön, M.; Bong, A.B.; Drewniok, C.; Herz, J.; Geilen, C.C.; Reifenberger, J.; Benninghoff, B.; Slade, H.B.; Gollnick, H.; Schön, M.P. Tumor-Selective Induction of Apoptosis and the Small-Molecule Immune Response Modifier Imiquimod. *J. Natl. Cancer Inst.* **2003**, *95*, 1138–1149. [CrossRef]
30. Tandon, Y.; Brodell, R.T. Local Reactions to Imiquimod in the Treatment of Basal Cell Carcinoma. *Dermatol. Online J.* **2012**, *18*, 1. [CrossRef]

31. Nemer, K.M.; Council, M.L. Topical and Systemic Modalities for Chemoprevention of Nonmelanoma Skin Cancer. *Dermatol. Clin.* **2019**, *37*, 287–295. [CrossRef] [PubMed]
32. Sterry, W.; Ruzicka, T.; Herrera, E.; Takwale, A.; Bichel, J.; Andres, K.; Ding, L.; Thissen, M.R.T.M. Imiquimod 5% Cream for the Treatment of Superficial and Nodular Basal Cell Carcinoma: Randomized Studies Comparing Low-Frequency Dosing with and without Occlusion. *Br. J. Dermatol.* **2002**, *147*, 1227–1236. [CrossRef]
33. Stockfleth, E. Actinic Keratoses. *Cancer Treat. Res.* **2009**, *146*, 227–239. [CrossRef] [PubMed]
34. Voiculescu, V.M.; Lisievici, C.V.; Lupu, M.; Vajaitu, C.; Draghici, C.C.; Popa, A.V.; Solomon, I.; Sebe, T.I.; Constantin, M.M.; Caruntu, C. Mediators of Inflammation in Topical Therapy of Skin Cancers. *Mediat. Inflamm.* **2019**, *2019*, 8369690. [CrossRef] [PubMed]
35. Cho, J.H.; Lee, H.-J.; Ko, H.-J.; Yoon, B.-I.; Choe, J.; Kim, K.-C.; Hahn, T.-W.; Han, J.A.; Choi, S.S.; Jung, Y.M.; et al. The TLR7 Agonist Imiquimod Induces Anti-Cancer Effects via Autophagic Cell Death and Enhances Anti-Tumoral and Systemic Immunity during Radiotherapy for Melanoma. *Oncotarget* **2017**, *8*, 24932–24948. [CrossRef]
36. Sisti, A.; Sisti, G.; Oranges, C.M. Topical Treatment of Melanoma Skin Metastases with Imiquimod: A Review. *Dermatol. Online J.* **2015**, *21*. [CrossRef]
37. Szeimies, R.-M.; Gerritsen, M.-J.P.; Gupta, G.; Ortonne, J.P.; Serresi, S.; Bichel, J.; Lee, J.H.; Fox, T.L.; Alomar, A. Imiquimod 5% Cream for the Treatment of Actinic Keratosis: Results from a Phase III, Randomized, Double-Blind, Vehicle-Controlled, Clinical Trial with Histology. *J. Am. Acad. Dermatol.* **2004**, *51*, 547–555. [CrossRef]
38. Marsden, J.R.; Fox, R.; Boota, N.M.; Cook, M.; Wheatley, K.; Billingham, L.J.; Steven, N.M.; on behalf of the NCRI Skin Cancer Clinical Studies Group, the U.K. Dermatology Clinical Trials Network and the LIMIT-1 Collaborative Group. Effect of Topical Imiquimod as Primary Treatment for Lentigo Maligna: The LIMIT-1 Study. *Br. J. Dermatol.* **2017**, *176*, 1148–1154. [CrossRef]
39. Price, N.M. The Treatment of Actinic Keratoses with a Combination of 5-Fluorouracil and Imiquimod Creams. *J. Drugs Dermatol. JDD* **2007**, *6*, 778–781.
40. Alomar, A.; Bichel, J.; McRae, S. Vehicle-controlled, Randomized, Double-blind Study to Assess Safety and Efficacy of Imiquimod 5% Cream Applied Once Daily 3 Days per Week in One or Two Courses of Treatment of Actinic Keratoses on the Head. *Br. J. Dermatol.* **2007**, *157*, 133–141. [CrossRef]
41. Chong, A.; Loo, W.J.; Banney, L.; Grant, J.W.; Norris, P.G. Imiquimod 5% Cream in the Treatment of Mycosis Fungoides—A Pilot Study. *J. Dermatol. Treat.* **2004**, *15*, 118–119. [CrossRef]
42. Sinclair, R.; Baker, C.; Spelman, L.; Supranowicz, M.; MacMahon, B. A Review of Actinic Keratosis, Skin Field Cancerisation and the Efficacy of Topical Therapies. *Australas. J. Dermatol.* **2021**, *62*, 119–123. [CrossRef] [PubMed]
43. Navarrete-Dechent, C.; Marghoob, A.A.; Marchetti, M.A. Contemporary Management of Actinic Keratosis. *J. Dermatol. Treat.* **2021**, *32*, 572–574. [CrossRef] [PubMed]
44. Ahmady, S.; Jansen, M.H.E.; Nelemans, P.J.; Kessels, J.P.H.M.; Arits, A.H.M.M.; de Rooij, M.J.M.; Essers, B.A.B.; Quaedvlieg, P.J.F.; Kelleners-Smeets, N.W.J.; Mosterd, K. Risk of Invasive Cutaneous Squamous Cell Carcinoma After Different Treatments for Actinic Keratosis: A Secondary Analysis of a Randomized Clinical Trial. *JAMA Dermatol.* **2022**, *158*, 634–640. [CrossRef] [PubMed]
45. Sotiriou, E.; Apalla, Z.; Vrani, F.; Lallas, A.; Chovarda, E.; Ioannides, D. Photodynamic Therapy vs. Imiquimod 5% Cream as Skin Cancer Preventive Strategies in Patients with Field Changes: A Randomized Intraindividual Comparison Study. *J. Eur. Acad. Dermatol. Venereol. JEADV* **2015**, *29*, 325–329. [CrossRef]
46. Chen, K.; Yap, L.M.; Marks, R.; Shumack, S. Short-Course Therapy with Imiquimod 5% Cream for Solar Keratoses: A Randomized Controlled Trial. *Australas. J. Dermatol.* **2003**, *44*, 250–255. [CrossRef]
47. Gebauer, K.; Shumack, S.; Cowen, P.S.J. Effect of Dosing Frequency on the Safety and Efficacy of Imiquimod 5% Cream for Treatment of Actinic Keratosis on the Forearms and Hands: A Phase II, Randomized Placebo-Controlled Trial. *Br. J. Dermatol.* **2009**, *161*, 897–903. [CrossRef]
48. Hanke, C.W.; Beer, K.R.; Stockfleth, E.; Wu, J.; Rosen, T.; Levy, S. Imiquimod 2.5% and 3.75% for the Treatment of Actinic Keratoses: Results of Two Placebo-Controlled Studies of Daily Application to the Face and Balding Scalp for Two 3-Week Cycles. *J. Am. Acad. Dermatol.* **2010**, *62*, 573–581. [CrossRef]
49. Jorizzo, J.; Dinehart, S.; Matheson, R.; Moore, J.K.; Ling, M.; Fox, T.L.; McRae, S.; Fielder, S.; Lee, J.H. Vehicle-Controlled, Double-Blind, Randomized Study of Imiquimod 5% Cream Applied 3 Days per Week in One or Two Courses of Treatment for Actinic Keratoses on the Head. *J. Am. Acad. Dermatol.* **2007**, *57*, 265–268. [CrossRef]
50. Korman, N.; Moy, R.; Ling, M.; Matheson, R.; Smith, S.; McKane, S.; Lee, J.H. Dosing with 5% Imiquimod Cream 3 Times per Week for the Treatment of Actinic Keratosis: Results of Two Phase 3, Randomized, Double-Blind, Parallel-Group, Vehicle-Controlled Trials. *Arch. Dermatol.* **2005**, *141*, 467–473. [CrossRef]
51. Stockfleth, E.; Meyer, T.; Benninghoff, B.; Salasche, S.; Papadopoulos, L.; Ulrich, C.; Christophers, E. A Randomized, Double-Blind, Vehicle-Controlled Study to Assess 5% Imiquimod Cream for the Treatment of Multiple Actinic Keratoses. *Arch. Dermatol.* **2002**, *138*, 1498–1502. [CrossRef]
52. Tanaka, N.; Ohata, C.; Ishii, N.; Imamura, K.; Ueda, A.; Furumura, M.; Yasumoto, S.; Kawakami, T.; Tsuruta, D.; Hashimoto, T. Comparative Study for the Effect of Photodynamic Therapy, Imiquimod Immunotherapy and Combination of Both Therapies on 40 Lesions of Actinic Keratosis in Japanese Patients. *J. Dermatol.* **2013**, *40*, 962–967. [CrossRef] [PubMed]

53. Shaffelburg, M. Treatment of Actinic Keratoses with Sequential Use of Photodynamic Therapy; and Imiquimod 5% Cream. *J. Drugs Dermatol. JDD* **2009**, *8*, 35–39.
54. Nahm, W.; Nichols, A.; Rapoport, E.; Kirsner, R.; Badiavas, E.; Wyant, W.; Arthur, A.; Shen, J. Keratinocyte Carcinoma Chemoprevention With a Combination of Imiquimod, 5-Fluorouracil, and Tretinoin. *J. Drugs Dermatol. JDD* **2023**, *22*, 486–490. [CrossRef] [PubMed]
55. Jorizzo, J.L.; Markowitz, O.; Lebwohl, M.G.; Bourcier, M.; Kulp, J.; Meng, T.-C.; Levy, S. A Randomized, Double-Blinded, Placebo-Controlled, Multicenter, Efficacy and Safety Study of 3.75% Imiquimod Cream Following Cryosurgery for the Treatment of Actinic Keratoses. *J. Drugs Dermatol. JDD* **2010**, *9*, 1101–1108. [PubMed]
56. Bostanci, S.; Kocyigit, P.; Vural, S.; Heper, A.O.; Botsali, A. Long-Term Follow-Up Results of Topical Imiquimod Treatment in Basal Cell Carcinoma. *Dermatol. Surg. Off. Publ. Am. Soc. Dermatol. Surg. Al* **2018**, *44*, 36–41. [CrossRef] [PubMed]
57. Geisse, J.K.; Rich, P.; Pandya, A.; Gross, K.; Andres, K.; Ginkel, A.; Owens, M. Imiquimod 5% Cream for the Treatment of Superficial Basal Cell Carcinoma: A Double-Blind, Randomized, Vehicle-Controlled Study. *J. Am. Acad. Dermatol.* **2002**, *47*, 390–398. [CrossRef]
58. Schulze, H.J.; Cribier, B.; Requena, L.; Reifenberger, J.; Ferrándiz, C.; Garcia Diez, A.; Tebbs, V.; McRae, S. Imiquimod 5% Cream for the Treatment of Superficial Basal Cell Carcinoma: Results from a Randomized Vehicle-Controlled Phase III Study in Europe. *Br. J. Dermatol.* **2005**, *152*, 939–947. [CrossRef]
59. Marks, R.; Gebauer, K.; Shumack, S.; Amies, M.; Bryden, J.; Fox, T.L.; Owens, M.L. Australasian Multicentre Trial Group Imiquimod 5% Cream in the Treatment of Superficial Basal Cell Carcinoma: Results of a Multicenter 6-Week Dose-Response Trial. *J. Am. Acad. Dermatol.* **2001**, *44*, 807–813. [CrossRef]
60. Ezughah, F.I.; Dawe, R.S.; Ibbotson, S.H.; Fleming, C.J. A Randomized Parallel Study to Assess the Safety and Efficacy of Two Different Dosing Regimens of 5% Imiquimod in the Treatment of Superficial Basal Cell Carcinoma. *J. Dermatol. Treat.* **2008**, *19*, 111–117. [CrossRef]
61. Eigentler, T.K.; Kamin, A.; Weide, B.M.; Breuninger, H.; Caroli, U.M.; Möhrle, M.; Radny, P.; Garbe, C. A Phase III, Randomized, Open Label Study to Evaluate the Safety and Efficacy of Imiquimod 5% Cream Applied Thrice Weekly for 8 and 12 Weeks in the Treatment of Low-Risk Nodular Basal Cell Carcinoma. *J. Am. Acad. Dermatol.* **2007**, *57*, 616–621. [CrossRef] [PubMed]
62. Messeguer, F.; Serra-Guillen, C.; Echeverria, B.; Requena, C.; Sanmartin, O.; Llombart, B.; Guillen, C.; Nagore, E. A Pilot Study of Clinical Efficacy of Imiquimod and Cryotherapy for the Treatment of Basal Cell Carcinoma with Incomplete Response to Imiquimod. *J. Eur. Acad. Dermatol. Venereol. JEADV* **2012**, *26*, 879–881. [CrossRef] [PubMed]
63. Spencer, J.M. Pilot Study of Imiquimod 5% Cream as Adjunctive Therapy to Curettage and Electrodesiccation for Nodular Basal Cell Carcinoma. *Dermatol. Surg. Off. Publ. Am. Soc. Dermatol. Surg. Al* **2006**, *32*, 63–69.
64. El-Khalawany, M.; Saudi, W.M.; Ahmed, E.; Mosbeh, A.; Sameh, A.; Rageh, M.A. The Combined Effect of CO_2 Laser, Topical Diclofenac 3%, and Imiquimod 5% in Treating High-Risk Basal Cell Carcinoma. *J. Cosmet. Dermatol.* **2022**, *21*, 2049–2055. [CrossRef] [PubMed]
65. Sinx, K.A.E.; Nelemans, P.J.; Kelleners-Smeets, N.W.J.; Winnepenninckx, V.J.L.; Arits, A.H.M.M.; Mosterd, K. Surgery versus Combined Treatment with Curettage and Imiquimod for Nodular Basal Cell Carcinoma: One-Year Results of a Noninferiority, Randomized, Controlled Trial. *J. Am. Acad. Dermatol.* **2020**, *83*, 469–476. [CrossRef] [PubMed]
66. Toren, K.L.; Parlette, E.C. Managing Melanoma in Situ. *Semin. Cutan. Med. Surg.* **2010**, *29*, 258–263. [CrossRef]
67. Leverkus, M. Imiquimod: Unexpected Killer. *J. Investig. Dermatol.* **2004**, *122*, XV. [CrossRef]
68. Mora, A.N.; Karia, P.S.; Nguyen, B.M. A Quantitative Systematic Review of the Efficacy of Imiquimod Monotherapy for Lentigo Maligna and an Analysis of Factors That Affect Tumor Clearance. *J. Am. Acad. Dermatol.* **2015**, *73*, 205–212. [CrossRef]
69. Tio, D.; van der Woude, J.; Prinsen, C.A.C.; Jansma, E.P.; Hoekzema, R.; van Montfrans, C. A Systematic Review on the Role of Imiquimod in Lentigo Maligna and Lentigo Maligna Melanoma: Need for Standardization of Treatment Schedule and Outcome Measures. *J. Eur. Acad. Dermatol. Venereol. JEADV* **2017**, *31*, 616–624. [CrossRef]
70. Globerson, J.A.; Nessel, T.; Basehore, B.M.; Saleeby, E.R. Novel Treatment of In-Transit Metastatic Melanoma with Shave Excision, Electrodesiccation and Curettage, and Topical Imiquimod 5% Cream. *J. Drugs Dermatol. JDD* **2021**, *20*, 555–557.
71. Rosenberg, S.A.; Rapp, H.J. Intralesional Immunotherapy of Melanoma with BCG. *Med. Clin. N. Am.* **1976**, *60*, 419–430. [CrossRef]
72. Radny, P.; Caroli, U.M.; Bauer, J.; Paul, T.; Schlegel, C.; Eigentler, T.K.; Weide, B.; Schwarz, M.; Garbe, C. Phase II Trial of Intralesional Therapy with Interleukin-2 in Soft-Tissue Melanoma Metastases. *Br. J. Cancer* **2003**, *89*, 1620–1626. [CrossRef] [PubMed]
73. Florin, V.; Desmedt, E.; Vercambre-Darras, S.; Mortier, L. Topical Treatment of Cutaneous Metastases of Malignant Melanoma Using Combined Imiquimod and 5-Fluorouracil. *Investig. New Drugs* **2012**, *30*, 1641–1645. [CrossRef]
74. Green, D.S.; Bodman-Smith, M.D.; Dalgleish, A.G.; Fischer, M.D. Phase I/II Study of Topical Imiquimod and Intralesional Interleukin-2 in the Treatment of Accessible Metastases in Malignant Melanoma. *Br. J. Dermatol.* **2007**, *156*, 337–345. [CrossRef] [PubMed]
75. Henriques, L.; Palumbo, M.; Guay, M.-P.; Bahoric, B.; Basik, M.; Kavan, P.; Batist, G. Imiquimod in the Treatment of Breast Cancer Skin Metastasis. *J. Clin. Oncol. Off. J. Am. Soc. Clin. Oncol.* **2014**, *32*, e22–e25. [CrossRef] [PubMed]
76. Morris, C.R.; Hurst, E.A. Extramammary Paget's Disease: A Review of the Literature Part II: Treatment and Prognosis. *Dermatol. Surg. Off. Publ. Am. Soc. Dermatol. Surg. Al* **2020**, *46*, 305–311. [CrossRef]

77. Sawada, M.; Kato, J.; Yamashita, T.; Yoneta, A.; Hida, T.; Horimoto, K.; Sato, S.; Uhara, H. Imiquimod 5% Cream as a Therapeutic Option for Extramammary Paget's Disease. *J. Dermatol.* **2018**, *45*, 216–219. [CrossRef]
78. Cowan, R.A.; Black, D.R.; Hoang, L.N.; Park, K.J.; Soslow, R.A.; Backes, F.J.; Gardner, G.J.; Abu-Rustum, N.R.; Leitao, M.M.; Eisenhauer, E.L.; et al. A Pilot Study of Topical Imiquimod Therapy for the Treatment of Recurrent Extramammary Paget's Disease. *Gynecol. Oncol.* **2016**, *142*, 139–143. [CrossRef]
79. Roccuzzo, G.; Mastorino, L.; Gallo, G.; Fava, P.; Ribero, S.; Quaglino, P. Folliculotropic Mycosis Fungoides: Current Guidance and Experience from Clinical Practice. *Clin. Cosmet. Investig. Dermatol.* **2022**, *15*, 1899–1907. [CrossRef]
80. Gordon, M.C.; Sluzevich, J.C.; Jambusaria-Pahlajani, A. Clearance of Folliculotropic and Tumor Mycosis Fungoides with Topical 5% Imiquimod. *JAAD Case Rep.* **2015**, *1*, 348–350. [CrossRef]
81. Deeths, M.J.; Chapman, J.T.; Dellavalle, R.P.; Zeng, C.; Aeling, J.L. Treatment of Patch and Plaque Stage Mycosis Fungoides with Imiquimod 5% Cream. *J. Am. Acad. Dermatol.* **2005**, *52*, 275–280. [CrossRef] [PubMed]
82. Su, O.; Dizman, D.; Onsun, N.; Bahali, A.G.; Biyik Ozkaya, D.; Tosuner, Z.; Demirkesen, C. Treatment of Localized Pagetoid Reticulosis with Imiquimod: A Case Report and Literature Review. *J. Eur. Acad. Dermatol. Venereol. JEADV* **2016**, *30*, 324–326. [CrossRef] [PubMed]
83. Chiam, L.Y.T.; Chan, Y.C. Solitary Plaque Mycosis Fungoides on the Penis Responding to Topical Imiquimod Therapy. *Br. J. Dermatol.* **2007**, *156*, 560–562. [CrossRef] [PubMed]
84. Brown, V.L.; Atkins, C.L.; Ghali, L.; Cerio, R.; Harwood, C.A.; Proby, C.M. Safety and Efficacy of 5% Imiquimod Cream for the Treatment of Skin Dysplasia in High-Risk Renal Transplant Recipients: Randomized, Double-Blind, Placebo-Controlled Trial. *Arch. Dermatol.* **2005**, *141*, 985–993. [CrossRef] [PubMed]

International Journal of *Molecular Sciences*

MDPI

Review

Genetic Influence on Treatment Response in Psoriasis: New Insights into Personalized Medicine

Emilio Berna-Rico [1,*], Javier Perez-Bootello [1], Carlota Abbad-Jaime de Aragon [1] and Alvaro Gonzalez-Cantero [1,2,*]

[1] Department of Dermatology, Hospital Universitario Ramón y Cajal, IRYCIS, Colmenar Viejo km 9.100, 28034 Madrid, Spain; jpbootello@gmail.com (J.P.-B.); carlotababbad@gmail.com (C.A.-J.d.A.)
[2] Faculty of Medicine, Universidad Francisco de Vitoria, 28223 Madrid, Spain
* Correspondence: emilioberna2a@gmail.com (E.B.-R.); alvarogc261893@hotmail.com (A.G.-C.); Tel.: +34-633-11-74-76 (E.B.-R.); +34-620-408-898 (A.G.-C.); Fax: +34-91373508 (E.B.-R. & A.G.-C.)

Abstract: Psoriasis is a chronic inflammatory disease with an established genetic background. The HLA-Cw*06 allele and different polymorphisms in genes involved in inflammatory responses and keratinocyte proliferation have been associated with the development of the disease. Despite the effectiveness and safety of psoriasis treatment, a significant percentage of patients still do not achieve adequate disease control. Pharmacogenetic and pharmacogenomic studies on how genetic variations affect drug efficacy and toxicity could provide important clues in this respect. This comprehensive review assessed the available evidence for the role that those different genetic variations may play in the response to psoriasis treatment. One hundred fourteen articles were included in this qualitative synthesis. *VDR* gene polymorphisms may influence the response to topical vitamin D analogs and phototherapy. Variations affecting the ABC transporter seem to play a role in methotrexate and cyclosporine outcomes. Several single-nucleotide polymorphisms affecting different genes are involved with anti-TNF-α response modulation (*TNF-α*, *TNFRSF1A*, *TNFRSF1B*, *TNFAIP3*, *FCGR2A*, *FCGR3A*, *IL-17F*, *IL-17R*, and *IL-23R*, among others) with conflicting results. HLA-Cw*06 has been the most extensively studied allele, although it has only been robustly related to the response to ustekinumab. However, further research is needed to firmly establish the usefulness of these genetic biomarkers in clinical practice.

Keywords: psoriasis; pharmacogenetics; pharmacogenomics; therapeutics; polymorphisms; toxicity

Citation: Berna-Rico, E.; Perez-Bootello, J.; Abbad-Jaime de Aragon, C.; Gonzalez-Cantero, A. Genetic Influence on Treatment Response in Psoriasis: New Insights into Personalized Medicine. *Int. J. Mol. Sci.* **2023**, *24*, 9850. https://doi.org/10.3390/ijms24129850

Academic Editor: Naoko Kanda

Received: 12 May 2023
Revised: 29 May 2023
Accepted: 31 May 2023
Published: 7 June 2023

1. Introduction

Psoriasis is an immune-mediated inflammatory disease that is highly prevalent worldwide, affecting approximately 2–3% of the world population [1,2]. According to the latest Global Burden of Disease study, there were 4.622.594 incident cases of psoriasis worldwide in 2019, with higher-income countries and territories having the highest incidence rate per 100,000 people (112.6, 95% uncertainty interval 108.9–116.1) [3]. Different clinical forms have been defined according to the type of lesions observed. The most common form is psoriasis vulgaris, which accounts for approximately 90% of the disease cases. Guttate, inverse, pustular, and erythrodermic psoriasis constitute other phenotypes of psoriasis [1]. Although it has been classically considered a skin disease, it is frequently associated with extracutaneous manifestations, such as psoriatic arthritis, mood disorders, inflammatory bowel disease, asthma, chronic obstructive pulmonary disease, cancer, metabolic syndrome, non-alcoholic fatty liver, cardiovascular disease, among others, reflecting the systemic nature of psoriasis [4–6]. Indeed, in addition to severely affecting the quality of life of the patient [7], psoriasis is associated with an increase in all-cause mortality [8,9].

Its etiopathogenesis remains unclear. It is probable that genetic, immunological, and environmental factors may play important roles in its development [10]. In this regard, different genetic variants have been associated with an increased risk of suffering from psoriasis. As with other autoimmune disorders, psoriasis manifests strong associations with human leucocyte antigen (HLA) molecules, which are involved in antigen presentation and help to identify exogenous proteins. Particularly, individuals carrying the HLA-Cw*06 allele (also known as HLA-C*06:02) have a 10–20-fold increased risk of psoriasis [11]. Other genes encoding cytokines such as TNF-α, IL-17, IL-23, or their receptors [12], as well as genes involved in keratinocyte proliferation, extracellular matrix remodeling, and angiogenesis [13,14] have been shown to increase the risk of its development. Disarrangements of both the innate and adaptative cutaneous immune system are the main drivers of the inflammatory cycle found in psoriatic lesions. Although not fully understood, the activation of keratinocytes, macrophages, neutrophils, and especially, plasmocytoid dendritic cells, leads to the secretion of different cytokines, including alpha and beta interferons (IFN-α and IFN-β), interleukin-1 beta (IL-1β), and tumor necrosis factor-α (TNF-α). In this cytokine milieu, myeloid dendritic cells are secondarily activated via Toll-like receptors (TLRs) and produce IL-12 and IL-23, which induce the proliferation of helper T lymphocytes (Th) and their differentiation toward a Th1 and Th17 profile. TNF-α and both Th17 (IL-17 and IL-22) and Th1 (IFN-γ) cytokines activate keratinocytes proliferation and angiogenesis, two key features in psoriasis pathogenesis. IL-17 also mediates the recruitment of neutrophils and its activation, degranulation, and neutrophil extracellular traps (NETs) formation, which contributes to the initial and maintenance phases of psoriasis [15,16].

Determining disease severity in medical practice requires a thorough evaluation of clinical and patient-reported factors. The Psoriasis Area and Severity Index (PASI) and body surface area (BSA) are frequently used metrics that provide objective assessments of disease severity. The absolute PASI and the percentage of improvement from baseline (e.g., PASI90 for a 90% reduction) are also used to evaluate the effectiveness of treatment. In addition to PASI and BSA, clinicians must consider other factors such as the impact on quality of life, clinical presentation, lesion location, and concurrent psoriatic arthritis to determine overall disease severity [17].

Moderate-to-severe psoriasis is defined by a PASI > 10, a BSA > 10, and/or a Dermatology Life Quality Index (DLQI) >10 [17]. Phototherapies or systemic treatments, such as conventional systemic drugs (methotrexate, acitretin, or cyclosporine) or small molecules (apremilast), are usually the first-line treatments for these patients, with biologics drugs used in cases of no response or contraindications. Biologics are the most effective treatments currently available [18], targeting the main disease effectors. They are classified according to their target in anti-TNF (infliximab, etanercept, adalimumab, and certolizumab), anti-IL12/23 (ustekinumab), anti-IL17 (secukinumab, ixekizumab, and bimekizumab), anti-IL17R (brodalumab), and anti IL23 drugs (guselkumab, tildrakizumab, and risankizumab). Despite its high effectiveness, not all patients achieve an acceptable response or sustain it in the long term [19]. Different genetic backgrounds, among others, have been involved in this heterogeneity of response [20].

Pharmacogenetic methods analyze the associations between patient responses to certain drugs and variants located in a selection of candidate genes. Most of these variants are single nucleotide polymorphisms (SNPs), which constitute substitutions of one nucleotide that occur in at least 1% of the population. Other variants far less frequently addressed are copy number variations (CNVs), which represent a decrease (deletion) or increase (insertions or duplications) in the number of copies of a DNA region. Pharmacogenomics is the field of genetics concerned with the identification of all human genes and the RNA and proteins encoded by them. In this regard, genome-wide association studies (GWASs) allow for an unbiased approach to examining the impact of genetic variants on the drug response by simultaneously testing hundreds of thousands of common polymorphic sites across many genomes [21].

This review aims to update the state of the art of psoriasis studies focusing on the influence of genetic variants on drug effectiveness. The identification of genetic markers of clinical response may aid patient selection for better cost-effective decisions.

2. Literature Search

PubMed and Embase searches were conducted using the terms: (psoriasis OR psoriatic OR psoriasis arthritis OR psoriasiform) AND (treatment OR acitretin OR cyclosporine OR methotrexate OR phototherapy OR biological therapy OR anti-tumor necrosis factor OR infliximab OR adalimumab OR etanercept OR certolizumab OR ustekinumab OR guselkumab OR risankizumab OR tildrakizumab OR secukinumab OR ixekizumab OR brodalumab OR bimekizumab) AND (polymorphism OR pharmacogenetic OR pharmacoepigenetic OR pharmacogenomic) AND (response OR loss of effect OR toxicity) on 17 February 2022.

Firstly, the titles and abstracts of the articles obtained in the first search were reviewed to assess relevant studies. The search was limited to (1) studies written in English or Spanish; (2) studies addressing the influence of genetic factors on the response to drugs used in psoriasis, including topical, phototherapy, conventional, and biologic therapies; and (3) any type of epidemiological study (meta-analysis, clinical trials, cohort studies, case-control, and cross-sectional studies). Systematic and narrative reviews, guidelines, protocols, conference abstracts, and case reports were excluded. Secondly, the full text of articles that met the inclusion criteria was reviewed. Previous systematic and narrative reviews were reviewed to ensure the accuracy of our search and to manually check their reference lists [16,20–23].

Figure 1 shows the literature search process.

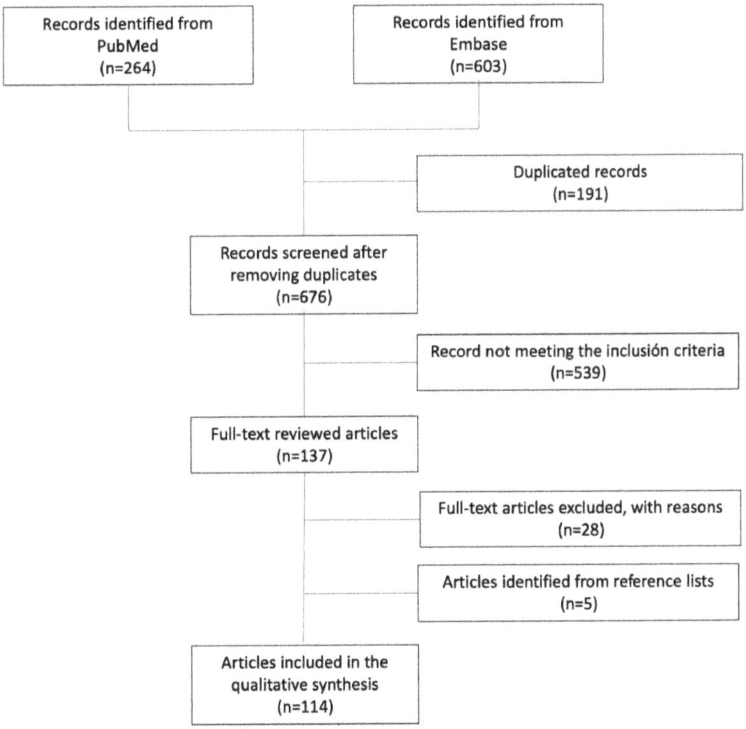

Figure 1. Flow chart showing the study selection process used in this narrative review.

3. Therapeutic Options

3.1. Topical Therapies

Topical therapy remains a cornerstone in the management of psoriasis. It is considered the first treatment option for milder forms of psoriasis, as well as serving as adjunctive therapy in patients undergoing systemic or biologic treatment. The effect on psoriasis is based on its anti-inflammatory and anti-proliferative capacity. Corticosteroids, vitamin D analogs (calcipotriol and tacalcitol), and calcineurin inhibitors are the most commonly used treatments. Most studies to date have focused on vitamin D analogs.

The rs1544410 (BsmI) polymorphism in the vitamin D receptor (*VDR*) gene did not influence the response to calcipotriol in 92 English patients with psoriasis [24]. However, the same polymorphism (Bb heterozygotic phenotype) predicted a significantly better response to topical tacalcitol in a later Italian study ($n = 25$) [25]. Saeki et al. found that the frequency of the F allele in the rs2228570-*VDR* gene polymorphism was lower in non-responders to tacalcitol compared to controls (47 vs. 64%, $p < 0.05$, Japan) [26]. Halshall et al. investigated other *VDR* gene SNPs, such as A-1012G, rs2228570 (FokI), and rs731236 (TaqI), and found that the A allele of the A-1012G variant and the rs731236-T allele were associated with a better response to calcipotriol (UK, $n = 205$) [27]. Conversely, the rs731236-T allele was associated with partial resistance to calcipotriol in a later Turkish study [28]. Another study on a Turkish population found that rs1544410 (BsmI) and rs7975232 (ApaI) showed no significant associations with response to calcipotriol, but patients with the rs2228570-Ff genotype had worse outcomes, while the rs2228570-ff and rs731236-TT genotypes were associated with a better response [29].

Nonetheless, there are discrepancies in these findings. Zhao et al., in 2015 ($n = 324$, China), found no effect of the SNPs mentioned above on calcipotriol response. Instead, the study found a significant association between a loss of response to this drug and the rs2228570-FF and rs11568820-AA genotypes. In addition, when analyzing the response to calcipotriol in combination with acitretin using the same SNPs, the rs11568820-AA genotype showed an increased response to the drug combination compared to the other SNPs [30].

To sum up, these studies suggest that *VDR* gene SNPs may be associated with the response to treatment with calcipotriol or other vitamin D analogs in psoriasis patients, although the studies are highly heterogeneous and showed scarce reproducibility. Further research is needed to clarify the role of these SNPs in clinical practice.

3.2. Phototherapy

Phototherapy, including narrowband ultraviolet B (NB-UVB) and psoralen ultraviolet A (PUVA), among others, is a treatment modality that is well-established in psoriasis treatment. Phototherapeutic regimens use repeated controlled ultraviolet exposures to alter cutaneous biology, aiming to induce remission of skin diseases [31].

There have been several studies searching for an association between genetic polymorphisms and the response to phototherapy in many different genes and populations: *PPARγ2* [32], *IL-12B*, *IL-17A*, *IL-23R*, *IL-23A* [33], *HLA-C* [34], *IL-17F* [35], *IL-6* [36], and *MC1R* [37], but all of them showed no effect on response.

The only associations found were on the *VDR* gene. Lesiak et al. analyzed 50 Polish patients treated with NB-UVB for 20 days and found that those carrying the TaaI/Cdx-2 (rs11568820) AA variant showed a worse response measured using the PASI. Other polymorphisms were analyzed, but no other associations were found [38]. In the study conducted by Ryan et al. ($n = 93$, Ireland), patients homozygous for the C allele in the TaqI (rs731236) *VDR* gene polymorphism, which is associated with decreased VDR activity, had a shorter remission duration after NB-UVB [39].

3.3. Conventional Systemic Drugs

3.3.1. Methotrexate

Methotrexate is a competitive inhibitor of dihydrofolate reductase, thus decreasing folate cofactors required for the synthesis of nucleic acids. Low-dose methotrexate (<25 mg per week) decreases the proliferation of lymphoid cells, which is considered to be the mechanism by which methotrexate improves psoriasis and psoriatic arthritis [40]. One of the first pharmacogenetic studies to determine the response to methotrexate in patients with psoriasis was conducted by Campalani et al. (UK, $n = 203$), which showed how at least one triplet (3R) in the 5′UTR of *TYMS* was significantly associated with both a poorer response to methotrexate and increased hepatotoxicity [41]. *TYMS* encodes thymidylate synthase, which is involved in pyrimidine synthesis and DNA synthesis/repair. Another study by the same research group (n = 374) showed how three variants of the *ABCC1* transporter predicted a better response (PASI75) to this drug: rs35592, rs2238476, and rs28364006, as well as two *ABCG2* SNPs: rs13120400 and rs17731538 [42]. These genes encode ATP-binding cassette (ABC) transporters, which have been involved in multidrug resistance [43]. A study on a South Indian Tamil population found that the HLA-Cw*06-positive allele and rs3761548 of the *FOXP3* gene were independent genetic predictors for the clinical response to methotrexate [44]. Other studies have validated the association between the HLA-Cw*06-positive allele and a greater response to this drug in English [45] and Chinese populations [46]. In this last study, a synergistic effect between the HLA-Cw*06-positive allele and the *ABCB1* rs1045742 SNP was also demonstrated [46]. Conversely, Chen et al. observed a worse response to methotrexate in psoriasis patients with the rs1045642 variant [47].

Carriers of the rs1801133-TT genotype of the *MTHFR* gene showed a better response rate (PASI75 and PASI90) to this drug at week 12 than carriers of the CT/CC genotypes and also a higher risk of ALT elevation. MTHFR encodes the methylenetetrahydrofolate reductase (MTHFR) enzyme, which is indirectly inhibited by methotrexate [48]. However, this association has not been replicated in other studies [41,42,49].

B7-H4 is located in genomic regions associated with susceptibility to type 1 diabetes. In a single-center, cross-sectional study including 265 Chinese psoriatic patients, carriers of the rs12025144-GG genotype had a higher prevalence of DM and worse response to methotrexate in the subgroup of diabetic patients [50]. Regarding annexin A6 (*ANxA6*), a susceptibility factor for psoriasis, the rs11960458-TT/CT genotype was significantly more likely to be unresponsive to MTX in both short (12 weeks) and long-term (1 year) treatment, whereas the rs960709 and rs13168551 polymorphisms were only associated with short-term efficacy [51]. Other polymorphisms have been associated with better (*IL-17F* rs2397084-T allele [52]; *TNIP1* rs10036748-TT genotype [53]) or worse responses (*GNMT* rs10948059-TT genotype; DNMT3b rs2424913-CT/TT genotype [49]) to methotrexate, although studies with larger sample sizes and on different populations will be needed to consolidate these data.

Lastly, there are studies that have used a pharmacogenomics approach to address this issue. A study that used a whole exon high-throughput sequencing technology to detect the DNA sequence of 22 Chinese patients with psoriasis identified 3 SNPs associated with methotrexate response: the T rs216195 variant of *SMG6* and C rs2285421 of *UPK1A* were associated with better outcomes, while the *IMMT* rs1050301 variant A was associated with a lower PASI75 achievement at week 12 [54]. A GWAS conducted by Zhang et al. on a Chinese cohort of patients with psoriasis (n = 333) revealed that the rs4713429 SNP, which has a significant impact on HLA-C expression, was significantly associated with methotrexate response [55].

3.3.2. Cyclosporine

Cyclosporine is a cyclic undecapeptide with a potent inhibitory action on T lymphocytes. It remains one of the most effective and rapidly acting treatments currently available for psoriasis. Virtually all the diverse manifestations of this disease can respond. The main side effects are nephrotoxicity and hypertension, which limit its usefulness as a long-term maintenance therapy [40].

Not many gene polymorphisms have been studied regarding cyclosporine response. The most studied gene is the *ABCB1*. Vasilopoulos et al. identified that the T allele on the C3435T polymorphism (rs1045642) was associated with a worse response to cyclosporine in a cohort of 84 Greek patients with psoriasis [56]. Chernov et al. came to the same conclusion regarding the same polymorphism, but they also found that the *ABCB1* C1236T (rs1128503) and G2677T/A (rs2032582) SNPs were significantly associated with a negative response to the cyclosporine therapy in the codominant, dominant, and recessive models (n = 168, Russia) [57].

Additionally, Antonatos et al. genotyped 27 SNPs mapped to 22 key protein nodes of the cyclosporine pathway in 200 Greek patients. Single-SNP analyses showed statistically significant associations between the rs12885713-T allele of *CALM1* (p = 0.0108) and the rs2874116-G allele of *MALT1* (p = 0.0006) genes with a positive response to cyclosporine after correction for multiple comparisons [58].

3.3.3. Acitretin

Acitretin's mechanism of action is not fully understood. It modulates keratinocyte proliferation and differentiation and also has anti-inflammatory and immunomodulatory effects. There is extensive experience in its use. Its main concern is teratogenicity, which severely limits its use in women of childbearing age [40].

One of the first genes studied in relation to acitretin response was the *VEGFA* gene. Its product, vascular endothelial growth factor (VEGF), induces angiogenesis in different settings, including psoriasis [59]. Young et al. analyzed the -460 SNP (rs833061), which is the most common SNP in the promoter region of the *VEGFA* gene (n = 106, United Kingdom). The -460 TT genotype was associated with non-response to oral acitretin, whereas the -460 TC genotype was associated with clearance/significant response to treatment [60]. However, this same polymorphism was subsequently studied by Chen et al. in 131 Chinese patients with psoriasis, who found no influence on acitretin response; they also found no association between different variants of the *EGF* gene and treatment effectiveness [61]. Finally, Bozduman et al. analyzed different *VEFGA* polymorphisms in 100 Turkish patients on acitretin. They found no significant associations except for the +405 G > C SNP (rs2010963), in which a subgroup of four patients with the GG genotype showed a better response [62].

In a study involving 105 Chinese patients treated with a combination of acitretin and topical calcipotriol, patients carrying the rs4149056-T allele in *SLCO1B1* and/or the rs2282143-C allele in *SLC22A1* showed a worse response based on PASI50 attainment at week 8 [63].

The relationship between mutations in certain interleukin genes and the response to acitretin has also been studied. Lin et al. conducted a study that included an acitretin-treated subgroup of 24 Chinese patients with the TG genotype in the rs3212227 SNP of the *IL12B* gene; these patients had a significantly better response (PASI50) to acitretin than patients with the GG genotype. Additionally, 19 secondary non-responders to anti-TNF-alpha treated with acitretin were included. In this setting, the presence of the rs112009032-A A genotype in the *IL23R* gene predicted a higher PASI75 achievement [64].

Borghi et al. studied the effect of a 14-base pair (bp) sequence insertion/deletion (INS/DEL) polymorphism in the *HLA-G* gene in psoriasis patients from Italy treated with acitretin (n = 21), cyclosporine, and anti-TNF-alfa. The investigators found a significantly higher frequency of the *HLA-G* DEL allele among the responders (PASI75 at week 16) in the acitretin group [65]. Zhou et al. also evaluated the influence of *HLA* gene variants on acitretin response (n = 100, China). After 8 weeks of treatment, the HLA-DQA1*0201 and HLA-DQB1*0202 alleles were independently associated with a better response to the drug [66]. The same research group conducted a study in which whole exome sequencing was performed on 116 Chinese patients. The *CRB2* rs1105223 CC (OR = 4.10, p = 0.007) and *ANKLE1* rs11086065 AG/GG (OR = 2.76, p = 0.003) genotypes were associated with no response to acitretin after 8-week treatment. Conversely, the *ARHGEF3* rs3821414 CT/CC (OR = 0.25, p = 0.006) and *SFRP4* rs1802073 GG/GT (OR =2.40, p = 0.011) genotypes were associated with a higher response rate [67].

Finally, other studies have evaluated the association between acitretin and SNPs on *ApoE* [68] and *IL36RN* [69] genes, but these did not show any effects on the response.

3.4. *Small Molecules*

Apremilast

Apremilast inhibits phosphodiesterase-4, which increases intracellular levels of cyclic adenosine monophosphate and subsequently downregulates inflammatory responses involving the Th1 and Th17 pathways [22,70]. To our knowledge, only the study by Verbenko et al. assessed the influence of a subset of 78 pre-selected SNPs strongly associated with psoriasis or psoriatic arthritis in apremilast effectiveness. Thirty-four Russian patients were included. Patients carrying the minor alleles rs1143633 (IL-1β), rs20541(*IL-4/IL-13*), rs2201841(*IL-23R*) and rs1800629(*TNF-α*) showed a higher PASI75 achievement [71].

3.5. *Biologics*

3.5.1. Anti-TNF-α Drugs

TNF-α inhibitors were the first biologic drugs available for psoriasis treatment. Etanercept acts as a soluble form of the TNF-α receptor and binds to both TNF-α and TNF-β, depleting these molecules. Conversely, infliximab and adalimumab are both monoclonal antibodies that directly target TNF-α. These molecules have been proven to be effective and safe in the treatment of moderate-to-severe psoriasis in randomized clinical trials controlled with a placebo and with conventional drugs [72–76]. Given their cost-effectiveness, for several authors, they may constitute the first line of biological treatment for the disease [77,78].

The influence of the HLA-Cw*06 allele in anti-TNF-α response has been extensively studied. In a recent study by Coto-Segura et al. (n = 169), HLA-Cw*06 positive patients showed a better response to adalimumab compared to those without the abovementioned allele (OR 2.35, $p = 0.018$) [79]. A previous study by the same Spanish research group (n = 116) observed that psoriasis patients who were carrying the HLA-Cw*06 allele together with the insertion-genotype of the two late cornified envelope genes (*LCE3B_LCE3C*) showed a higher probability of reaching PASI75 under anti-TNF-alfa at week 24 (OR 3.14, 95% CI 1.07–9.24, $p = 0.034$). However, when HLA-Cw*06 was assessed independently, statistical significance was not reached [80]. On the other hand, Gallo et al. (n = 109) observed that HLA-Cw*06 carriers were less likely to respond to adalimumab, infliximab, and etanercept than HLA-Cw*06-negative patients [81], and these results are in line with those found by Dand et al. in a study that included 839 patients treated with adalimumab and 487 treated with ustekinumab. A multivariable regression model was individually performed on each group of treatment: HLA-Cw*06 was associated with a worse response to adalimumab, defined as a failure to reach the PASI90 at 6 months (OR 0.54, $p = 1.67 \times 10^{-4}$) [82]. Similarly, Van den Reek et al. found a poorer response to adalimumab (PASI decline at 3 months) in the HLA-Cw*06-homozygous group of patients [83]. To add to this controversy, the HLA-Cw*06 status was not predictive of anti-TNF-α response in a study conducted in British and Irish patients (n = 138) [84], as well as in many other studies carried out in Spanish, Italian, and Chinese populations [85–89].

Apart from HLA-Cw*06, other HLA variants have also been analyzed. In a cohort of Greek patients with moderate-to-severe psoriasis (n = 228), the rs10484554 polymorphism in the *HLA-C* gene was associated with a better response to anti-TNF-α, as well as the *HLA-A*-rs610604 polymorphism with a better response to adalimumab [90]. The *HLA-B/MICA* rs13437088 polymorphism, which has been associated with early onset psoriasis [91], predicted a better response to etanercept in a study involving 81 Spanish patients [92]. Guarene et al. studied the effect of the *HLA-B* Bw4-80I and *HLA-A* Bw4-80I alleles on 48 Italian patients under biologic treatment including infliximab, etanercept, adalimumab, and ustekinumab. The abovementioned alleles present a greater binding affinity to killer-cell immunoglobulin-like receptors (KIRs), which modulate natural killer (NK) cell function. A significantly better response to etanercept was observed in the carriers of the *HLA-A* Bw80I allele [93]. The HLA-B*46 haplotype was not associated with biologic response in a study involving 74 Chinese patients (45 on etanercept) [85]. Finally, the *HLA-G* 14-base-pair insertion/deletion polymorphism (rs66554220) did not modify the anti-TNF-α response in a small group (n = 11) of Italian patients [65].

Given that TNF-α is the target of the drugs reviewed in this section (etanercept, adalimumab, and infliximab), several authors have raised the possibility that certain polymorphisms in the *TNF-α* gene may be biomarkers for the response to these therapies [21]. A meta-analysis by Song et al. explored the association between *TNF-α* gene polymorphisms and anti-TNF-α response in patients with autoimmune diseases including psoriasis. The analysis included 10 articles and 887 Caucasian and Asian patients. The *TNF-α* -238 (rs361525) G allele, the *TNF-α* -308 (rs1800629) G allele, and the *TNF-α* -857 (rs1799724) C allele were associated with a better response to these drugs. When stratifying by disease type, the *TNF-α* -857 C allele predicted a better response in psoriasis patients (OR = 2.238, 95% CI 1.319–3.790) [94]. However, only 2 studies with a total of 177 Caucasian patients were included [95,96]. In a Spanish study ($n = 109$), the *TNF-α* -238 G allele also predicted a better response to these drugs [81]. However, it was the *TNF-α* -857 T allele, not the C allele, that was associated with a better response to these treatments, and no association between the *TNF-α* -308 polymorphism and anti-TNF-α response was found. Patients carrying the TT genotype of the *TNF-α* rs1799964 polymorphism also showed a better response to anti-TNF-α both at 3 and 6 months [81]. However, the studies by Dapra et al. [97] and Ovejero-Benito et al. [98] found no effect of the four abovementioned polymorphisms on the response to etanercept in Italian and Spanish patients, respectively. A study including 49 Japanese patients with moderate-severe psoriasis also found no effect of the *TNF-α* -857 polymorphism on the response to adalimumab or infliximab [99].

Polymorphisms in other genes related to TNF-α signaling have also been studied. The tumor necrosis factor receptor superfamily member 1A (*TNFRSF1A*) and 1B (*TNFRSF1B*) genes encode two receptors (TNFRI/p55 and TNFRII/p75, respectively) that mediate the signaling of TNF-α. TNFRI mainly mediates inflammatory and pro-apoptotic responses, while TNFRII has been more implicated in immune regulation and tissue regeneration [100]. Chen et al. conducted a meta-analysis to investigate whether certain polymorphisms in these genes could predict the response to anti-TNF-α therapies in patients with autoimmune diseases (rheumatoid arthritis, psoriasis, and Crohn's disease). The analysis included 8 studies involving 929 subjects with the *TNFRSF1B* rs1061622 polymorphism and 564 subjects with the *TNFRSF1A* rs767455 polymorphism. Only 2 of the included studies were conducted on patients with psoriasis (a Greek and a Spanish cohort with 90 and 80 patients, respectively) [95,101]. Carriers of the rs1061622-T allele showed a better response to anti-TNF-α drugs (OR 0.62, 95% CI 0.40–0.97 for non-response T vs. G). When a subgroup analysis was conducted according to disease type, this association was maintained in the models for psoriasis (OR = 0.39, 95% CI 0.23–0.67) [102]. The influence of this polymorphism could be greater for Etanercept, as shown in the study by Vasilopoulos et al. [95].

The tumor necrosis factor-alpha-induced protein 3 (*TNFAIP3*) gene encodes a critical protein that functions as a negative regulator of the NF-κB signaling pathway, which is essential for the activation of the immune response. It is also involved in TNF-mediated apoptosis [16]. The influence of the *TNFAIP3* rs610604 and rs2230926 SNPs in the response to anti-TNF-α drugs was studied by Tejasvi et al. A total of 632 patients with psoriasis from the USA and Canada were included. The efficacy was measured with a visual scale. Patients that carried the rs610604-G allele responded better than those carrying the A allele (OR 1.50, $p = 0.05$). Stratifying by treatment, this difference was only significant for Etanercept (OR 1.64, $p = 0.016$). Although no association was found between treatment response and the rs2230926 SNPs, those who carried the rs2230926 T-rs610604 G haplotype showed better outcomes [103]. In a Spanish study that included 20 patients with psoriasis and psoriatic arthritis, both the AA-rs6920220 and the AC/CC-rs610604 genotypes were associated with a greater quality of life improvement after anti-TNF-α [98]. Conversely, Masouri et al. found that the A-allele and not the C-allele in the *TNFAIP3* rs610604 polymorphism was associated with a better response, which was only significant with Etanercept [90]. These findings are in line with those of an Iraqi study involving 100 patients with psoriasis [104]. Other authors have found no effect of *TNFAIP3* SNPs in response to these drugs [83,99].

Alongside TNF-α and related molecules genes polymorphisms, other potential biomarkers have been explored to predict anti-TNF-α response. The Fc fragment of IgG receptors IIA(*FCGR2A*) and IIIA(*FCGR3A*) are surface receptors that bind to the constant fraction of immunoglobulin G (IgG) and participate in antibody-dependent cellular toxicity mediated by phagocytic or cytotoxic cells. Genetic alterations in these genes can affect the receptor's affinity for the immune complex [16]. The presence of histidine (H) instead of asparagine (R) at position 131 (rs1801274) in *FCGR2A* and valine (V) instead of phenylalanine (F) at position 175 (rs396992) in *FCGR3A* results in higher-affinity receptors. In a Spanish study involving 70 patients with moderate-to-severe psoriasis, individuals carrying high-affinity genotypes (HH131 + HR131 and VV158 + VF158) showed a greater reduction in BSA at week 6 of anti-TNF-α treatment (beta = 0.372, $p = 0.3$ and beta = 0.425, $p = 0.02$, respectively). However, no significant differences were observed at week 12 or in terms of the PASI [105]. Another Spanish study involving 133 patients found that those harboring the low-affinity allele *FCGR2A* were 13.32 times more likely to be non-responders (PASI75 at week 6) to anti-TNF-α drugs [106]. Conversely, neither the study by Mendrinou et al. ($n = 100$, Greece) [107] nor the study by Batalla et al. ($n = 115$, Spain) [108] found an association between the *FCGR2A*-H131R polymorphism and anti-TNF-α response. Moreover, their results for the *FCGR3A*-V158F polymorphism were contradictory: while in the study by Mendrinou et al., the carriers of the high-affinity allele had a better response, especially to Etanercept [107], in the study of Batalla et al., those carrying the lower affinity allele had a greater response, which was only significant in the Etanercept subgroup [108].

Antonatos et al. recently conducted a meta-analysis addressing the role of these polymorphisms in the response to anti-TNF-α drugs. It included 37 papers with a total of 8398 Caucasian and Asian patients (4723 diagnosed with rheumatoid arthritis and/or spondyloarthritis, 780 with psoriasis, and 2895 with inflammatory bowel disease). No association was found between the *FCGR2A*-R131H SNP and response to anti-TNF-α overall and when stratified by disease (OR 0.959; 95% CI 0.46–2.02 in psoriasis), which are in line with the results for *FCGR3A*-V158F polymorphisms [109]. The authors also explored *TNF-alfa, TNFRSF1A, TNFRSD1B, TLR1, TLR5, IL12B, IL17A,* and *TRAILR1* SNPs. The results regarding *TNF-alpha* polymorphisms were analogous to those previously reported in the meta-analysis by Song et al. [94] and in the study by De Simone et al. [96]. The T-allele of *TNFRSF1B* rs1061622 was associated with the response to anti-TNF-α in the psoriasis subgroup (2 studies, $n = 162$, OR: 2.62, 95% CI 1.52–4.51). Null results were reported for the rest of the polymorphisms [109].

Other SNPs in *IL-17F, IL-17R, IL-23R, IL-12B, IL-1, IL-6, NFKBIZ,* and *CARD14* genes, among others, have been shown to modulate anti-TNF-α response in different settings. Table 1 summarizes them.

To date, most studies addressing this issue have used a candidate-gene approach, analyzing a limited number of genes previously linked to psoriasis or its treatments. A pharmacogenomic approach base on GWAS, on the other hand, has been used far less frequently. To our knowledge, only three studies were conducted following this methodology [110–112]. None of these studies were able to identify any SNP that reached genome-wide statistical significance ($p < 5 \times 10^{-8}$). Lowering the significance threshold to $p < 5 \times 10^{-5}$, Nishikawa et al. ($n = 65$) [110] found ten SNPs located in *SPEN, JAG2, MACC1, GUCY1B3, PDE6A, CDH23, SHOC2, LOC728724, ADRA2A,* and *KCNIP1* genes related to anti-TNF-α response; Ovejero-Benito et al. ($n = 243$) [111] identified nine polymorphisms that involved *AKAP13, SUPT3H, CDH12* (2), and *HNRNPKP3* (5) genes; and Ren et al. ($n = 209$) [112] found seven loci associated with the treatment response in the following genes: *IQGAP2-F2RL2, SDC3, IRF1-AS1, NPAP1, KRT31, CTSZ,* and *CNOT11*. Additionally, the authors of the latest work checked the associations for the 19 SNPs with $p < 5 \times 10^{-5}$ found in the 2 previous GWAS on anti-TNF-α. While two of these SNPs reached $p < 0.05$, none reached the significance thresholds required for these studies [112]. The different genetic backgrounds of the populations assessed in these studies (Japanese, Spanish, and Chinese, respectively) could be behind this lack of consistency. Anyway, GWAS requires a sample size of >1000 patients, so further studies with larger cohorts of patients will be needed in the coming years to validate these results.

In patients with sustained positive outcomes, a common clinical approach is to decrease the dosage or extend the time between administrations (off-label optimization) to minimize side effects and treatment costs. However, this de-intensification poses the risk of treatment loss. Ovejero-Benito et al. discovered that the rs1008953 *SDC4* SNP was linked to successful dose reduction without compromising the response, while certain polymorphisms in *IL28RA*, *TLR10*, *TRAF3IP2*, and *MICA-A9* predicted an inability to achieve it [113].

Finally, apart from predicting treatment efficacy, different genetic polymorphisms are involved with toxicity development, especially paradoxical psoriasis (PP). Bucalo et al. explored SNPs in the HLA-Cw*06, *IL23R*, *TNF-α*, and *IFIH1* genes in patients with inflammatory bowel disease or psoriasis and PP under anti-TNF-α. Although they found associations between PP and two SNPs in TNF-α and HLA-Cw*06 in patients with inflammatory bowel disease, no associations were found in patients with psoriasis [114]. Conversely, in the study by Cabaleiro et al. (n = 161, Spain), the following SNPs were associated with PP development in psoriasis patients under anti-TNF-α: the rs11209026 *IL23R*, rs10782001 *FBXL19*, rs3087243 *CTLA4*, rs651630 *SLC2A8*, and rs1800453 *TAP1* genes [115]. CNVs in regions involving the *ARNT2*, *LOC101929586*, and *MIR5572* genes have also been associated with the development of PP under infliximab or etanercept in a Spanish study (n = 70) [116].

3.5.2. Ustekinumab

Ustekinumab is a human monoclonal antibody directed at the common p40 subunit of IL-12 and IL-23, thereby blocking the Th1 and Th17 inflammatory pathways. It has been shown to be effective and safe for the short- and long-term treatment of psoriasis in both clinical trials and real-life studies [111,117–119].

In contrast to anti-TNF drugs, the influence of HLA-Cw*06 status on treatment response seems to be more consistent for ustekinumab. Talamonti et al. conducted a study that involved 51 Italian patients with moderate-to-severe psoriasis. The authors found striking differences in the rate of ustekinumab response between HLA-Cw*06-positive and -negative patients. A higher percentage of patients achieved PASI75 at week 12 in the HLA-Cw*06-positive group (96.4% vs. 65.2%, OR = 13.4). Carriers of the HLA-Cw*06 also showed a faster response at week 4 and longer disease control [120]. These results were replicated by the same research group in two larger cohorts. In the first one (n = 134), a significantly higher percentage of HLA-Cw*06-positive patients reached PASI75 at week 12 (82.9% vs. 54.2%), at week 52 (83.9% vs. 58.2%), and at week 104 (83.9% vs. 60.5%) [121]. A higher percentage of HLA-Cw*06-positive patients achieved not only PASI75 but also PASI90 and PASI100 at weeks 12, 28, 40, and 52 in the second study (n = 255) [122]. Taking together, HLA-Cw*06 may predispose to a better, faster, and longer-lasting response to ustekinumab in Caucasian patients.

Results from other investigations in both Asian and Caucasian populations have found results along the same lines. Chiu et al. studied the influence of different HLA-B and -C polymorphisms in a group of Chinese patients with psoriasis on biologic treatment, including ustekinumab (n = 29). Neither HLA-C*01, HLA-C*06, nor HLA-B*46 alleles were associated with a better response in the ustekinumab subgroup (PASI50 at week 12) [85]. However, in a later study by the same investigators (n = 66), HLA-Cw*06-positive patients showed a significantly higher mean PASI improvement (81.7% vs. 59.7%) and a higher achievement of PASI90 (62% vs. 26%) at week 28 [123], probably reflecting a lack of power in the former work. Additionally, in the previously discussed study by Dand et al. (n = 487 on ustekinumab), patients harboring HLA-Cw*06 were more likely to reach PASI90 at 6 months compared to HLA-Cw*06-negative patients (OR = 1.72, p = 0.018) [82]. HLA-Cw*06 was again a predictor of the response to ustekinumab at weeks 4, 28, 40, and 52 in a cohort of 64 Italian patients [124].

However, in the study conducted by Raposo et al. (n = 116, Portugal), the initial better response to ustekinumab in the HLA-Cw*06 patient subgroup (weeks 12 and 24) was lost at 52 weeks, raising doubts about the consistency of this biomarker across all time points [125]. Another US study determined the HLA-Cw*06 status from 601 participants in three phase III randomized clinical trials [117,118,126], 332 of whom received ustekinumab. A significantly higher percentage of HLA-Cw*06-positive patients achieved PASI75 at week 12 compared to HLA-Cw*06-negative patients (80.6% vs. 62.7%), but the association was again no longer significant in the long-term. Furthermore, there was no strong association between HLA-Cw*06 and the ustekinumab optimal response (PASI90 and PASI100), and the differences between the overall population and the HLA-Cw*06 positive subgroup were minimal (10% or less). In view of these findings, the authors suggested that HLA-Cw*06 status determination may have limited clinical utility in daily practice [127]. Van Vugt et al. outlined a similar conclusion in a meta-analysis that combined most of these individual studies. A total of 8 papers that involved 937 Caucasian and Asian patients were included for the primary analysis (PASI75 at 6 months). HLA-Cw*06-positive patients presented a higher response rate (OR 0.24, 95% CI 0.14–0.35). Indeed, the response rate in the HLA-Cw*06-positive group varied from 62% to 98% (median 92%), whereas it varied from 40% to 84% (median 67%) in the HLA-Cw*06-negative group. Nonetheless, in the authors' opinion, the actual clinical relevance of HLA genotyping might be questionable as the response rates in both groups were high [128]. Summarizing the evidence available, despite some studies reporting no association [83,90,129], most of the currently available evidence supports the positive influence of HLA-Cw*06 on ustekinumab response. However, further research is necessary to clarify the true clinical impact of HLA genotyping and its potential application in personalized medicine.

Alongside HLA-Cw*06, other gene polymorphisms have also been studied in relation to ustekinumab. A total of 62 SNPs in 44 different genes were evaluated in a Danish cohort of patients with psoriasis under biologic treatment, 230 with ustekinumab. Two variant alleles of the *IL1B* gene (rs1143623 and rs1143627, OR = 0.25 and OR = 0.24, respectively), which convey increased IL1B transcription, were associated with a significantly lower reduction in the PASI at 3 months of treatment. Conversely, *TLR5* rs5744174 and *TIRAP* rs8177374 polymorphisms, which are genetic variants related to an increased level of IFN-gamma, were associated with a better response (OR = 5.26 and OR = 9.42, respectively) [130]. Van den Reek et al. conducted a study on a Dutch population that included 66 episodes of ustekinumab treatment. The *IL12B* rs3213094-T allele was associated with a greater mean PASI reduction at 3 months, whereas the *TNFAIP3* rs610604-G allele predicted a worse outcome, with an even worse response in psoriatic arthritis patients [83]. Nonetheless, other studies have not been able to replicate the influence of *TNFAIP3* [90,120,124] or *IL12B* polymorphisms [125] in drug efficacy. *IL17-F* [131], *ERAP-1* [90], *CHUK, C17orf51, ZNF816A, STAT4, SLC22A4, Corf72, AGBL4, HTR2A, NFKB1A, ADAM33*, and *IL13* [132] polymorphisms have also been associated with the modulation of ustekinumab response. Table 2 summarizes the effect of these SNPs.

Table 1. Pharmacogenetic and pharmacogenomic studies on anti-TNF-α.

Author	Year	Country	Drug	Gen	SNP (Allele/Genotype)	Responsive Allele or Genotype	n	Follow-Up	Outcome	Response
Nani et al. [133]	2023	Greece	IFX, ADA and ETN	MIR155	rs767649	A	100	24 weeks	PASI75	(+)
Ren et al. γ [112]	2022	China	ETN ± MTX	IQGAP2-F2RL2	rs2431355	T	209	12 and 24 weeks	PASI75	(+)
				SDC3	rs11801616	G				(−)
				IRF1-AS1	rs13166823	G				(−)
				NPAP1	rs10220768	C				(+)
				KRT31	rs4796752	C				(+)
				CTSZ	rs4796752	T				(−)
				CNOT11	rs3754679	G				(−)
Sanz-Garcia et al. [116]	2021	Spain	IFX, ADA. and ETN	CPM	CVN	-	70	24 weeks	PASI90	(+) δ
Ovejero-Benito et al. γ [111]	2020	Spain	IFX, ADA, and ETN	AKAP13	rs28461892	A	243	3 months	PASI75	(+)
				SUPT3H	rs9472377	G				(+)
				CDH12	rs1487419	A				(+)
					rs77497886	T				(+)
				HNRNPKP3	rs11037360	A				(+)
					rs7481533	C				(+)
					rs11037342	C				(+)
					rs145304743	T				(+)
					rs1845821	C				(+)
Hassan Hadi et al. [104]	2020	Iraq	ETN	TNFAIP3	rs610604	C	100	6 months	Not specified	(−)
Coto-Segura et al. [79]	2019	Spain	ADA	NFKBIZ	rs3217713 (indel)	Ins/Del and Del/Del	169	24 weeks	PASI75	(+)
				HLA-C	HLA-Cw*06	Positive				(+)
Ovejero-Benito et al. [98]	2019	Spain	anti-TNF	TNFAIP3	rs610604	AC/CC	20	3 months	EQ-VAS	(+)
					rs6920220	AA				(+)
Dand et al. [82]	2019	United Kingdom and Ireland	ADA	HLA-C	HLA-Cw*06	Positive	1326 (839 ADA and 487 ustekinumab)	6 months	PASI90	(−)

Table 1. *Cont.*

Author	Year	Country	Drug	Gen	SNP (Allele/Genotype)	Responsive Allele or Genotype	n	Follow-Up	Outcome	Response
Guarene et al. [93]	2018	Italy	IFX, ADA, ETN, and UTK	HLA-A	HLA-A Bw480I	Positive	48	6 months	PASI75	(−)
Ovejero-Benito et al. [134]	2018	Spain	IFX and ADA	IVL	rs6661932	CT-TT	95	3 months	PASI75	(−)
				IL-12B	rs2546890	AG-AA				(+)
				NFKBIA	rs2145623	CG-GG				(−)
				ZNF816A	rs9304742	CT-CC				(+)
				SLC9A8	rs645544	GG				(−)
Batalla et al. [135]	2018	Spain	IFX, ADA, and ETN	IL17RA	rs4819554	A	238	24 weeks	PASI75	(+)
Prieto-Pérez et al. [106]	2018	Spain	IFX, ADA, and ETN	PGLYRP-4-24	rs2916205	AG/GG	144	3 months	PASI75	(−)
				ZNF816A	rs9304742	CC		3 months		(−)
				CTNNA2	rs11126740	AA		3 months		(−)
				IL-12B	rs2546890	AG/GG		3 months		(−)
								6 months		(−)
				MAP3K1	rs96844	CT/CC		3 months		(+)
								6 months		(+)
				HLA-C	rs12191877	CT/TT		3 months		(+)
				FCGR2A	rs1801274	CT/CC		6 months		(−)
				HTR2A	rs6311	CT/TT		6 months		(−)
				CDKAL1	rs6908425	CT/TT		6 months		(+)
Loft et al. [130]	2018	Denmark	IFX, ADA, and ETN	IL-1B	rs1143623	G/C	376	3 months	PASI75	(−)
					rs1143627	T/C				(−)
				LY96	rs11465996	C/G				(−)
				TLR2	rs11938228	C/A				(−)
					rs4696480	A/T				(−)
van den Reek et al. [83]	2017	Netherlands	ADA and ETN	CD84	rs6427528	GA	282 $^{\Phi}$	3 months	Change in PASI	(+)
				HLA-C	HLA-Cw*06	Positive				(−) $^{\delta}$

Table 1. *Cont.*

Author	Year	Country	Drug	Gen	SNP (Allele/ Genotype)	Responsive Allele or Genotype	*n*	Follow-Up	Outcome	Response
Ovejero-Benito et al. [92]	2017	Spain	ETN	HLA-B/MICA	rs13437088	TT	78	3 months	PASI75	(+)
				MAP3K1	rs96844	CT-CC				(+)
				PTTG1	rs2431697	CT-CC				(+)
				ZNF816A	rs9304742	CC				(+)
				IL12B	rs2546890	AG-GG		6 months		(−)
				GBP6	rs928655	AG-GG				(+)
Coto-Segura et al. [136]	2016	Spain	IFX, ADA and ETN	CARD14	rs11652075	CC	116	24 weeks	PASI75	(+)
				LCE3	indel	Ins				(+)
Nishikawa et al. [γ] [110]	2016	Japan	IFX and ADA	SPEN	rs6701290	G	65	12 weeks	PASI75	(−)
				JAG2	rs3784240	A				(−)
				MACC1	rs2390256	A				(−)
				GUCY1B3	rs2219538	A				(−)
				PDE6A	rs10515637	G				(−)
				CDH23	rs10823825	G				(−)
				SHOC2	rs1927159	A				(+)
				LOC728724	rs7820834	A				(−)
				ADRA2A	rs553668	A				(+)
				KCNIP1	rs4867965	C				(−)
Mendrinou et al. [107]	2016	Greek	IFX, ADA, and ETN	FCGR3A	rs396991	G	100	6 months	PASI75	(+) [ε]
Masouri et al. [90]	2016	Greece	IFX, ADA, and ETN	HLA-C	rs10484554	C	228	6 months	PASI75	(+)
				TRAF3IP2	rs13190932	G				(+) [λ]
				TNFAIP3	rs610604	A				(+) [ε]
				HLA-A	rs9260313	T				(+) [δ]
Coto-Segura et al. [137]	2015	Spain	IFX, ADA, and ETN	CDKAL12	rs6908435	CC	116	24 weeks	PASI75	(+)
Batalla et al. [108]	2015	Spain	IFX, ADA, and ETN	FCGR3A	rs396991	FF	115	6 months	PASI75	(+) [ε]

Table 1. *Cont.*

Author	Year	Country	Drug	Gen	SNP (Allele/ Genotype)	Responsive Allele or Genotype	*n*	Follow-Up	Outcome	Response
Prieto-Pérez et al. [131]	2015	Spain	IFX, ADA, and ETN	IL17F	rs763780	CT	180	28 weeks	PASI75	$(-)^{\delta}/(+)_{\lambda}$
De Simone et al. [96]	2015	Italy	ETN	TNF-alfa	rs361525 (-238)	GG	97	12 weeks	PASI75	(+)
					rs1800629 (-308)	GG				(+)
Batalla et al. [80]	2015	Spain	anti-TNF	LCE3C_LCE3B	indel	Del	116	24 weeks	PASI75	(−)
Julià et al. [138]	2015	Spain	IFX, ADA, and ETN	PDE3A-SLCO1C1	rs3794271	G	130	12 weeks	Change in PASI	(+)
González-Lara et al. [101]	2015	Spain	IFX, ADA, ETN, and UTK	TNFRSFB1	rs1061622	G	90	24 weeks	PASI75	(−)
Gallo et al. [81]	2013	Spain	IFX, ADA, and ETN	HLA-C	HLA-Cw*06	Positive	109	6 months	PASI75	(−)
				TNF-alfa	rs361525 (-238)	GG				(+)
					rs1799724 (-857)	CT/TT				(+)
					rs1799964 (-1031)	TT				(+)
				IL23R	rs11209026	GG				(+)
Julià et al. [105]	2013	Spain	IFX, ADA, and ETN	FCGR2A	rs1801274 (H131R)	HH	70	6 weeks	change in BSA	(+)
				FCGR3A	rs396991 (V158F)	VV				(+)
Vasilopoulos et al. [95]	2012	Greek	IFX, ADA, and ETN	TNFA	rs1799724 (-857)	C	80	6 months	PASI75	$(+)^{\varepsilon}$
				TNFRSF1B	rs1061622	T				(+)
Tejasvi et al. [103]	2012	USA and Canada	IFX, ADA, and ETN	TNFAIP3	rs610604	G	632	Not specified	Self-evaluated/ PASI50 *	$(+)^{\varepsilon}$
					rs2230926/rs610604 (haplotype analysis)	TG				(+)
Di Renzo et al. [139]	2012	Italy	IFX, ADA, and ETN	IL-6	rs1800795 (-174)	C	80	24 weeks	PASI75	(+)

Only studies that found statistically significant associations are included; ADA: adalimumab; CVN: copy number variation; ETN: etanercept; EQ-VAS: European Quality of Life Visual Analog Scale; IFX: infliximab; PASI: Psoriasis Area and Severity Index; $^{\gamma}$: genome-wide association study (GWAS); $^{\varepsilon}$: results for etanercept; $^{\delta}$: results for adalimumab; $^{\lambda}$: results for Infliximab; $^{\Phi}$: treatment episodes or cycles (one patient could receive more than one cycle of each drug); * self-evaluated using a 0–5 visual analog scale; good if scored from 3 to 5 and poor if scored 0 to 2; PASI50 Toronto cohort; (+): better response; (−) worse response.

The only GWAS evaluating the association between different genetic variants and the response to ustekinumab was recently published. It involved 439 European-descent psoriasis patients that had participated in at least one of the following randomized clinical trials: PHOENIX I [117], PHOENIX II [118], and ACCEPT [126]. SNP rs35569429, which is located on chromosome 4, was significantly associated with ustekinumab, effectivity (change in the PASI at week 12) exceeding the genome-wide significance threshold (beta = -15.83, $p = 2.42 \times 10^{-9}$). Specifically, patients carrying at least one deletion allele showed a worse response to the drug. This genetic variant is located in an intergenic region upstream of *WDR1*, whose protein regulates immune cell interactions and cell motility. The authors hypothesized that this variation may be involved in promoter/enhancer activities of proximal genes, but the functional effects of this variant still remain largely unknown. Interestingly, patients simultaneously carrying HLA-Cw*06 and the rs35569429-GG genotype presented the highest response to ustekinumab (84.4% achieved PASI75 at week 12), which was significantly higher than that obtained by patients harboring the HLA-Cw*06-negative/rs35569429-GG genotype (71.6%), the HLA-Cw*06-positive/rs35569429-deletion allele (65.5%), and the HLA-Cw*06-negative/rs35569429-deletion allele (38.8%) [140].

In this regard, Galluzo et al. also found that the *IL12B* rs6887695-GG genotype and the absence of the *IL12B* rs3212227-AA genotype predicted a better and a longer-lasting response only in patients that simultaneously carried the HLA-Cw*06 allele [124]. Morelli et al. further explored this question using their cohort of 152 Italian patients with psoriasis. As well as identifying different single SNPs associated with different responses to ustekinumab, the investigators found that HLA-Cw*06-positive and HLA-Cw*06-negative patients harbored distinct patterns of SNPs associated with varying clinical responses. Indeed, HLA-Cw*06-positive patients with an optimal response to ustekinumab were characterized by the co-presence of allelic variants of *CDSN*(rs33941312), *PSORS1C3*(rs1265181), *CCHCR1*(rs2073719, rs746647, and rs10484554), *HCP5*(rs2395029), the LCE3A-B intergenic region(rs12030223 and rs6701730), the and HLA-C promoter region(rs13207315 and rs13191343). Concerning SNPs that characterized HLA-Cw*06-negative patients, those present in *MICA*(rs2523497) and *CDSN*(rs1042127 and rs4713436) were associated with a worse response. The authors hypothesized that multi-gene markers, instead of the classical single-SNP biomarker approach, could gain importance in the coming years for informing clinical decisions [141].

Table 2. Pharmacogenetic and pharmacogenomic studies on ustekinumab.

Author	Year	Country	Gen	Allele/SNP	Responsive Allele or Genotype	n	Follow-Up	Outcome	Response
Morelli et al. [141]	2022	Italy	CCHCR1	rs2073719	Not provided	152	12, 28, 64, 76, and 88 weeks	PASI90	(+)
			TNFA	rs1800610			64, 76, 88, and 100 weeks	PASI100	(−)
			Intergenic region upstream of HLA-C	rs12189871 (HLA-Cw*06_LD1)			12, 28, 76, and 88 weeks	PASI90	(+)
				rs4406273 (HLA-Cw*06_LD3)			12, 28, 76, and 88 weeks	PASI90	(+)
				rs9348862			12, 28, 40, and 52	PASI90	(−)
				rs9368670			12, 28, 40, and 52	PASI90	(−)
			PSORS1C3	rs1265181			12, 28, 52, 76, and 88 weeks	PASI90	(+)
			MICA	rs2523497			64, 76, 88, and 100 weeks	PASI100	(−)
			Intergenic region between LCE3B and LCE3A	rs12030223			12, 40,52, and 64 weeks	PASI100	(+)
				rs6701730			12, 40, 52, and 64 weeks	PASI100	(+)
			CDSN	rs1042127			52, 64, 88, and 100 weeks	PASI100	(−)
				rs4713436			52, 64, 88, and 100 weeks	PASI100	(−)
Connell et al. [140] γ	2022	Europe	Intergenic region upstream WDR1	rs35569429	Deletion allele	439	12 weeks	Change in PASI	(−)

Table 2. *Cont.*

Author	Year	Country	Gen	Allele/SNP	Responsive Allele or Genotype	*n*	Follow-Up	Outcome	Response
Dand et al. [82]	2019	UK and Ireland	HLA-C	HLA-Cw*06	Positive	487	6 months	PASI90	(+)
Loft et al. [130]	2018	Denmark	IL1B	rs1143623	G/C	230	12 weeks	PASI reduction	(−)
			IL1B	rs1143627	T/C				(−)
			TIRAP	rs8177374	C/T				(+)
			TLR5	rs5744174	T/C				(+)
Prieto-Pérez et al. [132]	2017	Spain	AGBL4	rs191190	TT	69	16 weeks	PASI75	(−)
			HTR2A	rs6311	TT				(−)
			NFKB1A	rs2145623	CC				(−)
			ADAM33	rs2787094	CC				(−)
			IL13	rs848	TT				(−)
			CHUK	rs11591741	GC				(+)
			C17orf51	rs1975974	AG				(+)
			ZNF816A	rs9304742	CT				(+)
			STAT4	rs7574865	GT				(+)
			SLCC22A4	rs1050152	CT				(+)
			C9orf72	rs774359	CT				(+)
van den Reek et al. [83]	2017	Netherlands	IL12B	rs3213094	CT	66 $^{\Phi}$	3 months	Change in PASI	(+)
			TNFAIP3	rs610604	GG			Change in PASI	(−)
Raposo et al. [125]	2017	Portugal	HLA-C	HLA-Cw*06	Positive	116	12 and 24	PASI75	(+)
Talamonti et al. [122]	2017	Italy	HLA-C	HLA-Cw*06	Positive	255	4, 12, 28, 40, and 52	PASI50, PASI75, PASI90 and PASI100	(+)
Talamonti et al. [121]	2016	Italy	HLA-C	HLA-Cw*06	Positive	134	12, 28, 52, and104	PASI75	(+)
Galluzo et al. [124]	2016	Italy	HLA-C	HLA-Cw*06	Positive	64	4, 28, 40, and 52	PASI75	(+)
Li et al. [127]	2016	USA	HLA-C	HLA-Cw*96	Positive	332	4 and 12 weeks	PASI50 and PASI75	(+)
Masouri et al. [90]	2016	Greece	ERAP1	rs151823	CC	22	24 weeks	PASI75	(+)
				rs26653	GG				(+)
Prieto-Pérez et al. [131]	2015	Spain	IL-17F	rs763780	TC	70	12 and 24 weeks	PASI75	(−)
Chiu et al. [123]	2014	China	HLA-C	HLA-Cw*06	Positive	66	4 and 28 weeks	PASI75 and PASI90	(+)
Talamonti et al. [120]	2013	Italy	HLA-C	HLA-Cw*06	Positive	51	4, 12, 28, and 40 weeks	PASI75	(+)

Only studies that found statistically significant associations are included; PASI: Psoriasis Area and Severity Index; $^{\Upsilon}$: genome-wide association study (GWAS); $^{\Phi}$: treatment episodes or cycles (one patient could receive more than one cycle of each drug); (+): better response; (−) worse response.

3.5.3. Other Biologics

A recent network meta-analysis involving 167 studies and 58.912 patients with psoriasis analyzed the efficacy of systemic pharmacological treatments for chronic plaque psoriasis, including anti-TNF-α and cytokine inhibitors. Anti-IL17 and anti-IL-23 biologics showed a higher proportion of patients achieving PASI90 compared to all the interventions. These results are in line with other meta-analyses that addressed this issue [142,143]. However, despite being the most effective drugs to date, there have been few studies exploring the influence of genetic background on their efficacy. All of them have focused on the pharmacogenetics of anti-IL17 and anti-IL17R drugs.

The influence of HLA-Cw*06 on secukinumab response was analyzed in the SUPREME study, a 24-week phase IIIb trial that included 434 patients with moderate-to-severe psoriasis. No differences were found in either PASI90 or absolute PASI at 16 and 24 weeks of treatment between HLA-Cw*06-positive and -negative patients. There were also no differences in effectiveness and safety in the open-label extension of the trial (n = 384), in which the proportion of patients that reached PASI75/PASI90/PASI100 was comparable across both groups throughout the 72 weeks of treatment [144,145]. A study involving 18 Swiss patients also failed to find differences in secukinumab response based on HLA-Cw*06 status, although the sample size was not powered to identify differences similar to those observed in ustekinumab works [146].

On the other side, in a retrospective study involving 151 Italian patients with moderate-to-severe psoriasis treated with secukinumab, HLA-Cw*06 predicted a higher PASI90 achievement from week 16 to week 72. However, this association lost significance when other variables were considered in multivariable models [147]. Another study by Morelli et al. examined 62 Italian patients receiving secukinumab and also observed that HLA-Cw*06-positive patients were more likely to achieve PASI90 at weeks 24, 40, and 56, and PASI100 at weeks 8, 16, and 24 compared to HLA-Cw*06-negative patients. The authors explored the impact of 417 genetic variants previously associated with psoriasis risk or response to biologics. Apart from HLA-Cw*06, different SNPs located in the *HLA-C* promoter region and upstream *HLA-C* were associated with better a response to this drug. The authors hypothesized that these non-coding genetic variants could regulate *HLA-C* transcription. The absence of rs9267325 SNP in *MICB-DT* and the presence of rs909253 and rs1800683 in *LTA* also predicted a stronger response to secukinumab. Interestingly, rs34085293 in *DDX58* and rs2304255 in *TYK2* may identify a subgroup of super-responder patients, as a high proportion of patients carrying these alleles achieved PASI100 both at short- and long-term follow-ups. Both *TYK2* and *DDX58* encode proteins recently involved in the IL-23/IL-17 axis by inducing IL-23 and regulating IL-23-mediated pathways. Interestingly, as with ustekinumab, the authors divided the patients into clusters according to HLA-Cw*06 status and response to secukinumab. Certain SNPs in *DDX58*, the upstream region of *HLA-C*, the *HLA-C* promoter region, or *CCHR1* significantly clustered with HLA-Cw*06 and identified a subgroup of HLA-Cw*06 carriers with a better response. Conversely, different polymorphisms in *MICB-DT, ERAP1*, and *MICA* might identify a subgroup with low response among HLA-Cw*06-negative patients [148].

Finally, van Vugt et al. investigated the effect of *IL-17A* gene polymorphisms on secukinumab and ixekizumab response in a cohort of 134 Dutch patients with psoriasis. Although five SNPs in non-coding regions (rs2275913, rs8193037, rs3819025, rs7747909, and rs3748067) were identified, none of them were associated with drug response when evaluating change in PASI or PASI75/90 achievement at 12 and 24 weeks [149].

4. Conclusions and Future Directions

As reviewed in this article, more than a hundred papers have addressed the influence of different genetic variants on the response to most of the treatments that currently compose the therapeutic arsenal for psoriasis, from topical treatments to biologic drugs. However, despite this huge effort to identify genetic biomarkers that help predict drug response, these biomarkers have barely reached daily clinical practice. Most of the findings of these studies have not been replicated in other series, which are generally of small sample size and mainly include Caucasian and, to a lesser extent, Asian patients. Indeed, the association between different genetic polymorphisms and drug response varies among different populations, which may indicate the existence of population-specific genetic biomarkers. Further research with larger cohorts of patients and including different ethnicities and races will be needed in the coming years to fully establish the role of these polymorphisms on a daily-clinical basis.

The most widely studied drugs are the anti-TNF-α. While some polymorphisms in the *TNF-α* and *TNFRSF1B* gene have been associated with a better response to these drugs using meta-analyses, these generally include few studies, and the evidence remains conflicting. Examining the response to these drugs as a homogeneous group may have contributed to the heterogeneity in results. As their mechanism of action differs, the polymorphisms evaluated may not exert the same effect with different biologics. Indeed, some studies have found different results when stratifying for etanercept, adalimumab, or infliximab [81,95]. The influence of the HLA-Cw*06 allele on the response to ustekinumab appears to be more robust. Nonetheless, given the high rate of response to the drug regardless of the presence of the allele, some authors question the practical usefulness of its determination. Conducting pharmaco-economic studies could shed light on this issue [150]. Furthermore, pharmacogenetic and pharmacoeconomic studies aimed not only at predicting effectiveness but also at predicting toxicity or effective drug optimization could also provide valuable information on treatment selection. To date, very few studies have addressed this issue.

Finally, epigenetic modifications have also been shown to explain inter-individual differences in response to therapy [151] and have also been involved in psoriasis development [152]. A Spanish research group found that differences in DNA and histone methylation could influence the anti-TNF-α response [153,154]. This largely unexplored genetic field could also provide important clues for identifying predictors for response in this complex heterogeneous disease.

5. Limitations

The limitations of the present review include its narrative design. In addition, the search strategy may have limited the scope of this study, as the search terms did not include drugs that are rarely used in our setting but may be frequently used in other regions, such as etretinate or retinoids other than acitretin. This could have made it difficult for us to find studies evaluating the effect of genetic variations in the response to these drugs.

Author Contributions: Conceptualization, E.B.-R. and A.G.-C.; methodology, E.B.-R. and A.G.-C.; software, E.B.-R.; validation, A.G.-C., J.P.-B. and C.A.-J.d.A.; formal analysis, E.B.-R. and J.P.-B.; investigation, E.B.-R., J.P.-B. and C.A.-J.d.A.; resources, A.G.-C.; data curation, E.B.-R.; writing—original draft preparation, E.B.-R., J.P.-B. and C.A.-J.d.A.; writing—review and editing, A.G.-C.; supervision, A.G.-C. All authors have read and agreed to the published version of the manuscript.

Funding: This research received no external funding.

Institutional Review Board Statement: Not applicable.

Informed Consent Statement: Not applicable.

Data Availability Statement: The data that support the findings of this study are available from the corresponding author upon reasonable request. The data are not publicly available due to privacy or ethical restrictions.

Conflicts of Interest: Gonzalez-Cantero has served as a consultant for Abbie, Janssen, Novartis, Lilly, Almirall, Celgene, and Leo Pharma receiving grants/other payments. The rest authors declare no conflict of interest.

References

1. Boehncke, W.H.; Schön, M.P. Psoriasis. *Lancet* **2015**, *386*, 983–994. [CrossRef]
2. Parisi, R.; Symmons, D.P.M.; Griffiths, C.E.M.; Ashcroft, D.M. Global Epidemiology of Psoriasis: A Systematic Review of Incidence and Prevalence. *J. Investig. Dermatol.* **2013**, *133*, 377–385. [CrossRef]
3. Damiani, G.; Bragazzi, N.L.; Aksut, C.K.; Wu, D.; Alicandro, G.; McGonagle, D.; Guo, C.; Dellavalle, R.; Grada, A.; Wong, P.; et al. The Global, Regional, and National Burden of Psoriasis: Results and Insights From the Global Burden of Disease 2019 Study. *Front. Med.* **2021**, *8*, 743180. [CrossRef] [PubMed]
4. Santus, P.; Rizzi, M.; Radovanovic, D.; Airoldi, A.; Cristiano, A.; Conic, R.; Petrou, S.; Pigatto, P.D.M.; Bragazzi, N.; Colombo, D.; et al. Psoriasis and Respiratory Comorbidities: The Added Value of Fraction of Exhaled Nitric Oxide as a New Method to Detect, Evaluate, and Monitor Psoriatic Systemic Involvement and Therapeutic Efficacy. *BioMed Res. Int.* **2018**, *2018*, 3140682. [CrossRef] [PubMed]
5. Conic, R.R.; Damiani, G.; Schrom, K.P.; Ramser, A.E.; Zheng, C.; Xu, R.; McCormick, T.S.; Cooper, K.D. Psoriasis and Psoriatic Arthritis Cardiovascular Disease Endotypes Identified by Red Blood Cell Distribution Width and Mean Platelet Volume. *J. Clin. Med.* **2020**, *9*, 186. [CrossRef] [PubMed]
6. Takeshita, J.; Grewal, S.; Langan, S.M.; Mehta, N.N.; Ogdie, A.; Van Voorhees, A.S.; Gelfand, J.M. Psoriasis and comorbid diseases. *J. Am. Acad. Dermatol.* **2017**, *76*, 377–390. [CrossRef]

7. Feldman, S.R. Psoriasis causes as much disability as other major medical diseases. *J. Am. Acad. Dermatol.* **2020**, *82*, 256–257. [CrossRef] [PubMed]
8. Dhana, A.; Yen, H.; Yen, H.; Cho, E. All-cause and cause-specific mortality in psoriasis: A systematic review and meta-analysis. *J. Am. Acad. Dermatol.* **2019**, *80*, 1332–1343. [CrossRef] [PubMed]
9. Abuabara, K.; Azfar, R.S.; Shin, D.B.; Neimann, A.L.; Troxel, A.B.; Gelfand, J.M. Cause-specific mortality in patients with severe psoriasis: A population-based cohort study in the U.K.: Cause-specific mortality in patients with severe psoriasis. *Br. J. Dermatol.* **2010**, *163*, 586–592. [CrossRef]
10. Harden, J.L.; Krueger, J.G.; Bowcock, A.M. The immunogenetics of Psoriasis: A comprehensive review. *J. Autoimmun.* **2015**, *64*, 66–73. [CrossRef]
11. Nair, R.P.; Stuart, P.E.; Nistor, I.; Hiremagalore, R.; Chia, N.V.; Jenisch, S.; Weichenthal, M.; Abecasis, G.R.; Lim, H.W.; Christophers, E.; et al. Sequence and Haplotype Analysis Supports HLA-C as the Psoriasis Susceptibility 1 Gene. *Am. J. Hum. Genet.* **2006**, *78*, 827–851. [CrossRef] [PubMed]
12. Lee, Y.H.; Song, G.G. Associations between interleukin-23R and interleukin-12B polymorphisms and psoriasis susceptibility: A meta-analysis. *Immunol. Investig.* **2013**, *42*, 726–736. [CrossRef] [PubMed]
13. Caputo, V.; Strafella, C.; Termine, A.; Dattola, A.; Mazzilli, S.; Lanna, C.; Cosio, T.; Campione, E.; Novelli, G.; Giardina, E.; et al. Overview of the molecular determinants contributing to the expression of Psoriasis and Psoriatic Arthritis phenotypes. *J. Cell. Mol. Med.* **2020**, *24*, 13554–13563. [CrossRef] [PubMed]
14. Prieto-Pérez, R.; Cabaleiro, T.; Daudén, E.; Ochoa, D.; Roman, M.; Abad-Santos, F. Genetics of Psoriasis and Pharmacogenetics of Biological Drugs. *Autoimmune Dis.* **2013**, *2013*, 613086. [CrossRef] [PubMed]
15. Rendon, A.; Schäkel, K. Psoriasis Pathogenesis and Treatment. *Int. J. Mol. Sci.* **2019**, *20*, 1475. [CrossRef]
16. Membrive Jiménez, C.; Pérez Ramírez, C.; Sánchez Martín, A.; Vieira Maroun, S.; Arias Santiago, S.A.; Ramírez Tortosa, M.D.C.; Jiménez Morales, A. Influence of Genetic Polymorphisms on Response to Biologics in Moderate-to-Severe Psoriasis. *J. Pers. Med.* **2021**, *11*, 293. [CrossRef] [PubMed]
17. Daudén, E.; Puig, L.; Ferrándiz, C.; Sánchez-Carazo, J.L.; Hernanz-Hermosa, J.M.; the Spanish Psoriasis Group of the Spanish Academy of Dermatology and Venereology. Consensus document on the evaluation and treatment of moderate-to-severe psoriasis: Psoriasis Group of the Spanish Academy of Dermatology and Venereology. *J. Eur. Acad. Dermatol. Venereol.* **2016**, *30*, 1–18. [CrossRef]
18. Sbidian, E.; Chaimani, A.; Garcia-Doval, I.; Do, G.; Hua, C.; Mazaud, C.; Droitcourt, C.; Hughes, C.; Ingram, J.R.; Naldi, L.; et al. Systemic pharmacological treatments for chronic plaque psoriasis: A network meta-analysis. Cochrane Skin Group, editor. *Cochrane Database Syst. Rev.* **2022**, *8*, CD011535.
19. Farhangian, M.E.; Feldman, S.R. Immunogenicity of Biologic Treatments for Psoriasis: Therapeutic Consequences and the Potential Value of Concomitant Methotrexate. *Am. J. Clin. Dermatol.* **2015**, *16*, 285–294. [CrossRef]
20. Muñoz-Aceituno, E.; Martos-Cabrera, L.; Ovejero-Benito, M.C.; Reolid, A.; Abad-Santos, F.; Daudén, E. Pharmacogenetics Update on Biologic Therapy in Psoriasis. *Medicina* **2020**, *56*, 719. [CrossRef]
21. Ovejero-Benito, M.C.; Muñoz-Aceituno, E.; Reolid, A.; Saiz-Rodríguez, M.; Abad-Santos, F.; Daudén, E. Pharmacogenetics and Pharmacogenomics in Moderate-to-Severe Psoriasis. *Am. J. Clin. Dermatol.* **2018**, *19*, 209–222. [CrossRef] [PubMed]
22. Caputo, V.; Strafella, C.; Cosio, T.; Lanna, C.; Campione, E.; Novelli, G.; Giardina, E.; Cascella, R. Pharmacogenomics: An Update on Biologics and Small-Molecule Drugs in the Treatment of Psoriasis. *Genes* **2021**, *12*, 1398. [CrossRef] [PubMed]
23. Van Vugt, L.J.; Van Den Reek, J.M.P.A.; Coenen, M.J.H.; De Jong, E.M.G.J. A systematic review of pharmacogenetic studies on the response to biologics in patients with psoriasis. *Br. J. Dermatol.* **2018**, *178*, 86–94. [CrossRef] [PubMed]
24. Mee, J.B.; Cork, M.J. Vitamin D Receptor Polymorphism and Calcipotriol Response in Patients with Psoriasis. *J. Investig. Dermatol.* **1998**, *110*, 301–302. [CrossRef]
25. Giomi, B.; Ruggiero, M.; Fabbri, P.; Gulisano, M.; Peruzzi, B.; Caproni, M.; Pacini, S. Does the determination of the Bb vitamin D receptor genotype identify psoriasis vulgaris patients responsive to topical tacalcitol? *J. Dermatol. Sci.* **2005**, *37*, 180–181. [CrossRef]
26. Saeki, H.; Asano, N.; Tsunemi, Y.; Takekoshi, T.; Kishimoto, M.; Mitsui, H.; Tada, Y.; Torii, H.; Komine, M.; Asahina, A.; et al. Polymorphisms of vitamin D receptor gene in Japanese patients with psoriasis vulgaris. *J. Dermatol. Sci.* **2002**, *30*, 167–171. [CrossRef]
27. Halsall, J.A.; Osborne, J.E.; Pringle, J.H.; Hutchinson, P.E. Vitamin D receptor gene polymorphisms, particularly the novel A-1012G promoter polymorphism, are associated with vitamin D3 responsiveness and non-familial susceptibility in psoriasis. *Pharm. Genom.* **2005**, *15*, 349–355. [CrossRef]
28. Dayangac-Erden, D.; Karaduman, A.; Erdem-Yurter, H. Polymorphisms of vitamin D receptor gene in Turkish familial psoriasis patients. *Arch. Dermatol. Res.* **2007**, *299*, 487–491. [CrossRef]
29. Acikbas, I.; Sanlı, B.; Tepeli, E.; Ergin, S.; Aktan, S.; Bagci, H. Vitamin D receptor gene polymorphisms and haplotypes (Apa I, Bsm I, Fok I, Taq I) in Turkish psoriasis patients. *Med. Sci. Monit.* **2012**, *18*, CR661–CR666. [CrossRef]
30. Zhao, Y.; Chen, X.; Li, J.; He, Y.; Su, J.; Chen, M.; Zhang, W.; Chen, W.; Zhu, W. VDR gene polymorphisms are associated with the clinical response to calcipotriol in psoriatic patients. *J. Dermatol. Sci.* **2015**, *79*, 305–307. [CrossRef]

31. Elmets, C.A.; Lim, H.W.; Stoff, B.; Connor, C.; Cordoro, K.M.; Lebwohl, M.; Armstrong, A.W.; Davis, D.M.; Elewski, B.E.; Gelfand, J.M.; et al. Joint American Academy of Dermatology–National Psoriasis Foundation guidelines of care for the management and treatment of psoriasis with phototherapy. *J. Am. Acad. Dermatol.* **2019**, *81*, 775–804. [CrossRef] [PubMed]
32. Seleit, I.; Bakry, O.; Abd El Gayed, E.; Ghanem, M. Peroxisome proliferator-activated receptor-γ gene polymorphism in psoriasis and its relation to obesity, metabolic syndrome, and narrowband ultraviolet B response: A case–control study in Egyptian patients. *Indian J. Dermatol.* **2019**, *64*, 192. [PubMed]
33. Youssef, R.; Abdel-Halim, M.R.; Kamel, M.; Khorshied, M.; Fahim, A. Effect of polymorphisms in IL-12B p40, IL-17A and IL-23 A/G genes on the response of psoriatic patients to narrowband UVB. *Photodermatol. Photoimmunol. Photomed.* **2018**, *34*, 347–349. [CrossRef] [PubMed]
34. Bojko, A.; Ostasz, R.; Białecka, M.; Klimowicz, A.; Malinowski, D.; Budawski, R.; Bojko, P.; Drozdzik, M.; Kurzawski, M. IL12B, IL23A, IL23R and HLA-C*06 genetic variants in psoriasis susceptibility and response to treatment. *Hum. Immunol.* **2018**, *79*, 213–217. [CrossRef]
35. Białecka, M.; Ostasz, R.; Kurzawski, M.; Klimowicz, A.; Fabiańczyk, H.; Bojko, P.; Dziedziejko, V.; Safranow, K.; Machoy-Mokrzyńska, A.; Droździk, M. ***IL17A*** and ***IL17F*** Gene Polymorphism Association with Psoriasis Risk and Response to Treatment in a Polish Population. *Dermatology* **2016**, *232*, 592–596. [CrossRef]
36. Białecka, M.; Ostasz, R.; Kurzawski, M.; Klimowicz, A.; Fabiańczyk, H.; Bojko, P.; Dziedziejko, V.; Safranow, K.; Droździk, M. *IL6* −174G>C polymorphism is associated with an increased risk of psoriasis but not response to treatment. *Exp. Dermatol.* **2015**, *24*, 146–147. [CrossRef]
37. Smith, G.; Wilkie, M.; Deeni, Y.; Farr, P.; Ferguson, J.; Wolf, C.; Ibbotson, S. Melanocortin 1 receptor (MC1R) genotype influences erythemal sensitivity to psoralen–ultraviolet A photochemotherapy. *Br. J. Dermatol.* **2007**, *157*, 1230–1234. [CrossRef]
38. Lesiak, A.; Wódz, K.; Ciążyńska, M.; Skibinska, M.; Waszczykowski, M.; Ciążyński, K.; Olejniczak-Staruch, I.; Sobolewska-Sztychny, D.; Narbutt, J. TaaI/Cdx-2 AA Variant of VDR Defines the Response to Phototherapy amongst Patients with Psoriasis. *Life* **2021**, *11*, 567. [CrossRef]
39. Ryan, C.; Renfro, L.; Collins, P.; Kirby, B.; Rogers, S. Clinical and genetic predictors of response to narrowband ultraviolet B for the treatment of chronic plaque psoriasis: Predictors of response to NB-UVB for psoriasis. *Br. J. Dermatol.* **2010**, *163*, 1056–1063. [CrossRef]
40. Menter, A.; Gelfand, J.M.; Connor, C.; Armstrong, A.W.; Cordoro, K.M.; Davis, D.M.; Elewski, B.E.; Gordon, K.B.; Gottlieb, A.B.; Kaplan, D.H.; et al. Joint American Academy of Dermatology–National Psoriasis Foundation guidelines of care for the management of psoriasis with systemic nonbiologic therapies. *J. Am. Acad. Dermatol.* **2020**, *82*, 1445–1486. [CrossRef]
41. Campalani, E.; Arenas, M.; Marinaki, A.M.; Lewis, C.; Barker, J.; Smith, C.H. Polymorphisms in Folate, Pyrimidine, and Purine Metabolism Are Associated with Efficacy and Toxicity of Methotrexate in Psoriasis. *J. Investig. Dermatol.* **2007**, *127*, 1860–1867. [CrossRef] [PubMed]
42. Warren, R.B.; Smith, R.L.; Campalani, E.; Eyre, S.; Smith, C.H.; Barker, J.N.; Worthington, J.; Griffiths, C.E. Genetic Variation in Efflux Transporters Influences Outcome to Methotrexate Therapy in Patients with Psoriasis. *J. Investig. Dermatol.* **2008**, *128*, 1925–1929. [CrossRef] [PubMed]
43. Duan, C.; Yu, M.; Xu, J.; Li, B.-Y.; Zhao, Y.; Kankala, R.K. Overcoming Cancer Multi-drug Resistance (MDR): Reasons, mechanisms, nanotherapeutic solutions, and challenges. *Biomed. Pharmacother.* **2023**, *162*, 114643. [CrossRef] [PubMed]
44. Indhumathi, S.; Rajappa, M.; Chandrashekar, L.; Ananthanarayanan, P.H.; Thappa, D.M.; Negi, V.S. Pharmacogenetic markers to predict the clinical response to methotrexate in south Indian Tamil patients with psoriasis. *Eur. J. Clin. Pharmacol.* **2017**, *73*, 965–971. [CrossRef]
45. West, J.; Ogston, S.; Berg, J.; Palmer, C.; Fleming, C.; Kumar, V.; Foerster, J. HLA-Cw6-positive patients with psoriasis show improved response to methotrexate treatment. *Clin. Exp. Dermatol.* **2017**, *42*, 651–655. [CrossRef]
46. Mao, M.; Kuang, Y.; Chen, M.; Yan, K.; Lv, C.; Liu, P.; Lu, Y.; Chen, X.; Zhu, W.; Chen, W. The HLA-Cw*06 allele may predict the response to methotrexate (MTX) treatment in Chinese arthritis-free psoriasis patients. *Arch. Dermatol. Res.* **2023**, *315*, 1241–1247. [CrossRef]
47. Chen, M.; Chen, W.; Liu, P.; Yan, K.; Lv, C.; Zhang, M.; Lu, Y.; Qin, Q.; Kuang, Y.; Zhu, W.; et al. The impacts of gene polymorphisms on methotrexate in Chinese psoriatic patients. *J. Eur. Acad. Dermatol. Venereol.* **2020**, *34*, 2059–2065. [CrossRef]
48. Giletti, A.; Esperon, P. Genetic markers in methotrexate treatments. *Pharmacogenom. J.* **2018**, *18*, 689–703. [CrossRef]
49. Grželj, J.; Mlinarič-Raščan, I.; Marko, P.B.; Marovt, M.; Gmeiner, T.; Šmid, A. Polymorphisms in GNMT and DNMT3b are associated with methotrexate treatment outcome in plaque psoriasis. *Biomed. Pharmacother.* **2021**, *138*, 111456. [CrossRef]
50. Yang, W.; Huang, Q.; Han, L.; Wang, B.; Yawalkar, N.; Zhang, Z.; Yan, K. B7-H4 Polymorphism Influences the Prevalence of Diabetes Mellitus and Pro-Atherogenic Dyslipidemia in Patients with Psoriasis. *J. Clin. Med.* **2022**, *11*, 6235. [CrossRef]
51. Fan, Z.; Zhang, Z.; Huang, Q.; Han, L.; Fang, X.; Yang, K.; Wu, S.; Zheng, Z.; Yawalkar, N.; Wang, Z.; et al. The Impact of ANxA6 Gene Polymorphism on the Efficacy of Methotrexate Treatment in Psoriasis Patients. *Dermatology* **2021**, *237*, 579–587. [CrossRef] [PubMed]
52. Hamza, A.; Abo Elwafa, R.; Ramadan, N.; Omar, S. Il17A (rs2275913 G>A) and IL17F (rs2397084 T>C) gene polymorphisms: Relation to psoriasis risk and response to methotrexate. *J. Egypt. Womens Dermatol. Soc.* **2021**, *18*, 167.
53. Yan, K.X.; Zhang, Y.J.; Han, L.; Huang, Q.; Zhang, Z.H.; Fang, X.; Zheng, Z.Z.; Yawalkar, N.; Chang, Y.L.; Zhang, Q.; et al. TT genotype of rs10036748 in TNIP *1* shows better response to methotrexate in a Chinese population: A prospective cohort study. *Br. J. Dermatol.* **2019**, *181*, 778–785. [CrossRef] [PubMed]

54. Kuang, Y.H.; Lu, Y.; Yan, K.X.; Liu, P.P.; Chen, W.Q.; Shen, M.X.; He, Y.J.; Wu, L.S.; Qin, Q.S.; Zhou, X.C.; et al. Genetic polymorphism predicting Methotrexate efficacy in Chinese patients with psoriasis vulgaris. *J. Dermatol. Sci.* **2019**, *93*, 8–13. [CrossRef] [PubMed]
55. Zhang, Y.; Ding, X.; Meng, Z.; Chen, M.; Zheng, X.; Cai, M.; Wu, J.; Chang, Y.; Zhang, Q.; Jin, L.; et al. A Genome-wide association study identified *HLA-C* associated with the effectiveness of methotrexate for psoriasis treatment. *J. Eur. Acad. Dermatol. Venereol.* **2021**, *35*, e898–e900. [CrossRef]
56. Vasilopoulos, Y.; Sarri, C.; Zafiriou, E.; Patsatsi, A.; Stamatis, C.; Ntoumou, E.; Fassos, I.; Tsalta, A.; Karra, A.; Roussaki-Schulze, A.; et al. A pharmacogenetic study of ABCB1 polymorphisms and cyclosporine treatment response in patients with psoriasis in the Greek population. *Pharmacogenom. J.* **2014**, *14*, 523–525. [CrossRef]
57. Chernov, A.; Kilina, D.; Smirnova, T.; Galimova, E. Pharmacogenetic Study of the Impact of ABCB1 Single Nucleotide Polymorphisms on the Response to Cyclosporine in Psoriasis Patients. *Pharmaceutics* **2022**, *14*, 2441. [CrossRef]
58. Antonatos, C.; Patsatsi, A.; Zafiriou, E.; Stavrou, E.F.; Liaropoulos, A.; Kyriakoy, A.; Evangelou, E.; Digka, D.; Roussaki-Schulze, A.; Sotiriadis, D.; et al. Protein network and pathway analysis in a pharmacogenetic study of cyclosporine treatment response in Greek patients with psoriasis. *Pharmacogenom. J.* **2023**, *23*, 8–13. [CrossRef]
59. Nofal, A.; Al-Makhzangy, I.; Attwa, E.; Nassar, A.; Abdalmoati, A. Vascular endothelial growth factor in psoriasis: An indicator of disease severity and control. *J. Eur. Acad. Dermatol. Venereol.* **2009**, *23*, 803–806. [CrossRef]
60. Young, H.S.; Summers, A.M.; Read, I.R.; Fairhurst, D.A.; Plant, D.J.; Campalani, E.; Smith, C.H.; Barker, J.N.; Detmar, M.J.; Brenchley, P.E.; et al. Interaction between Genetic Control of Vascular Endothelial Growth Factor Production and Retinoid Responsiveness in Psoriasis. *J. Investig. Dermatol.* **2006**, *126*, 453–459. [CrossRef]
61. Chen, W.; Wu, L.; Zhu, W.; Chen, X. The polymorphisms of growth factor genes (*VEGFA* & EGF) were associated with response to acitretin in psoriasis. *Pers. Med.* **2018**, *15*, 181–188.
62. Bozduman, T.; Evans, S.E.; Karahan, S.; Hayran, Y.; Akbiyik, F.; Lay, I. Genetic Risk Factors for Psoriasis in Turkish Population: -1540 C/A, -1512 Ins18, and +405 C/G Polymorphisms within the Vascular Endothelial Growth Factor Gene. *Ann. Dermatol.* **2016**, *28*, 30. [CrossRef] [PubMed]
63. Chen, W.; Zhang, X.; Zhang, W.; Peng, C.; Zhu, W.; Chen, X. Polymorphisms of SLCO1B1 rs4149056 and SLC22A1 rs2282143 are associated with responsiveness to acitretin in psoriasis patients. *Sci. Rep.* **2018**, *8*, 13182. [CrossRef] [PubMed]
64. Lin, L.; Wang, Y.; Lu, X.; Wang, T.; Li, Q.; Wang, R.; Wu, J.; Xu, J.; Du, J. The Inflammatory Factor SNP May Serve as a Promising Biomarker for Acitretin to Alleviate Secondary Failure of Response to TNF-a Monoclonal Antibodies in Psoriasis. *Front. Pharmacol.* **2022**, *13*, 937490. [CrossRef] [PubMed]
65. Borghi, A.; Rizzo, R.; Corazza, M.; Bertoldi, A.M.; Bortolotti, D.; Sturabotti, G.; Virgili, A.; Di Luca, D. HLA-G 14-bp polymorphism: A possible marker of systemic treatment response in psoriasis vulgaris? Preliminary results of a retrospective study: HLA-G 14-bp polymorphism and therapy in psoriasis. *Dermatol. Ther.* **2014**, *27*, 284–289. [CrossRef] [PubMed]
66. Zhou, X.; He, Y.; Kuang, Y.; Chen, W.; Zhu, W. HLA-DQA1 and DQB1 Alleles are Associated with Acitretin Response in Patients with Psoriasis. *Front. Biosci.-Landmark* **2022**, *27*, 266. [CrossRef]
67. Zhou, X.; He, Y.; Kuang, Y.; Li, J.; Zhang, J.; Chen, M.; Chen, W.; Su, J.; Zhao, S.; Liu, P.; et al. Whole Exome Sequencing in Psoriasis Patients Contributes to Studies of Acitretin Treatment Difference. *Int. J. Mol. Sci.* **2017**, *18*, 295. [CrossRef] [PubMed]
68. Campalani, E.; Allen, M.H.; Fairhurst, D.; Young, H.S.; Mendonca, C.O.; Burden, A.D.; Griffiths, C.E.; Crook, M.A.; Barker, J.N.; Smith, C.H. Apolipoprotein E gene polymorphisms are associated with psoriasis but do not determine disease response to acitretin: ApoE gene polymorphisms, psoriasis and acitretin. *Br. J. Dermatol.* **2006**, *154*, 345–352. [CrossRef]
69. Zhu, T.; Jin, H.; Shu, D.; Li, F.; Wu, C. Association of IL36RN mutations with clinical features, therapeutic response to acitretin, and frequency of recurrence in patients with generalized pustular psoriasis. *Eur. J. Dermatol.* **2018**, *28*, 217–224. [CrossRef]
70. Papp, K.; Reich, K.; Leonardi, C.L.; Kircik, L.; Chimenti, S.; Langley, R.G.; Hu, C.; Stevens, R.M.; Day, R.M.; Gordon, K.B.; et al. Apremilast, an oral phosphodiesterase 4 (PDE4) inhibitor, in patients with moderate to severe plaque psoriasis: Results of a phase III, randomized, controlled trial (Efficacy and Safety Trial Evaluating the Effects of Apremilast in Psoriasis [ESTEEM] 1). *J. Am. Acad. Dermatol.* **2015**, *73*, 37–49. [CrossRef]
71. Verbenko, D.A.; Karamova, A.E.; Artamonova, O.G.; Deryabin, D.G.; Rakitko, A.; Chernitsov, A.; Krasnenko, A.; Elmuratov, A.; Solomka, V.S.; Kubanov, A.A. Apremilast Pharmacogenomics in Russian Patients with Moderate-to-Severe and Severe Psoriasis. *J. Pers. Med.* **2020**, *11*, 20. [CrossRef] [PubMed]
72. Reich, K.; Nestle, F.O.; Papp, K.; Ortonne, J.P.; Evans, R.; Guzzo, C.; Li, S.; Dooley, L.T.; Griffiths, C.E.; EXPRESS study investigators. Infliximab induction and maintenance therapy for moderate-to-severe psoriasis: A phase III, multicentre, double-blind trial. *Lancet* **2005**, *366*, 1367–1374. [CrossRef] [PubMed]
73. Papp, K.A.; Armstrong, A.W.; Reich, K.; Karunaratne, M.; Valdecantos, W. Adalimumab Efficacy in Patients with Psoriasis Who Received or Did Not Respond to Prior Systemic Therapy: A Pooled Post Hoc Analysis of Results from Three Double-Blind, Placebo-Controlled Clinical Trials. *Am. J. Clin. Dermatol.* **2016**, *17*, 79–86. [CrossRef] [PubMed]
74. Menter, A.; Tyring, S.K.; Gordon, K.; Kimball, A.B.; Leonardi, C.L.; Langley, R.G.; Strober, B.E.; Kaul, M.; Gu, Y.; Okun, M.; et al. Adalimumab therapy for moderate to severe psoriasis: A randomized, controlled phase III trial. *J. Am. Acad. Dermatol.* **2008**, *58*, 106–115. [CrossRef] [PubMed]
75. Saurat, J.-H.; Stingl, G.; Dubertret, L.; Papp, K.A.; Langley, R.G.; Ortonne, J.-P.; Unnebrink, K.; Kaul, M.; Camez, A.; for the CHAMPION Study Investigators. Efficacy and safety results from the randomized controlled comparative study of adalimumab

vs. methotrexate vs. placebo in patients with psoriasis (CHAMPION): Adalimumab vs. methotrexate in psoriasis. *Br. J. Dermatol.* **2007**, *158*, 558–566. [CrossRef] [PubMed]
76. Papp, K.; Tyring, S.; Lahfa, M.; Prinz, J.; Griffiths, C.; Nakanishi, A.; Zitnik, R.; van de Kerkhof, P. A global phase III randomized controlled trial of etanercept in psoriasis: Safety, efficacy, and effect of dose reduction. *Br. J. Dermatol.* **2005**, *152*, 1304–1312. [CrossRef]
77. Carrascosa, J.M.; Puig, L.; Belinchón Romero, I.; Salgado-Boquete, L.; del Alcázar, E.; Andrés Lencina, J.J.; Moreno, D.; Cueva, P.D.L. Actualización práctica de las recomendaciones del Grupo de Psoriasis de la Academia Española de Dermatología y Venereología (GPS) para el tratamiento de la psoriasis con terapia biológica. Parte 1. «Conceptos y manejo general de la psoriasis con terapia biológica». *Actas Dermo-Sifiliográficas* **2022**, *113*, 261–277.
78. Amin, M.; No, D.J.; Egeberg, A.; Wu, J.J. Choosing First-Line Biologic Treatment for Moderate-to-Severe Psoriasis: What Does the Evidence Say? *Am. J. Clin. Dermatol.* **2018**, *19*, 1–13. [CrossRef]
79. Coto-Segura, P.; González-Lara, L.; Batalla, A.; Eiris, N.; Quiero, R.; Coto, E. NFKBIZ and CW6 in Adalimumab Response among Psoriasis Patients: Genetic Association and Alternative Transcript Analysis. *Mol. Diagn. Ther.* **2019**, *23*, 627–633. [CrossRef]
80. Batalla, A.; Coto, E.; González-Fernández, D.; González-Lara, L.; Gómez, J.; Santos-Juanes, J.; Quiero, R.; Coto-Segura, P. The Cw6 and late-cornified envelope genotype plays a significant role in anti-tumor necrosis factor response among psoriatic patients. *Pharmacogenet. Genom.* **2015**, *25*, 313–316. [CrossRef]
81. Gallo, E.; Cabaleiro, T.; Román, M.; Solano-López, G.; Abad-Santos, F.; García-Díez, A.; Daudén, E. The relationship between tumour necrosis factor (TNF)-α promoter and *IL12B/IL-23R* genes polymorphisms and the efficacy of anti-TNF-α therapy in psoriasis: A case-control study. *Br. J. Dermatol.* **2013**, *169*, 819–829. [CrossRef]
82. Dand, N.; Duckworth, M.; Baudry, D.; Russell, A.; Curtis, C.J.; Lee, S.H.; Evans, I.; Mason, K.J.; Alsharqi, A.; Becher, G.; et al. HLA-C*06:02 genotype is a predictive biomarker of biologic treatment response in psoriasis. *J. Allergy Clin. Immunol.* **2019**, *143*, 2120–2130. [CrossRef]
83. van den Reek, J.M.P.A.; Coenen, M.J.H.; van de L'Isle Arias, M.; Zweegers, J.; Rodijk-Olthuis, D.; Schalkwijk, J.; Vermeulen, S.H.; Joosten, I.; van de Kerkhof, P.C.M.; Seyger, M.M.B.; et al. Polymorphisms in *CD84*, *IL12B* and *TNFAIP3* are associated with response to biologics in patients with psoriasis. *Br. J. Dermatol.* **2017**, *176*, 1288–1296. [CrossRef]
84. Ryan, C.; Kelleher, J.; Fagan, M.F.; Rogers, S.; Collins, P.; Barker, J.N.; Allen, M.; Hagan, R.; Renfro, L.; Kirby, B. Genetic markers of treatment response to tumour necrosis factor-α inhibitors in the treatment of psoriasis. *Clin. Exp. Dermatol.* **2014**, *39*, 519–524. [CrossRef]
85. Chiu, H.Y.; Huang, P.Y.; Jee, S.H.; Hu, C.Y.; Chou, C.T.; Chang, Y.T.; Hwang, C.Y.; Tsai, T.F. HLA polymorphism among Chinese patients with chronic plaque psoriasis: Subgroup analysis: HLA polymorphism among Chinese patients with psoriasis. *Br. J. Dermatol.* **2012**, *166*, 288–297. [CrossRef]
86. Talamonti, M.; Galluzzo, M.; Zangrilli, A.; Papoutsaki, M.; Egan, C.G.; Bavetta, M.; Tambone, S.; Fargnoli, M.C.; Bianchi, L. HLA-C*06:02 Does Not Predispose to Clinical Response Following Long-Term Adalimumab Treatment in Psoriatic Patients: A Retrospective Cohort Study. *Mol. Diagn. Ther.* **2017**, *21*, 295–301. [CrossRef]
87. Talamonti, M.; Galluzzo, M.; Botti, E.; Pavlidis, A.; Spallone, G.; Chimenti, S.; Antonio, C. Potential role of HLA-Cw6 in clinical response to anti-tumour necrosis factor alpha and T-cell targeting agents in psoriasis patients. *Clin. Drug. Investig.* **2013**, *33*, S71–S73.
88. Caldarola, G.; Sgambato, A.; Fanali, C.; Moretta, G.; Farina, M.; Lucchetti, D.; Peris, K.; De Simone, C. HLA-Cw6 allele, NFkB1 and NFkBIA polymorphisms play no role in predicting response to etanercept in psoriatic patients. *Pharmacogenet. Genom.* **2016**, *26*, 423–427. [CrossRef]
89. Burlando, M.; Russo, R.; Clapasson, A.; Carmisciano, L.; Stecca, A.; Cozzani, E.; Parodi, A. The HLA-Cw6 Dilemma: Is It Really an Outcome Predictor in Psoriasis Patients under Biologic Therapy? A Monocentric Retrospective Analysis. *J. Clin. Med.* **2020**, *9*, 3140. [CrossRef]
90. Masouri, S.; Stefanaki, I.; Ntritsos, G.; Kypreou, K.P.; Drakaki, E.; Evangelou, E.; Nicolaidou, E.; Stratigos, A.J.; Antoniou, C. A Pharmacogenetic Study of Psoriasis Risk Variants in a Greek Population and Prediction of Responses to Anti-TNF-α and Anti-IL-12/23 Agents. *Mol. Diagn. Ther.* **2016**, *20*, 221–225. [CrossRef]
91. Prieto-Pérez, R.; Solano-López, G.; Cabaleiro, T.; Román, M.; Ochoa, D.; Talegón, M.; Baniandrés, O.; López-Estebaranz, J.L.; de la Cueva, P.; Daudén, E.; et al. Polymorphisms Associated with Age at Onset in Patients with Moderate-to-Severe Plaque Psoriasis. *J. Immunol. Res.* **2015**, *2015*, 101879. [CrossRef] [PubMed]
92. Ovejero-Benito, M.C.; Prieto-Pérez, R.; Llamas-Velasco, M.; Belmonte, C.; Cabaleiro, T.; Román, M.; Ochoa, D.; Talegón, M.; Saiz-Rodríguez, M.; Daudén, E.; et al. Polymorphisms associated with etanercept response in moderate-to-severe plaque psoriasis. *Pharmacogenomics* **2017**, *18*, 631–638. [CrossRef] [PubMed]
93. Guarene, M.; Pasi, A.; Bolcato, V.; Cananzi, R.; Piccolo, A.; Sbarsi, I.; Klersy, C.; Cacciatore, R.; Brazzelli, V. The Presence of HLA-A Bw4-80I KIR Ligands Could Predict "Difficult-to-Treat" Psoriasis and Poor Response to Etanercept. *Mol. Diagn. Ther.* **2018**, *22*, 471–474. [CrossRef] [PubMed]
94. Song, G.G.; Seo, Y.H.; Kim, J.H.; Choi, S.J.; Ji, J.D.; Lee, Y.H. Association between *TNF-α* (-308 A/G, -238 A/G, -857 C/T) polymorphisms and responsiveness to TNF-α blockers in spondyloarthropathy, psoriasis and Crohn's disease: A meta-analysis. *Pharmacogenomics* **2015**, *16*, 1427–1437. [CrossRef]

95. Vasilopoulos, Y.; Manolika, M.; Zafiriou, E.; Sarafidou, T.; Bagiatis, V.; Krüger-Krasagaki, S.; Tosca, A.; Patsatsi, A.; Sotiriadis, D.; Mamuris, Z.; et al. Pharmacogenetic Analysis of TNF, TNFRSF1A, and TNFRSF1B Gene Polymorphisms and Prediction of Response to Anti-TNF Therapy in Psoriasis Patients in the Greek Population. *Mol. Diagn. Ther.* **2012**, *16*, 29–34. [CrossRef]
96. De Simone, C.; Farina, M.; Maiorino, A.; Fanali, C.; Perino, F.; Flamini, A.; Caldarola, G.; Sgambato, A. TNF-alpha gene polymorphisms can help to predict response to etanercept in psoriatic patients. *J. Eur. Acad. Dermatol. Venereol.* **2015**, *29*, 1786–1790. [CrossRef]
97. Daprà, V.; Ponti, R.; Lo Curcio, G.; Archetti, M.; Dini, M.; Gavatorta, M.; Quaglino, P.; Fierro, M.T.; Bergallo, M. Functional study of TNF-α as a promoter of polymorphisms in psoriasis. *Ital. J. Dermatol. Venereol.* **2022**, *157*, 146–153. [CrossRef]
98. Ovejero-Benito, M.C.; Muñoz-Aceituno, E.; Reolid, A.; Fisas, L.H.; Llamas-Velasco, M.; Prieto-Pérez, R.; Abad-Santos, F.; Daudén, E. Polymorphisms associated with anti-TNF drugs response in patients with psoriasis and psoriatic arthritis. *J. Eur. Acad. Dermatol. Venereol.* **2019**, *33*, e175–e177. [CrossRef]
99. Ito, M.; Hirota, T.; Momose, M.; Ito, T.; Umezawa, Y.; Fukuchi, O.; Asahina, A.; Nakagawa, H.; Tamari, M.; Saeki, H. Lack of association of *TNFA*, *TNFRSF1B* and *TNFAIP3* gene polymorphisms with response to anti-tumor necrosis factor therapy in Japanese patients with psoriasis. *J. Dermatol.* **2020**, *47*, e110–e111. [CrossRef]
100. Fischer, R.; Kontermann, R.E.; Pfizenmaier, K. Selective Targeting of TNF Receptors as a Novel Therapeutic Approach. *Front. Cell Dev. Biol.* **2020**, *8*, 401. [CrossRef]
101. González-Lara, L.; Batalla, A.; Coto, E.; Gómez, J.; Eiris, N.; Santos-Juanes, J.; Queiro, R.; Coto-Segura, P. The TNFRSF1B rs1061622 polymorphism (p.M196R) is associated with biological drug outcome in Psoriasis patients. *Arch. Dermatol. Res.* **2015**, *307*, 405–412. [CrossRef]
102. Chen, W.; Xu, H.; Wang, X.; Gu, J.; Xiong, H.; Shi, Y. The tumor necrosis factor receptor superfamily member 1B polymorphisms predict response to anti-TNF therapy in patients with autoimmune disease: A meta-analysis. *Int. Immunopharmacol.* **2015**, *28*, 146–153. [CrossRef]
103. Tejasvi, T.; Stuart, P.E.; Chandran, V.; Voorhees, J.J.; Gladman, D.D.; Rahman, P.; Elder, J.T.; Nair, R.P. TNFAIP3 Gene Polymorphisms Are Associated with Response to TNF Blockade in Psoriasis. *J. Investig. Dermatol.* **2012**, *132*, 593–600. [CrossRef]
104. Hassan Hadi, A.M.; Abbas, A.A.; Abdulamir, A.S.; Fadheel, B.M. The effect of TNFAIP3 gene polymorphism on disease susceptibility and response of etanercept in psoriatic patients. *Eur. J. Mol. Clin. Med.* **2020**, *7*, 240–246.
105. Julià, M.; Guilabert, A.; Lozano, F.; Suarez-Casasús, B.; Moreno, N.; Carrascosa, J.M.; Ferrándiz, C.; Pedrosa, E.; Alsina-Gibert, M.; Mascaró, J.M., Jr. The Role of Fcγ Receptor Polymorphisms in the Response to Anti–Tumor Necrosis Factor Therapy in Psoriasis: A Pharmacogenetic Study. *JAMA Dermatol.* **2013**, *149*, 1033. [CrossRef]
106. Prieto-Pérez, R.; Solano-López, G.; Cabaleiro, T.; Román, M.; Ochoa, D.; Talegón, M.; Baniandrés, O.; López-Estebaranz, J.L.; de la Cueva, P.; Daudén, E.; et al. New polymorphisms associated with response to anti-TNF drugs in patients with moderate-to-severe plaque psoriasis. *Pharmacogenom. J.* **2018**, *18*, 70–75. [CrossRef]
107. Mendrinou, E.; Patsatsi, A.; Zafiriou, E.; Papadopoulou, D.; Aggelou, L.; Sarri, C.; Mamuris, Z.; Kyriakou, A.; Sotiriadis, D.; Roussaki-Schulze, A.; et al. FCGR3A-V158F polymorphism is a disease-specific pharmacogenetic marker for the treatment of psoriasis with Fc-containing TNFα inhibitors. *Pharmacogenom. J.* **2017**, *17*, 237–241. [CrossRef]
108. Batalla, A.; Coto, E.; Coto-Segura, P. Influence of Fcγ Receptor Polymorphisms on Response to Anti–Tumor Necrosis Factor Treatment in Psoriasis. *JAMA Dermatol.* **2015**, *151*, 1376. [CrossRef]
109. Antonatos, C.; Stavrou, E.F.; Evangelou, E.; Vasilopoulos, Y. Exploring pharmacogenetic variants for predicting response to anti-TNF therapy in autoimmune diseases: A meta-analysis. *Pharmacogenomics* **2021**, *22*, 435–445. [CrossRef]
110. Nishikawa, R.; Nagai, H.; Bito, T.; Ikeda, T.; Horikawa, T.; Adachi, A.; Matsubara, T.; Nishigori, C. Genetic prediction of the effectiveness of biologics for psoriasis treatment. *J. Dermatol.* **2016**, *43*, 1273–1277 [CrossRef]
111. Ovejero-Benito, M.C.; Muñoz-Aceituno, E.; Sabador, D.; Almoguera, B.; Prieto-Pérez, R.; Hakonarson, H.; Coto-Segura, P.; Carretero, G.; Reolid, A.; Llamas-Velasco, M.; et al. Genome-wide association analysis of psoriasis patients treated with anti-TNF drugs. *Exp. Dermatol.* **2020**, *29*, 1225–1232. [CrossRef]
112. Ren, Y.; Wang, L.; Dai, H.; Qiu, G.; Liu, J.; Yu, D.; Liu, J.; Lyu, C.Z.; Liu, L.; Zheng, M. Genome-wide association analysis of anti-TNF-α treatment response in Chinese patients with psoriasis. *Front. Pharmacol.* **2022**, *13*, 968935. [CrossRef]
113. Ovejero-Benito, M.C.; Muñoz-Aceituno, E.; Sabador, D.; Reolid, A.; Llamas-Velasco, M.; Prieto-Pérez, R.; Abad-Santos, F.; Daudén, E. Polymorphisms associated with optimization of biological therapy through drug dose reduction in moderate-to-severe psoriasis. *J. Eur. Acad. Dermatol. Venereol.* **2020**, *34*, e271–e275. [CrossRef]
114. Bucalo, A.; Rega, F.; Zangrilli, A.; Silvestri, V.; Valentini, V.; Scafetta, G.; Marraffa, F.; Grassi, S.; Rogante, E.; Piccolo, A.; et al. Paradoxical Psoriasis Induced by Anti-TNFα Treatment: Evaluation of Disease-Specific Clinical and Genetic Markers. *Int. J. Mol. Sci.* **2020**, *21*, 7873. [CrossRef]
115. Cabaleiro, T.; Prietoperez, R.; Navarro, R.M.; Solano, G.; Roman, M.J.; Ochoa, D.; Abad-Santos, F.; Dauden, E. Paradoxical psoriasiform reactions to anti-TNFα drugs are associated with genetic polymorphisms in patients with psoriasis. *Pharmacogenom. J.* **2016**, *16*, 336–340. [CrossRef]
116. Sanz-Garcia, A.; Reolid, A.; Fisas, L.; Muñoz-Aceituno, E.; Llamas-Velasco, M.; Sahuquillo-Torralba, A.; Botella-Estrada, R.; García-Martínez, J.; Navarro, R.; Daudén, E.; et al. DNA Copy Number Variation Associated with Anti-tumour Necrosis Factor Drug Response and Paradoxical Psoriasiform Reactions in Patients with Moderate-to-severe Psoriasis. *Acta Derm. Venereol.* **2021**, *101*, adv00448. [CrossRef]

117. Leonardi, C.L.; Kimball, A.B.; Papp, K.A.; Yeilding, N.; Guzzo, C.; Wang, Y.; Li, S.; Dooley, L.T.; Gordon, K.B.; PHOENIX 1 study investigators. Efficacy and safety of ustekinumab, a human interleukin-12/23 monoclonal antibody, in patients with psoriasis: 76-week results from a randomised, double-blind, placebo-controlled trial (PHOENIX 1). *Lancet* **2008**, *371*, 1665–1674. [CrossRef]
118. Papp, K.A.; Langley, R.G.; Lebwohl, M.; Krueger, G.G.; Szapary, P.; Yeilding, N.; Guzzo, C.; Hsu, M.C.; Wang, Y.; Li, S.; et al. Efficacy and safety of ustekinumab, a human interleukin-12/23 monoclonal antibody, in patients with psoriasis: 52-week results from a randomised, double-blind, placebo-controlled trial (PHOENIX 2). *Lancet* **2008**, *371*, 1675–1684. [CrossRef]
119. Zweegers, J.; Groenewoud, J.M.M.; van den Reek, J.M.P.A.; Otero, M.E.; van de Kerkhof, P.C.M.; Driessen, R.J.B.; van Lümig, P.P.M.; Njoo, M.D.; Ossenkoppele, P.M.; Mommers, J.M.; et al. Comparison of the 1- and 5-year effectiveness of adalimumab, etanercept and ustekinumab in patients with psoriasis in daily clinical practice: Results from the prospective BioCAPTURE registry. *Br. J. Dermatol.* **2017**, *176*, 1001–1009. [CrossRef]
120. Talamonti, M.; Botti, E.; Galluzzo, M.; Teoli, M.; Spallone, G.; Bavetta, M.; Chimenti, S.; Costanzo, A. Pharmacogenetics of psoriasis: *HLA-Cw6* but not *LCE3B/3C* deletion nor *TNFAIP3* polymorphism predisposes to clinical response to interleukin 12/23 blocker ustekinumab. *Br. J. Dermatol.* **2013**, *169*, 458–463. [CrossRef]
121. Talamonti, M.; Galluzzo, M.; Chimenti, S.; Costanzo, A. HLA-C*06 and response to ustekinumab in Caucasian patients with psoriasis: Outcome and long-term follow-up. *J. Am. Acad. Dermatol.* **2016**, *74*, 374–375. [CrossRef]
122. Talamonti, M.; Galluzzo, M.; van den Reek, J.M.; de Jong, E.M.; Lambert, J.L.W.; Malagoli, P.; Bianchi, L.; Costanzo, A. Role of the *HLA-C*06* allele in clinical response to ustekinumab: Evidence from real life in a large cohort of European patients. *Br. J. Dermatol.* **2017**, *177*, 489–496. [CrossRef]
123. Chiu, H.-Y.; Wang, T.-S.; Chan, C.-C.; Cheng, Y.-P.; Lin, S.-J.; Tsai, T.-F. Human leucocyte antigen-Cw6 as a predictor for clinical response to ustekinumab, an interleukin-12/23 blocker, in C hinese patients with psoriasis: A retrospective analysis. *Br. J. Dermatol.* **2014**, *171*, 1181–1188. [CrossRef]
124. Galluzzo, M.; Boca, A.N.; Botti, E.; Potenza, C.; Malara, G.; Malagoli, P.; Vesa, S.; Chimenti, S.; Buzoianu, A.D.; Talamonti, M.; et al. IL12B (p40) Gene Polymorphisms Contribute to Ustekinumab Response Prediction in Psoriasis. *Dermatology* **2016**, *232*, 230–236. [CrossRef]
125. Raposo, I.; Carvalho, C.; Bettencourt, A.; Da Silva, B.M.; Leite, L.; Selores, M.; Torres, T. Psoriasis pharmacogenetics: HLA-Cw*0602 as a marker of therapeutic response to ustekinumab. *Eur. J. Dermatol.* **2017**, *27*, 528–530. [CrossRef]
126. Griffiths, C.E.M.; Strober, B.E.; van de Kerkhof, P.; Ho, V.; Fidelus-Gort, R.; Yeilding, N.; Guzzo, C.; Xia, Y.; Zhou, B.; Li, S.; et al. Comparison of Ustekinumab and Etanercept for Moderate-to-Severe Psoriasis. *N. Engl. J. Med.* **2010**, *362*, 118–128. [CrossRef]
127. Li, K.; Huang, C.C.; Randazzo, B.; Li, S.; Szapary, P.; Curran, M.; Campbell, K.; Brodmerkel, C. HLA-C*06:02 Allele and Response to IL-12/23 Inhibition: Results from the Ustekinumab Phase 3 Psoriasis Program. *J. Investig. Dermatol.* **2016**, *136*, 2364–2371. [CrossRef]
128. van Vugt, L.J.; van den Reek, J.M.P.A.; Hannink, G.; Coenen, M.J.H.; de Jong, E.M.G.J. Association of *HLA-C*06:02* Status with Differential Response to Ustekinumab in Patients with Psoriasis: A Systematic Review and Meta-analysis. *JAMA Dermatol.* **2019**, *155*, 708. [CrossRef]
129. Anzengruber, F.; Ghosh, A.; Maul, J.T.; Drach, M.; Navarini, A.A. Limited clinical utility of HLA-Cw6 genotyping for outcome prediction in psoriasis patients under ustekinumab therapy: A monocentric, retrospective analysis. *Psoriasis Targets Ther.* **2018**, *8*, 7–11. [CrossRef]
130. Loft, N.D.; Skov, L.; Iversen, L.; Gniadecki, R.; Dam, T.N.; Brandslund, I.; Hoffmann, H.J.; Andersen, M.R.; Dessau, R.; Bergmann, A.C.; et al. Associations between functional polymorphisms and response to biological treatment in Danish patients with psoriasis. *Pharmacogenom. J.* **2018**, *18*, 494–500. [CrossRef]
131. Prieto-Pérez, R.; Solano-López, G.; Cabaleiro, T.; Román, M.; Ochoa, D.; Talegón, M.; Baniandrés, O.; Estebaranz, J.L.L.; de la Cueva, P.; Daudén, E.; et al. The polymorphism rs763780 in the *IL-17F* gene is associated with response to biological drugs in patients with psoriasis. *Pharmacogenomics* **2015**, *16*, 1723–1731. [CrossRef] [PubMed]
132. Prieto-Pérez, R.; Llamas-Velasco, M.; Cabaleiro, T.; Solano-López, G.; Márquez, B.; Román, M.; Ochoa, D.; Talegón, M.; Daudén, E.; Abad-Santos, F. Pharmacogenetics of ustekinumab in patients with moderate-to-severe plaque psoriasis. *Pharmacogenomics* **2017**, *18*, 157–164. [CrossRef] [PubMed]
133. Nani, P.; Ladopoulou, M.; Papaioannou, E.H.; Papagianni, E.D.; Antonatos, C.; Xiropotamos, P.; Kapsoritakis, A.; Potamianos, P.S.; Karmiris, K.; Tzathas, C.; et al. Pharmacogenetic Analysis of the *MIR146A* rs2910164 and *MIR155* rs767649 Polymorphisms and Response to Anti-TNF Treatment in Patients with Crohn's Disease and Psoriasis. *Genes* **2023**, *14*, 445. [CrossRef]
134. Ovejero-Benito, M.C.; Prieto-Pérez, R.; Llamas-Velasco, M.; Muñoz-Aceituno, E.; Reolid, A.; Saiz-Rodríguez, M.; Belmonte, C.; Román, M.; Dolores Ochoa, D.; Talegón, M.; et al. Polymor-phisms associated with adalimumab and infliximab response in moderate-to-severe plaque psoriasis. *Pharmacogenomics* **2018**, *19*, 7–16. [CrossRef]
135. Batalla, A.; Coto, E.; Gómez, J.; Eiris, N.; González-Fernández, D.; Castro, C.G.-D.; Daudén, E.; Llamas-Velasco, M.; Prieto-Perez, R.; Abad-Santos, F.; et al. IL17RA gene variants and anti-TNF response among psoriasis patients. *Pharmacogenom. J.* **2018**, *18*, 76–80. [CrossRef] [PubMed]
136. Coto-Segura, P.; González-Fernández, D.; Batalla, A.; Gómez, J.; González-Lara, L.; Queiro, R.; Alonso, B.; Iglesias, S.; Coto, E. Common and rare *CARD14* gene variants affect the antitumour necrosis factor response among patients with psoriasis. *Br. J. Dermatol.* **2016**, *175*, 134–141. [CrossRef] [PubMed]

137. Coto-Segura, P.; Batalla, A.; González-Fernández, D.; Gómez, J.; Santos-Juanes, J.; Queiro, R.; Alonso, B.; Iglesias, S.; Coto, E. CDKAL1 gene variants affect the anti-TNF response among Psoriasis patients. *Int. Immunopharmacol.* **2015**, *29*, 947–949. [CrossRef] [PubMed]
138. Julià, A.; Ferrándiz, C.; Dauden, E.; Fonseca, E.; Fernández-López, E.; Sanchez-Carazo, J.L.; Vanaclocha, F.; Puig, L.; Moreno-Ramírez, D.; Lopez-Estebaranz, J.L.; et al. Association of the PDE3A-SLCO1C1 locus with the response to anti-TNF agents in psoriasis. *Pharmacogenom. J.* **2015**, *15*, 322–325. [CrossRef]
139. Di Renzo, L.; Bianchi, A.; Saraceno, R.; Calabrese, V.; Cornelius, C.; Iacopino, L.; Chimenti, S.; De Lorenzo, A. −174G/C IL-6 gene promoter polymorphism predicts therapeutic response to TNF-α blockers. *Pharm. Genom.* **2012**, *22*, 134–142. [CrossRef]
140. Connell, W.T.; Hong, J.; Liao, W. Genome-Wide Association Study of Ustekinumab Response in Psoriasis. *Front. Immunol.* **2022**, *12*, 815121. [CrossRef]
141. Morelli, M.; Galluzzo, M.; Scarponi, C.; Madonna, S.; Scaglione, G.L.; Girolomoni, G.; Talamonti, M.; Bianchi, L.; Albanesi, C. Allelic Variants of HLA-C Upstream Region, PSORS1C3, MICA, TNFA and Genes Involved in Epidermal Homeostasis and Barrier Function Influence the Clinical Response to Anti-IL-12/IL-23 Treatment of Patients with Psoriasis. *Vaccines* **2022**, *10*, 1977. [CrossRef]
142. Sawyer, L.M.; Malottki, K.; Sabry-Grant, C.; Yasmeen, N.; Wright, E.; Sohrt, A.; Borg, E.; Warren, R.B. Assessing the relative efficacy of interleukin-17 and interleukin-23 targeted treatments for moderate-to-severe plaque psoriasis: A systematic review and network meta-analysis of PASI response. *PLoS ONE* **2019**, *14*, e0220868. [CrossRef]
143. Bai, F.; Li, G.G.; Liu, Q.; Niu, X.; Li, R.; Ma, H. Short-Term Efficacy and Safety of IL-17, IL-12/23, and IL-23 Inhibitors Brodalumab, Secukinumab, Ixekizumab, Ustekinumab, Guselkumab, Tildrakizumab, and Risankizumab for the Treatment of Moderate to Severe Plaque Psoriasis: A Systematic Review and Network Meta-Analysis of Randomized Controlled Trials. *J. Immunol. Res.* **2019**, *2019*, 2546161.
144. Costanzo, A.; Bianchi, L.; Flori, M.L.; Malara, G.; Stingeni, L.; Bartezaghi, M.; Carraro, L.; Castellino, G. Secukinumab shows high efficacy irrespective of *HLA-Cw6* status in patients with moderate-to-severe plaque-type psoriasis: SUPREME study. *Br. J. Dermatol.* **2018**, *179*, 1072–1080. [CrossRef]
145. Papini, M.; Cusano, F.; Romanelli, M.; Burlando, M.; Stinco, G.; Girolomoni, G.; Peris, K.; Potenza, C.; Offidani, A.; Bartezaghi, M.; et al. Secukinumab shows high efficacy irrespective of *HLA-Cw6* status in patients with moderate-to-severe plaque-type psoriasis: Results from extension phase of the SUPREME study. *Br. J. Dermatol.* **2019**, *181*, 413–414. [CrossRef]
146. Anzengruber, F.; Drach, M.; Maul, J.-T.; Kolios, A.; Meier, B.; Navarini, A.A. Therapy response was not altered by HLA-Cw6 status in psoriasis patients treated with secukinumab: A retrospective case series. *J. Eur. Acad. Dermatol. Venereol.* **2018**, *32*, e274–e276. [CrossRef]
147. Galluzzo, M.; D'Adamio, S.; Silvaggio, D.; Lombardo, P.; Bianchi, L.; Talamonti, M. In which patients the best efficacy of secukinumab? Update of a real-life analysis after 136 weeks of treatment with secukinumab in moderate-to-severe plaque psoriasis. *Expert Opin. Biol. Ther.* **2020**, *20*, 173–182. [CrossRef]
148. Morelli, M.; Galluzzo, M.; Madonna, S.; Scarponi, C.; Scaglione, G.L.; Galluccio, T.; Andreani, M.; Pallotta, S.; Girolomoni, G.; Bianchi, L.; et al. *HLA-Cw6* and other HLA-C alleles, as well as *MICB-DT, DDX58,* and *TYK2* genetic variants associate with optimal response to anti-IL-17A treatment in patients with psoriasis. *Expert Opin. Biol. Ther.* **2021**, *21*, 259–270. [CrossRef]
149. Van Vugt, L.; Reek, J.V.D.; Meulewaeter, E.; Hakobjan, M.; Heddes, N.; Traks, T.; Kingo, K.; Galluzzo, M.; Talamonti, M.; Lambert, J.; et al. Response to IL -17A inhibitors secukinumab and ixekizumab cannot be explained by genetic variation in the protein-coding and untranslated regions of the IL -17A gene: Results from a multicentre study of four European psoriasis cohorts. *J. Eur. Acad. Dermatol. Venereol.* **2020**, *34*, 112–118. [CrossRef]
150. Verbelen, M.; Weale, M.E.; Lewis, C.M. Cost-effectiveness of pharmacogenetic-guided treatment: Are we there yet? *Pharmacogenom. J.* **2017**, *17*, 395–402. [CrossRef]
151. Ivanov, M.; Barragan, I.; Ingelman-Sundberg, M. Epigenetic mechanisms of importance for drug treatment. *Trends Pharmacol. Sci.* **2014**, *35*, 384–396. [CrossRef]
152. Zhou, F.; Wang, W.; Shen, C.; Li, H.; Zuo, X.; Zheng, X.; Yue, M.; Zhang, C.; Yu, L.; Chen, M.; et al. Epigenome-Wide Association Analysis Identified Nine Skin DNA Methylation Loci for Psoriasis. *J. Investig. Dermatol.* **2016**, *136*, 779–787. [CrossRef]
153. Ovejero-Benito, M.C.; Cabaleiro, T.; Sanz-García, A.; Llamas-Velasco, M.; Saiz-Rodríguez, M.; Prieto-Pérez, R.; Talegón, M.; Román, M.; Ochoa, D.; Reolid, A.; et al. Epigenetic biomarkers associated with antitumour necrosis factor drug response in moderate-to-severe psoriasis. *Br. J. Dermatol.* **2018**, *178*, 798–800. [CrossRef]
154. Ovejero-Benito, M.C.; Reolid, A.; Sánchez-Jiménez, P.; Saiz-Rodríguez, M.; Muñoz-Aceituno, E.; Llamas-Velasco, M.; Martín-Vílchez, S.; Cabaleiro, T.; Román, M.; Ochoa, D.; et al. Histone modifications associated with biological drug response in moderate-to-severe psoriasis. *Exp. Dermatol.* **2018**, *27*, 1361–1371. [CrossRef]

International Journal of *Molecular Sciences*

MDPI

Article

Innovative Rocuronium Bromide Topical Formulation for Targeted Skin Drug Delivery: Design, Comprehensive Characterization, In Vitro 2D/3D Human Cell Culture and Permeation

Victor H. Ruiz [1], David Encinas-Basurto [1,2], Bo Sun [1,3], Basanth Babu Eedara [1,4], Eunmiri Roh [5,6], Neftali Ortega Alarcon [1], Clara Curiel-Lewandrowski [3,7,8], Ann M. Bode [5] and Heidi M. Mansour [1,4,9,10,*]

1 Skaggs Pharmaceutical Sciences Center, College of Pharmacy, The University of Arizona, Tucson, AZ 85721, USA
2 Department of Physics, Mathematics and Engineering, Campus Navojoa, Universidad de Sonora, Sonora 85880, Mexico
3 The University of Arizona Cancer Center, Skin Cancer Institute, Tucson, AZ 85721, USA
4 Center for Translational Science, Florida International University, Port St. Lucie, FL 34987, USA
5 The Hormel Institute, University of Minnesota, Austin, MN 55912, USA
6 Department of Cosmetic Science, Kwangju Women's University, Gwangju 62396, Republic of Korea
7 University of Arizona Cancer Center, University of Arizona, Tucson, AZ 85724, USA
8 Department of Medicine, Division of Dermatology, The University of Arizona College of Medicine, Tucson, AZ 85724, USA
9 Department of Medicine, Division of Translational & Regenerative Medicine, College of Medicine, The University of Arizona, Tucson, AZ 85724, USA
10 BIO5 Institute, The University of Arizona, Tucson, AZ 85721, USA
* Correspondence: hmansour@fiu.edu; Tel.: +1-772-345-4731

Citation: Ruiz, V.H.; Encinas-Basurto, D.; Sun, B.; Eedara, B.B.; Roh, E.; Alarcon, N.O.; Curiel-Lewandrowski, C.; Bode, A.M.; Mansour, H.M. Innovative Rocuronium Bromide Topical Formulation for Targeted Skin Drug Delivery: Design, Comprehensive Characterization, In Vitro 2D/3D Human Cell Culture and Permeation. *Int. J. Mol. Sci.* **2023**, *24*, 8776. https://doi.org/10.3390/ijms24108776

Academic Editor: Antonio Di Stefano

Received: 5 March 2023
Revised: 9 May 2023
Accepted: 10 May 2023
Published: 15 May 2023

Abstract: Cutaneous squamous cell carcinoma (cSCC) is the second-most common type of non-melanoma skin cancer and is linked to long-term exposure to ultraviolet (UV) radiation from the sun. Rocuronium bromide (RocBr) is an FDA-approved drug that targets p53-related protein kinase (PRPK) that inhibits the development of UV-induced cSCC. This study aimed to investigate the physicochemical properties and in vitro behavior of RocBr. Techniques such as thermal analysis, electron microscopy, spectroscopy and in vitro assays were used to characterize RocBr. A topical oil/water emulsion lotion formulation of RocBr was successfully developed and evaluated. The in vitro permeation behavior of RocBr from its lotion formulation was quantified with Strat-M® synthetic biomimetic membrane and EpiDerm™ 3D human skin tissue. Significant membrane retention of RocBr drug was evident and more retention was obtained with the lotion formulation compared with the solution. This is the first systematic and comprehensive study to report these findings.

Keywords: drug flux; Franz cell diffusion system; Strat-M® synthetic biomimetic membrane; HaCaT human skin cell line; NHEK human primary skin cells; EpiDerm® 3D human skin tissue

1. Introduction

The incidence of cutaneous squamous cell carcinoma (cSCC), a non-melanoma skin cancer, rises 2–4% per year in the United States [1]. A significant challenge in estimating accurate incidence rate of cSCC is the lack of reliable registries for non-melanoma skin cancer. Recent reports indicate that, if we apply the increase in incidences seen when multiple cSCCs per patient are included with the first cSCC, it is possible that the incidences could be as large as 112.8 per 100,000 person-years for male patients and 92.7 per 100,000 person-years for female patients. These incidences would be greater than the incidence of prostate cancer in males and approach the incidence of breast cancer in females in the US [2,3].

In addition, health care costs and morbidity associated with skin cancer have continued to increase in recent years [4]. Therefore, development of effective, preventive and therapeutic techniques is imperative. Ultraviolet (UV) radiation from the sun (sUV) is a significant environmental carcinogen that induces inflammation and skin cancer. Long-term exposure to sUV can trigger inflammatory reactions, oxidative stress, DNA damage and gene alterations in the skin, which have been linked to various skin conditions, including an increased risk of skin cancers [5]. Hence, identifying the primary signaling molecules involved in cSCC development for more precise treatments would be advantageous. Roh, Lee et al. have reported that the T-LAK cell-originated protein kinase (TOPK) and p53-related protein kinase (PRPK) are critical players in the development of skin malignancy and that targeting PRPK with rocuronium bromide (RocBr) could inhibit the development of cSCC [5].

For patients with localized cSCC, complete surgical resection is indicated, followed by radiotherapy in those with non-resectable tumors [6,7]. Localized cSCC is the most common clinical presentation for cSCC and, therefore, surgical, topical and intralesional approaches are considered the primary types of therapeutic interventions. Importantly, cSCC can also be prevented through therapeutic prevention approaches for pre-cancerous lesions such as actinic keratoses (AKs) and/or cSCC. These options range from topical products such as retinoids, 5-fluoruracil, chemical peels and photodynamic therapy to systemic agents such as acitretin and capecitabine. These interventions have strengths and weakness in efficacy and associated side effects, limiting their application in the general population with the largest cSCC incidence/AK prevalence. The vast majority of patients with increased burden of AKs and cSCCs require combination and rotational therapy. Based on experimental studies, RocBr may have the potential to become another alternative for topical treatment of AK/cSCC, especially in patients of advanced age and with multiple comorbidities. Treatment choice is based on staging, risk stratification and pathological findings, per the National Comprehensive Cancer Network (NCCN) clinical practice guidelines [7]. Other studies have examined alternative therapies, such as epidermal growth factor receptor (EGFR) inhibitors, but are not currently recommended for treatment [6,8,9].

RocBr is an FDA-approved aminosteroid neuromuscular blocking drug administered by injection (Zemoron®) and works by decreasing or suppressing the depolarization of acetylcholine on the terminal disc of the muscle cell [10]. A rational approach to utilize RocBr for the targeted non-invasive therapy of cSCC would be a topical skin formulation and, in this work, we have successfully developed a new oil/water emulsion lotion of RocBr for topical skin drug delivery that can be used as an alternative to the intravenous route to potentiate its beneficial effect. Comprehensive physicochemical characterization, such as thermal analysis, imaging by electron microscopy with energy dispersive spectroscopy X-ray spectroscopy, imaging by hot-stage microscopy, molecular fingerprinting by spectroscopy and in vitro properties of RocBr, were conducted in vitro to determine the oil/water partition coefficient that can be used to optimize the formulation, ensuring that the drug is delivered to the skin effectively and achieves the desired therapeutic effect for the first time. Additionally, in vitro cell viability using 2D cell culture of HaCaT and normal human epidermal keratinocytes (NHEK®) primary cells was used to determine the toxicity of the RocBr formulations by measuring their proliferation, to determine the safe and effective concentration of RocBr in the topical formulation. Moreover, cell viability studies also provide insights into the permeation behavior of the drug in the skin. Finally, the RocBr lotion was tested for drug permeation and membrane drug retention using Strat-M® synthetic biomimetic membrane with a Franz cell diffusion system. In addition, a reconstructed human epidermis tissue (EpiDerm®) was used to evaluate the membrane drug retention and drug diffusion behavior of RocBr through this human skin tissue model. To the authors' knowledge, this comprehensive and systematic study is the first to report these findings.

2. Results

2.1. Physicochemical Characterization of Raw Rocuronium Bromide

Scanning Electron Microscopy (SEM) and Energy-Dispersive X-ray (EDX) Spectroscopy

Raw RocBr showed an irregular shape (Figure 1) under SEM; as such, it proved difficult to determine its average geometric size. For chemical identification of RocBr (Figure 2), the characteristic Kα lines (peaks) of bromide (Br) were seen at 1.7 keV. The Kα line of carbon (C) was observed at 0.3 keV and the Kα of oxygen (O) and nitrogen (N) were both seen at 0.5 keV. The peaks corresponding to Br, C, O, N and atoms from elemental analysis of RocBr are shown in Figure 2.

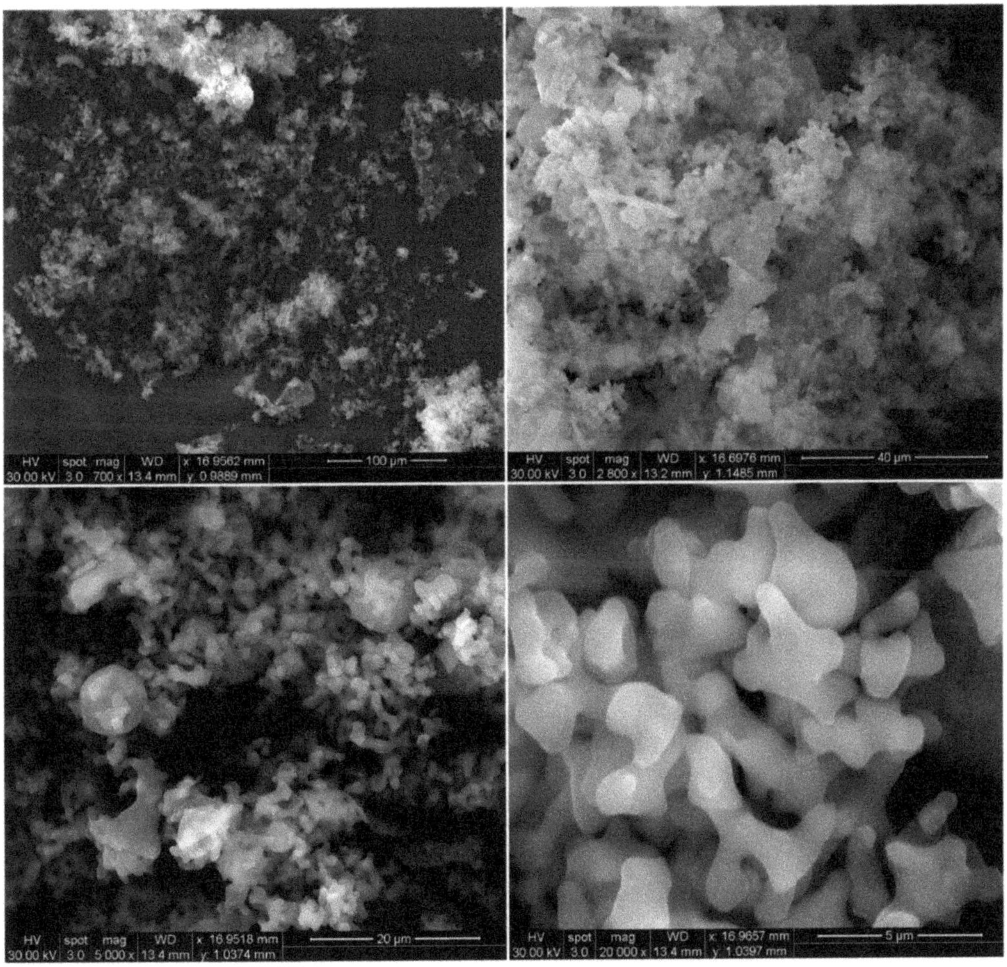

Figure 1. SEM micrographs of RocBr at 700×, 2800×, 5000× and 20,000× resolution.

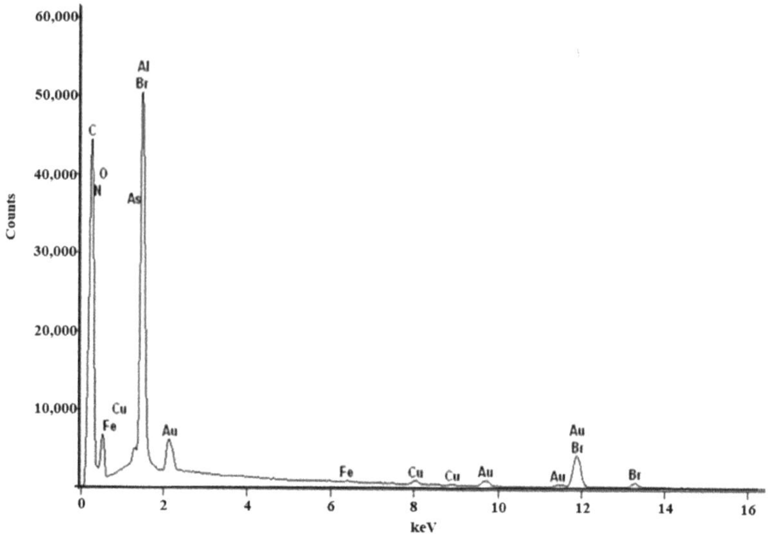

Figure 2. EDX spectra of raw RocBr powder showing characteristic peaks.

2.2. X-ray Powder Diffraction (XRPD)

XRPD is a non-destructive technique to evaluate the solid-state nature of samples [11]. The XRPD spectrum of raw RocBr (Figure 3) showed only a background hump without any characteristic diffraction peaks, indicating the absence of long-range molecular order, i.e., non-crystalline, amorphous nature of the drug [12].

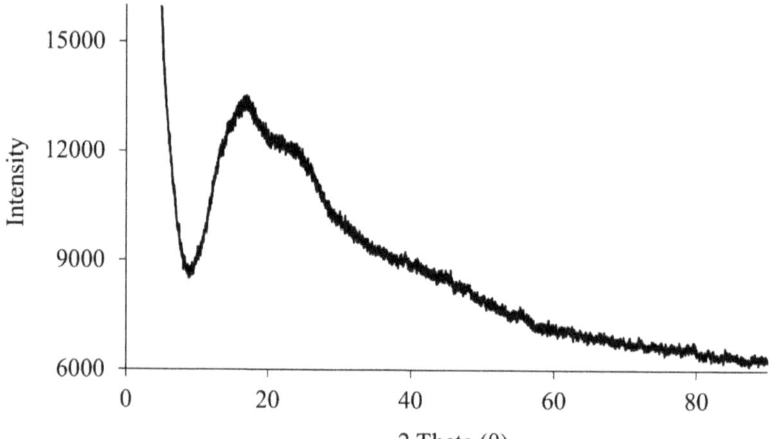

Figure 3. XRPD diffraction patterns of raw RocBr.

2.3. Differential Scanning Calorimetry (DSC)

The DSC thermograms of raw RocBr (Figure 4) exhibited broad endothermic peaks at 53.6 °C, 96.9 °C and 173.2 °C, representing a glass transition (T_g) step followed by water loss and melting decomposition, respectively. The enthalpy and temperature values are summarized in Table 1. The predicted melting point of RocBr is ~169 °C.

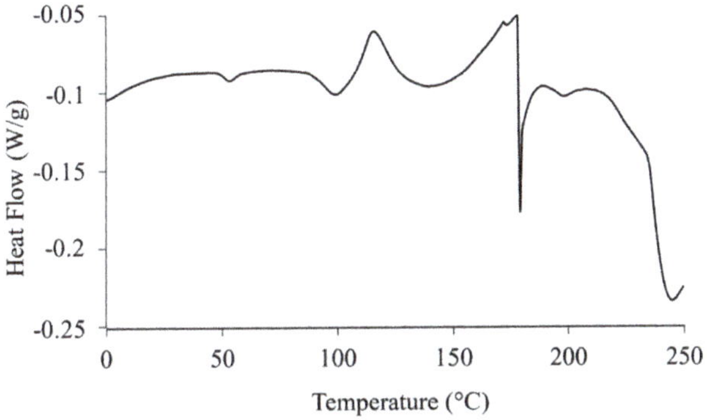

Figure 4. DSC thermogram of raw RocBr.

Table 1. DSC thermal analysis of RocBr (n = 3, mean ± standard deviation).

Sample	Peak 1		Peak 2		Peak 3	
	T_{peak} (°C)	Enthalpy (J/g)	T_{peak} (°C)	Enthalpy (J/g)	T_{peak} (°C)	Enthalpy (J/g)
Raw RocBr	53.6 ± 0.2	0.3 ± 0.1	96.9 ± 3.8	5.6 ± 0.8	173.2 ± 8.3	4.0 ± 0.3

2.4. Hot-Stage Microscopy (HSM)

Raw RocBr showed irregularly shaped aggregated particles without birefringence, indicating the non-crystalline nature of the solid-state drug, which was consistent with its XRPD diffractogram (Figure 5). At 164–166 °C, raw RocBr solid-state particles started to show a solid-to-liquid phase first-order transition, characteristic of melting, at ~175 °C. As temperature increased, RocBr remained in a liquid state, with possible decomposition shown at 250 °C. The transitions observed during HSM were consistent with DSC thermograms (Figure 4).

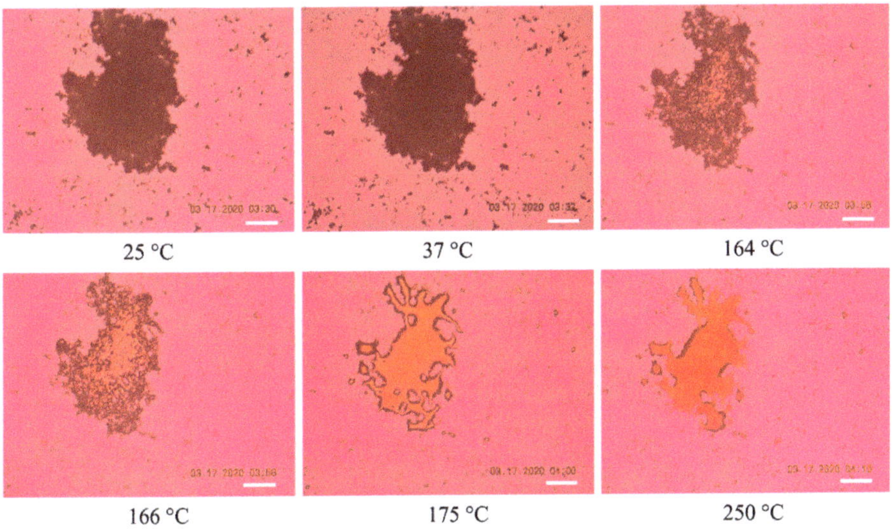

Figure 5. Representative HSM images of raw RocBr. The scale bar represents 100 μm.

2.5. Karl Fisher Titration (KFT)

The residual water content of raw RocBr was quantified by Karl Fisher coulometric titration. Raw RocBr powder had an average residual water content of 0.086 % $w/w \pm 0.023$ (Table 2).

Table 2. Residual water content in raw RocBr powder quantified by KFT (n = 3, mean ± standard deviation).

Sample Identification	Residual Water Content (% *w/w*)
RocBr1	0.065
RocBr2	0.084
RocBr3	0.110
Average ± SD	0.086 ± 0.023

2.6. Raman Spectroscopy

The Raman spectrum (Figure 6) of RocBr showed characteristic peaks (cm^{-1}) at 3125 (ν O–H, weak), 2994, 2871, 2825 (ν C–H, strong), 2354 (ν C=C, strong), 1749, 1641 (ν C=O, medium), 1446, 1310 (δ CH_2, medium), 1252, 1211, 1121, 1036, 856, 773, 716 and 655 (ν C–C, medium), as previously reported [13–15].

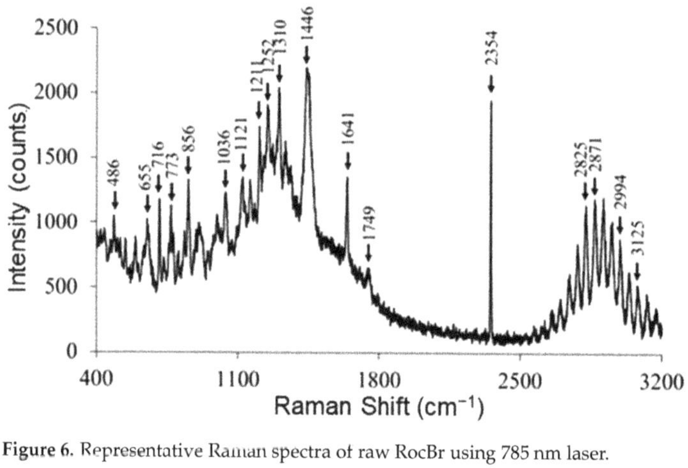

Figure 6. Representative Raman spectra of raw RocBr using 785 nm laser.

2.7. Attenuated Total Reflectance (ATR)–Fourier-Transform Infrared (FTIR) Spectroscopy

Figure 7 shows the ATR–FTIR spectrum of RocBr. The FTIR spectrum showed characteristic peaks (cm^{-1}) at 3360 (ν O–H, phenolic), 2928, 2858 (ν C–H, alkane), 1748 (ν C=O, ester), 1646 (ν C=C, alkene), 1451 (δ O–H, phenolic), 1376, 1219 (ν C–N), 1119 and 1024 (ν C–O, ester), as previously reported [14,15]. The spectral pattern seen in the fingerprint region (<1000 cm^{-1}) was consistently observed in raw RocBr.

2.8. In Vitro and In Silico Oil/Water Partitioning Coefficient (Log P) of RocBr

The in silico predicted pKa values of RocBr were 7.2 and 14.5 using ChemDraw™ (Ver. 16.0.; Cambridge Soft, Cambridge, MA, USA). The in silico calculated/computed Log P (cLog P) of RocBr was 2.43 using ChemDraw™ Ver. 16.0 (Cambridge Soft, Cambridge, MA, USA) and 1.72 using Swiss ADME (Swiss Institute of Bioinformatics, Switzerland). The experimental partition coefficient of RocBr was measured at pH 7.1 and 12.9. Log P of RocBr at 35 °C ranged from −0.61 to 0.90 and from −0.20 to 0.56 at room temperature (Table 3).

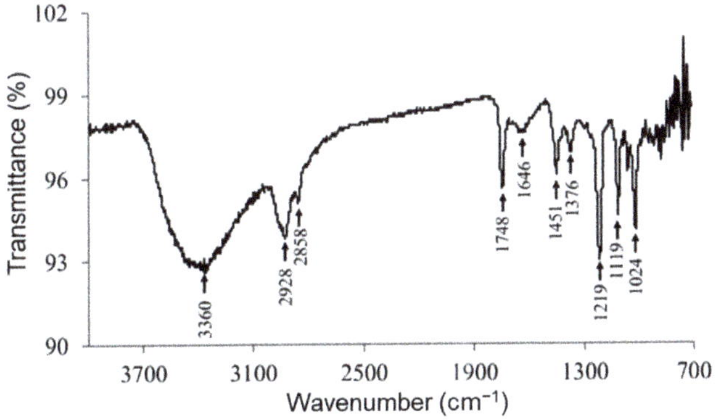

Figure 7. ATR–FTIR spectrum of raw RocBr.

Table 3. Summary of partition coefficient (Log P) for RocBr at various pH values (n = 3, mean ± standard deviation).

Experimental (Log P)	**Average ± SD**
At 35 °C, pH = 7.1	−0.61 ± 1.10
At Room temperature/ambient temperature, pH = 7.1	−0.20 ± 0.30
Experimental (Log P)	**Avg. Log P ± SD**
At 35 °C, pH = 12.9	0.90 ± 0.15
At Room temperature/ambient temperature, pH = 12.9	0.56 ± 0.48
Predicted (cLog P)	**Predicted Value**
ChemDraw Version 16.0	2.43
Swiss ADME	1.72

2.9. Ultraviolet (UV)/Visible (Vis) Spectroscopy

An absorption below wavelength of 200–250 nm (UVA) with a lambda maximum was observed in the UVA region at 210 nm, in both 0.1% (*w*/*v*) and 0.5% (*w*/*v*) RocBr solutions, when compared to methanol as a blank (Figure 8).

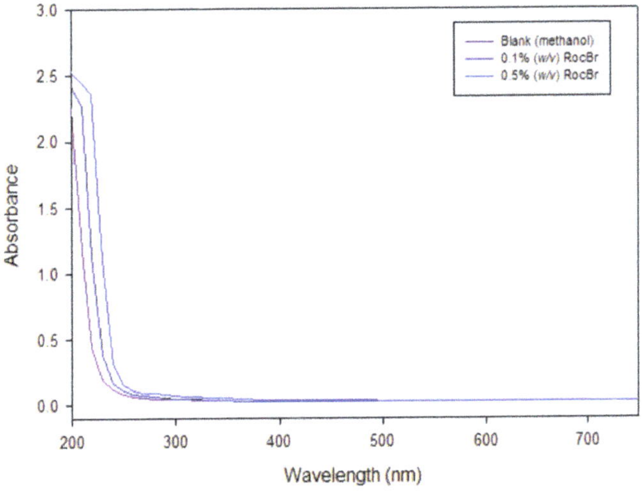

Figure 8. UV/Vis of 0.1% and 0.5% (*w*/*v*) RocBr in HPLC-grade methanol, as compared to HPLC-grade methanol alone over a range of 200 nm to 750 nm.

2.10. *High Performance Liquid Chromatography (HPLC) Analysis*

RocBr showed an average retention time of 7.02 ± 0.04 min (Figure 9B) when compared with acetonitrile (Figure 9A).

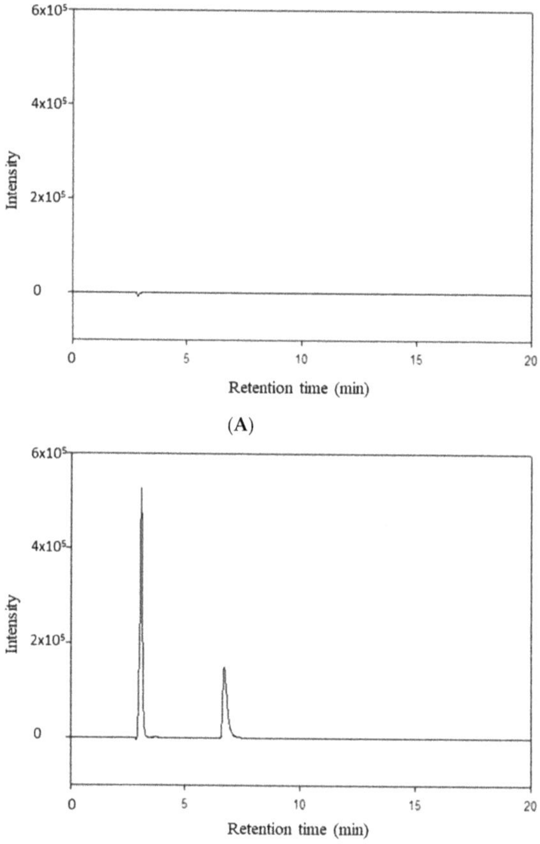

(**B**)

Figure 9. HPLC chromatogram of (**A**) HPLC-grade acetonitrile; (**B**) RocBr.

2.11. *In Silico ADME Prediction*

The Lipinski Rule of Five is a widely used guideline in drug design and development that predicts a compound's likelihood of being bioavailable. A set of rules known as the Lipinski Rule of Five is frequently applied in the drug discovery process to assess the possibility that a drug candidate would be successful in terms of being absorbed by the body. The rule is founded on the idea that substances which have particular physicochemical characteristics are more likely to have good oral bioavailability, which refers to a drug's capacity to enter the bloodstream.

A quaternary ammonium chemical called rocuronium bromide was first employed as a skeletal muscle relaxant. Its physicochemical characteristics are crucial to its active ingredient cutaneous and transdermal distribution. RocBr has a 610.78 g/mol molecular weight, which is a high value. Due to their large size, high-MW drugs are usually considered to have poor skin permeability. However, because rocuronium bromide is a charged chemical, ions could partner with skin lipids, which could increase skin penetration. Important factors in predicting skin permeation include the quantity of H-bond donors (NHD) and acceptors (NHA). With one H-bond donor and four H-bond acceptors, RocBr may be able to form a hydrogen bond with the skin molecules, improving its permeability. In general, RocBr physicochemical characteristics indicate that, depending on the particular skin conditions and formulation employed, it may have moderate-to-high skin permeability.

2.12. *In Vitro Cell Dose–Response Assay in 2D Cell Culture*

RocBr did not show any significant reduction in cell viability in either HaCaT or NHEK cells after 48 h of exposure to varying dose concentrations of drug, comparing experimental groups to control groups without RocBr (Figure 10A,B). The viability of NHEK primary cells was ~100% at all drug dose concentrations except 1000 µM. At 1000 µM drug concentration, the NHEK primary cell viability decreased significantly ($p < 0.0001$) compared to the other concentrations tested. The viability of HaCaT skin cells was ~100% when treated with RocBr at dose concentrations of 0.01 µM, 1 µM or 10 µM. The viability of HaCaT cells decreased significantly at 100 µM ($p < 0.05$) and 1000 µM ($p < 0.0001$) drug concentrations, compared to the lower concentrations tested.

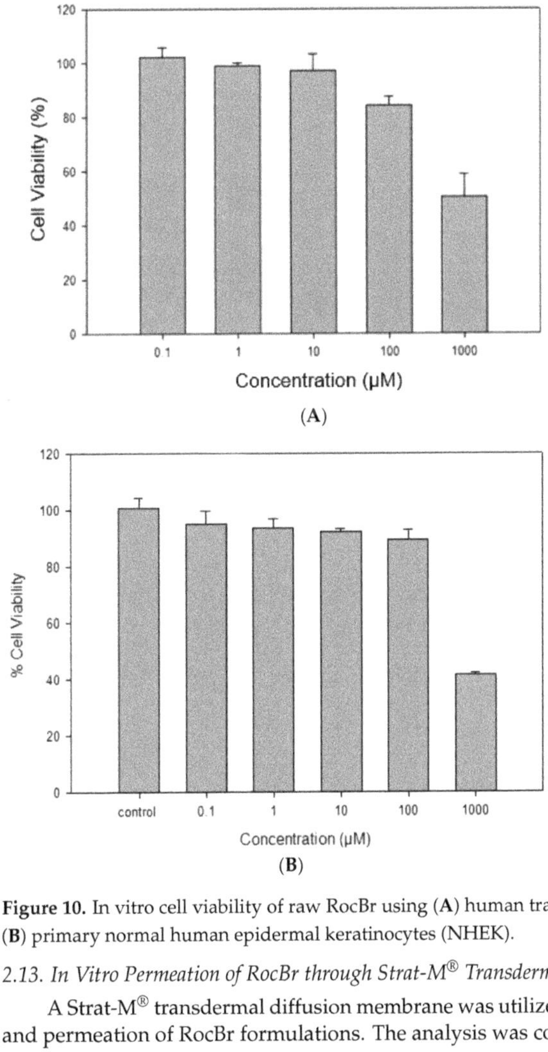

Figure 10. In vitro cell viability of raw RocBr using (**A**) human transformed keratinocytes (HaCaT), (**B**) primary normal human epidermal keratinocytes (NHEK).

2.13. *In Vitro Permeation of RocBr through Strat-M® Transdermal Diffusion Membrane*

A Strat-M® transdermal diffusion membrane was utilized to evaluate in vitro diffusion and permeation of RocBr formulations. The analysis was conducted with 1% (*w*/*v*) RocBr lotion and 1% (*w*/*v*) RocBr solution. RocBr in 1% (*w*/*v*) solution and lotion exhibited no measurable permeation through/diffusion out of the Strat-M® membrane at all the timepoints. As expected, RocBr lotion showed significantly ($p < 0.0001$) higher retention (953.9 ± 17.9 μg) on the membrane than that of solution (768.3 ± 12.6 μg) (Table 4).

Table 4. In vitro skin permeation parameters of RocBr 1% (*w*/*v*) lotion and 1% (*w*/*v*) solution through Strat-M® transdermal diffusion membrane (n = 3, mean ± standard deviation).

Sample	Flux (μg/cm²/h)	Lag Time (h)	Drug Retention (μg)
1% (*w*/*v*) solution in PBS (pH = 7.4)		-	768.3 ± 12.6
1% (*w*/*v*) RocBr lotion	-	-	953.9 ± 17.9

Diffusion through the 3D cell model is relevant, as it helps to predict RocBr skin depth penetration capacity and drug accumulation in the human tissue, which are essential for topical delivery for skin carcinogenesis treatment. Epiderm™ was used to study drug permeation of 1% (*w*/*v*) RocBr lotion and solution over the course of 6 h (Figure 11). Flux (J) value from 1% (*w*/*v*) lotion was lower than that of drug solution. On the other hand, RocBr lotion (29.2 ± 6.76 μg) showed less retention than RocBr solution (Table 5).

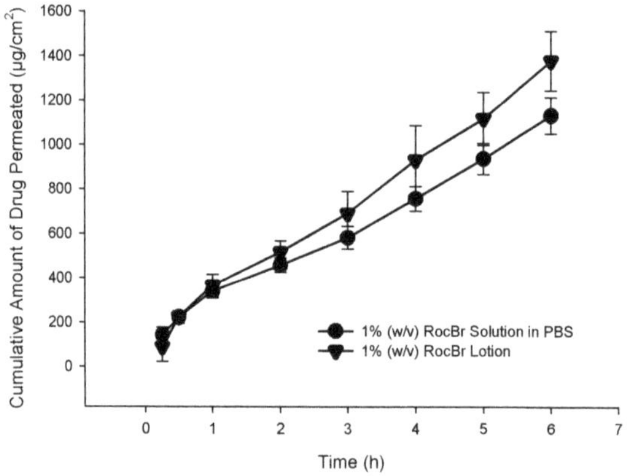

Figure 11. In vitro EpiDerm™ permeation profile of RocBr. 1% (*w*/*v*) PBS (pH = 7.4) solution and 1% (*w*/*v*) RocBr lotion.

Table 5. In vitro skin permeation parameters of RocBr 1% (*w*/*v*) lotion and 1% (*w*/*v*) solution through EpiDerm™ 3D normal human-derived epidermal keratinocytes (n = 3, mean ± standard deviation).

Sample	Flux (μg/cm²/h)	Lag Time (h)	Drug Retention (μg)
1% (*w*/*v*) solution in PBS (pH = 7.4)	177.2 ± 9.25	-	63.5 ± 19.8
1% (*w*/*v*) RocBr lotion	112.0 ± 12.0	-	29.2 ± 6.76

3. Discussion

RocBr is a steroidal neuromuscular blocking agent and is commonly used as a muscle relaxant during surgery or mechanical ventilation [16]. Recently, RocBr was identified as an inhibitor of PRPK, attenuating the development of solar-simulated light-induced cSCC and expression of proliferation and oncogenesis markers in SKH1 hairless mice [5]. A preformulation study to understand the physicochemical and solid-state nature of the drug is important. Thus, an in-depth physicochemical characterization and solid-state analysis of raw RocBr was conducted. Comprehensive physicochemical characterization—thermal analysis, imaging by electron microscopy with energy dispersive spectroscopy X-ray spectroscopy, imaging by hot-stage microscopy, molecular fingerprinting by spectroscopy and in vitro properties of RocBr—was conducted and reported for the first time. RocBr powder appears to be non-crystalline at room and biological temperatures, as indicated by the lack of sharp diffraction peaks which are characteristic of long-range molecular order in crystalline powders in XRPD, the lack of crystalline birefringence in HSM and the exothermic peak indicative of a disorder-to-order solid-state first-order phase transition followed by melting in DSC, which is also a first-order phase transition. RocBr powder has a measurable first-order phase transition of melting at a high temperature well above 100 °C. The very low residual water content of the RocBr powder is consistent with hydrophobicity. In addition, we have successfully developed, for the first time, a RocBr lotion with biocompatible excipients that are commonly used in the cosmetics industry.

In vitro cell viability was evaluated with 2D human cell culture of HaCaT skin cells and 2D normal human epidermal keratinocytes (NHEK®). Keratinocytes play a vital role in providing functions and structure to the skin [17]. Normal human epidermal keratinocytes (NHEK) are primary cells collected from the epidermis of adult donors, which have been widely used as a model for inflammatory skin diseases and skin responses to ultraviolet radiation or oxidative stress [18–22]. HaCaT is a spontaneously immortalized keratinocyte line derived from adult trunk skin and has been widely used as a reliable in vitro model for studies of epidermal architecture, inflammatory responses and skin metabolism [23–26]. In addition, HaCaT cells have p53 mutations that are characteristic of cutaneous squamous cell carcinomas and, thus, are considered as a relevant model for analyzing skin cancer development [27]. In vitro toxicity of RocBr on human skin cells was successfully demonstrated over a wide drug concentration dose range using 2D cell culture. This was evident for both the HaCaT human keratinocyte cell line and NHEK primary cells. The findings indicate that the viability of NHEK primary cells and HaCaT cells remained high at all tested drug dose concentrations, except for the highest concentration (1000 μM). At this concentration, the NHEK primary cell viability decreased significantly compared to the other concentrations tested. The significant difference in viability at the highest dose concentration compared to the others indicates that there is likely a dose-dependent effect on cell viability. The high cell viability observed in this study at the lower drug concentrations indicates that the drug may be safe to use at therapeutic doses.

In vitro oil/water partition coefficient at two different temperatures (representing ambient and skin temperature) were successfully completed and reported for the first time. In vitro Log P was measured under various conditions and was found to be ~0, which is consistent with amphiphilic drugs which demonstrate near-equal partitioning of drug molecules into both the hydrophobic octanol phase and hydrophilic aqueous phase.

In vitro models are very important for predicting drug permeation through skin in the early stage of formulation development. Strat-M® membrane is a synthetic model designed to mimic the structure and lipid composition of human skin, which has been widely used to evaluate topical formulations [28–32] and screen between different formulations for their optimization. While the Strat-M® membrane can be used for studying drug permeation across the skin, it is not identical to the complex structure and properties of the skin. Another in vitro model, EpiDerm®, was used as a three-dimensional tissue model, consisting of multiple layers of normal human epidermal keratinocytes on inserts [33]. EpiDerm® model exhibits similar morphology, lipid profile, metabolic activity and barrier functions of normal human skin and, thus, it has been used for assessing skin irritancy, phototoxicity and drug transport [34]. The new RocBr lotion formulation was successfully tested for drug permeation and membrane drug retention using Strat-M® synthetic biomimetic membrane with the in vitro Franz cell diffusion system. No measurable drug flux was observed for RocBr lotion nor RocBr solution using the in vitro Strat-M® synthetic biomimetic membrane/Franz cell diffusion system. RocBr lotion provided significantly ($p < 0.0001$) higher retention in the Strat-M® membrane compared to the RocBr solution using the in vitro Strat-M® synthetic biomimetic membrane/Franz cell diffusion system. This demonstrates that both formulations are suitable for targeted skin drug delivery with relatively high tissue retention, with the lotion being superior to the solution under these conditions.

In addition to the in vitro Strat-M® synthetic biomimetic membrane/Franz cell diffusion system, EpiDerm® 3D human tissue was successfully used to evaluate the membrane drug retention and drug diffusion behavior of RocBr in vitro. Both RocBr lotion and solution formulations demonstrated measurable drug flux and membrane retention. However, RocBr solution demonstrated relatively higher values of both flux and tissue membrane retention than the RocBr lotion when using EpiDerm® 3D human tissue. One advantage of using EpiDerm® tissue for drug permeation studies is its close resemblance to human skin, which can provide more accurate and representative results compared to synthetic membranes such as Strat-M®. However, EpiDerm™ tissue typically has a thickness of 0.3 to 0.4 mm, which can limit its use for studying the permeation of drugs with regard to deeper skin penetration. Another plausible explanation for the difference in results in both Strat-M® and EpiDerm™ is the potential for RocBr skin penetration. Molecular modeling showed how RocBr may have poor penetration given its molecular weight being >500 g/mol, despite its low Log P, as shown in Table 3. Furthermore, other factors which could have impacted penetration are pH of formulation, hydration of membranes and concentration of dissolved drug.

This again demonstrates that both formulations are suitable for targeted skin drug delivery with relatively high tissue retention, with the lotion being superior to the solution under these conditions.

4. Materials and Methods

4.1. Materials

Rocuronium bromide (purity 99%, molecular weight 529.79 g/mol, $C_{32}H_{53}N_2O_4{}^+Br^-$) was purchased from MuseChem (Fairfield, NJ, USA), with structure as shown in Figure 12 (ChemDraw™ Ver. 16.0.; Cambridge Soft, Cambridge, MA, USA). Sodium bromide (purity 99%), tetramethylammonium hydroxide pentahydrate (purity > 97%), phosphoric acid for HPLC (purity 85–90%) and Hydranal®-Coulomat AD and resazurin sodium salt were purchased from Sigma-Aldrich (St. Louis, MO, USA). Sodium chloride (purity 99%, salt, crystal, reagent, A.C.S) was purchased from Spectrum Chemical MFG Corp. (Gardena, CA, USA). The digital thermometer/hygrometer LSCs were purchased from Veanic (Shenzhen-shi Aoyu Keji Co., Ltd., Shenzhen, China). The 0.2 µm nylon membranes (25 mm) were purchased from VWR (Radnor, PA, USA).

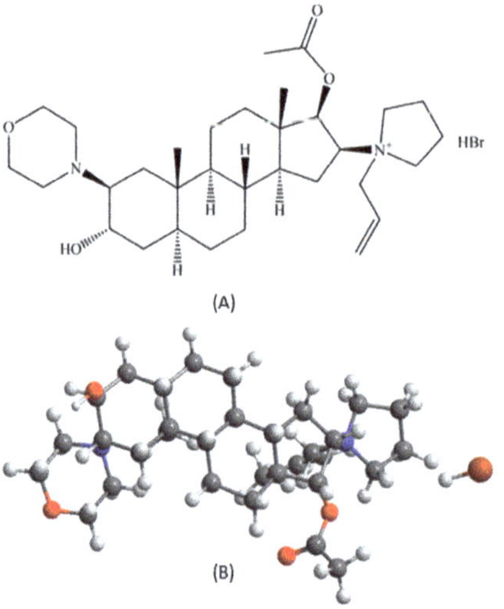

Figure 12. Rocuronium bromide (RocBr): (**A**) chemical structure (**B**) 3D ball-and-stick chemical structure (ChemDraw™ Ver. 16.0.; Cambridge Soft, Cambridge, MA, USA).

The human keratinocyte immortal cell line (HaCaT, AddexBio® T0020001) was purchased from AddexBio (San Diego, CA, USA). The Dulbecco's modified Eagle's medium (DMEM), optimized 1X was obtained from AddexBio (San Diego, CA, USA). Fetal bovine serum (FBS), Pen-Strep (5000 U/mL) and Fungizone® were obtained from Gibco™ Life Technologies (Thermo Fisher Inc, Waltham, MA, USA). Normal human epidermal keratinocytes (NHEK®), which are primary adult cells, and their growth media (NHEK-GM®) were both purchased from MatTek Life Sciences (Ashland, MA, USA). EpiDerm™, a 3D tissue model consisting of normal human-derived epidermal keratinocytes, and its EpiDerm™ special growth medium were purchased from MatTek Life Sciences (Ashland, MA, USA). The Strat-M® membrane (Transdermal Diffusion Test Model, 47 mm) was purchased from Millipore Sigma (Danvers, MA, USA).

4.2. Preparation of the Topical Oil/Water Emulsion Formulation

The rocuronium bromide (RocBr) 1% (*w*/*v*) oil/water emulsion lotion was prepared by the Dr. Ann Bode lab at The Hormel Institute at the University of Minnesota (Austin, MN, USA) [35]. Briefly, oil-in-water lotion of RocBr was prepared by mixing Phase A and B at 70 °C. All ingredients in Phase A and B were melted at 75–80 °C before mixing. Phase A comprised 0.05 g sodium salt of ethylenediamine tetra-acetic acid (nonallergenic preservative and stabilizer), 3 mL 1,3-butylene glycol (humectant), 4 mL glycerin (humectant), 2 mL pentylene glycol (skin conditioning agent) and distilled water to prepare 100 mL; phase B comprised 1.2 g cetyl alcohol (emulsion stabilizer), 1.5 g glyceryl stearate (emulsifying agent) and 8 mL hydrogenated polydecene (skin conditioning agent). RocBr powder was slowly added during continuous mixing of phase A and phase B at 70 °C and then the mixture was allowed to cool down to 30–35 °C. RocBr lotion was stored at 4 °C until further evaluation.

4.3. Scanning Electron Microscopy (SEM) and Energy-Dispersive X-ray (EDX) Spectroscopy

Surface morphology of raw RocBr powder was visualized under scanning electron microscopy (SEM) (FEI, Brno, Czech Republic). The sample was mounted on the stub with double-sided adhesive carbon tape (TedPatella, Inc., Redding, CA, USA) and coated with a 7 nm thin film of gold palladium alloy under argon plasma in the Anatech Hummer 6.2 sputtering system (Union City, CA, USA). SEM micrographs were captured under 30 kV accelerating voltage at a working distance of approximately 9–12 mm. Mean size, standard deviation and size range of the particles were determined digitally in SEM micrographs using SigmaScan™ Pro 5.0.0 (Systat, Inc., San Jose, CA, USA). At least 60 particles were measured in the representative micrographs of raw RocBr powder at 400–5000× magnification.

EDX for elemental fingerprinting was performed on raw RocBr powder with Thermo Noran System Six (Thermo Scientific, Waltham, MA, USA) at an accumulation voltage of 30 keV. The spot size was increased until a dead time of 20–30 s was reached.

4.4. X-ray Powder Diffraction (XRPD)

The crystalline nature of raw RocBr powder was determined by a PANalytical X'pert diffractometer (PANalytical Inc., Westborough, MA, USA) equipped with a programmable incident beam slit and an X'celerator detector. The X-ray radiation used was Ni-filtered Cu Kα (45 kV, 40 Ma and λ = 1.5444 Å). Measurements were taken between 5° and 89.9° (2θ) with a scan rate of 2.00°/min. The powder samples were loaded on a zero-background silicon sample holder.

4.5. Differential Scanning Calorimetry (DSC)

A TA Q1000 differential scanning calorimeter, with autosampler and RSC autocooling system (TA Instruments, New Castle, DE, USA), was used to analyze the thermal transition of raw RocBr powder. Approximately 1–3 mg of raw RocBr were weighed and hermetically sealed in a DSC pan (TA Instruments, New Castle, DE, USA). An empty hermetically sealed aluminum pan was used as a reference. UHP nitrogen gas was used as the purging gas at a flow rate of 40 mL/min. The samples were heated from 0.00 °C to 250.00 °C at a scanning rate of 5.00 °C/min. All measurements were conducted in triplicate.

4.6. Hot-Stage Microscopy (HSM)

Thermal changes of raw RocBr powder during heating were observed under a Leica DMLP cross-polarized microscope (Wetzlar, Germany) equipped with a Mettler FP 80 central processor heating unit and a Mettler FP82 hot stage (Columbus, OH, USA). Raw RocBr powder was mounted onto a glass slide and heated from 25 °C to 250 °C at a heating rate of 5.00 °C/min. The images were digitally captured with a Nikon Coolpix 8800 digital camera (Nikon, Tokyo, Japan) under 10× optical objective and 10× digital zoom.

4.7. Karl Fisher Titration (KFT)

Coulometric KFT was utilized to determine the residual water content of raw RocBr powder. Briefly, RocBr was dissolved in anhydrous methanol at 1 µg/mL (0.1% *w*/*v*) and 1 mL of solution was added to the titration cell containing Hydranal® Coulomat AD reagent in a TitroLine 750 trace titrator (SI Analytics, Weilheim, Germany).

4.8. Raman Spectroscopy

Raman spectra for molecular fingerprinting of raw RocBr powder were obtained using Renishaw inVia Reflex (Gloucestershire, United Kingdom) at exciting laser wavelength of 785 nm, under Leica DM2700 optical microscope (Wetzlar, Germany) at 20× magnification. The scans were obtained with 1% of laser power and 10 s exposure time. Baseline correction was made in the spectra prior to analysis with Renishaw WiRE 3.4 software.

4.9. Attenuated Total Reflectance (ATR)–Fourier-Transform Infrared (FTIR) Spectroscopy

ATR–FTIR spectra for molecular fingerprinting of raw RocBr powder were obtained using a Nicolet Avatar 360 FTIR spectrometer (Varian, Inc.,Palo Alto, CA, USA) to determine the molecular fingerprint and presence of functional groups of RocBr. Each spectrum was collected over the wavenumber range of 4000–700 cm^{-1} after 32 scans at a resolution of 2 cm^{-1}. A background spectrum was obtained under the same conditions. EZ-OMNIC software version 7.3 was used to acquire and analyze the spectra.

4.10. Ultraviolet (UV)/Visible (Vis) Spectroscopy

UV/Vis spectra of raw RocBr were obtained with Molecular Devices® SpectraMax® M3 Multi-Mode Microplate Reader (Sunnyvale, CA, USA) from 200 nm to 750 nm. RocBr was dissolved in methanol at 0.1% and 0.5% (*w*/*v*) and analyzed in a 96-well plate.

4.11. High Performance Liquid Chromatography (HPLC) Analysis

The HPLC analysis was performed on a Shimadzu LC-2010A HT liquid chromatograph (Torrance, CA, USA) coupled with a UV–Vis dual wavelength detector and a Luna Silica, 5 µm column (250 mm × 4.6 mm) (Phenomenex, Torrance, CA, USA). RocBr was detected at 210 nm. The mobile phase was 60:40 (*v*/*v*) acetonitrile:tetramethylammonium hydroxide pentahydrate (0.025M), with pH adjusted to approximately 7.4 with 1:9 (*v*/*v*) phosphoric acid:acetonitrile solution. The flow rate was set to 1.0 mL/min and injection volume was 10 µL, as previously reported [36,37]. The retention time for RocBr was ~7 min. Drug concentration was determined with a five-point standard curve (0.03125 mg/mL to 1 mg/mL, R^2 = 0.9998). Standards were prepared by serial dilution of RocBr bulk solution with acetonitrile and stored at 4 °C, protected from light.

4.12. In Vitro and In Silico Oil/Water Partition Coefficient (Log P) of RocBr

For in vitro measurements, 3 mg of RocBr powder was added to an amber glass vial containing equal volume (1.5 mL) of 1-octanol and phosphate buffered saline (PBS, 1×, pH 7.4) to make a 1 mg/mL solution. The pH was adjusted to 7.1 and 12.9 with

0.1 M hydrochloric acid (HCl) solution and 0.1 M sodium hydroxide (NaOH) solution, respectively. Log P of RocBr was determined using Equation (1):

$$\text{Log P} = \text{Log}\{[\text{RocBr}]_{\text{oil}}/[\text{RocBr}]_{\text{water}}\} \quad (1)$$

Two temperatures—ambient room temperature and 35 °C, which is the widely reported and generally accepted average human skin temperature—were used. The vials were rotated for 24 h and then left undisturbed in a vertical position for phase separation for the next 24 h. A volume of 200 µL of the organic and aqueous layer were sampled very carefully without disturbing the interface and analyzed using the HPLC method described above.

For in silico predictive modeling, ChemDraw™ Ver. 16.0 (Cambridge Soft, Cambridge, MA, USA) and Swiss ADME (Swiss Institute of Bioinformatics, Switzerland) web server were used. The purpose of molecular modeling was to have theoretical values for the physicochemical properties, lipophilicity and water solubility of rocuronium bromide. Theoretical Log P was compared to the in vitro results.

4.13. In Silico ADME Prediction

Lipinski's Rule of Five and skin permeation RocBr were all tested utilizing the SwissADME web server.

4.14. In Vitro Cell Viability by 2D Cell Culture of a Human Skin Cell Line and Human Primary Skin Cells

The cell viability of RocBr on human epidermis was evaluated with the HaCaT human keratinocyte immortal cell line and NHEK (normal human epidermal keratinocyte) primary cells as 2D cell culture. The HaCaT cells were grown in Dulbecco's modified Eagle's medium (DMEM, Optimized 1X), supplemented with 10% (*v*/*v*) fetal bovine serum (FBS) and Pen-Strep (100 units/mL penicillin, 100 µg/mL) in a humidified incubator at 37 °C and 5% CO_2. NHEK primary cells were grown in the medium provided by MatTek (Ashland, MA, USA) in a humidified incubator at 37 °C and 5% CO_2.

HaCaT and NHEK cells were seeded into 96-black well plates at 5000 cells in 100 µL medium per well. After 48 h, cells were exposed to RocBr at concentrations of 1000 µM, 100 µM, 10 µM, 1 µM or 0.1 µM. Drug solutions were prepared by dissolving raw RocBr powder in 1 mL of HPLC-grade ethanol (EtOH) and diluted with 9 mL of growth media. A volume of 100 µL of drug solution was added to each well. After 48 h, 20 µL of 20 µM resazurin sodium salt was added to each well and incubated for 4 h. Fluorescence intensity of resofurin was detected at 544 nm (excitation) and 590 nm (emission) using the Molecular Devices® SpectraMax® M3 Multi-Mode Microplate Reader (Sunnyvale, CA, USA). The relative viability of the cells was calculated by Equation (2) as follows:

$$\text{Relative Viability\%} = \frac{\text{Sample flourescence intensity}}{\text{Control flourescece intensity}} \times 100\% \quad (2)$$

4.15. In Vitro Permeation of RocBr Using Strat-M® Synthetic Biomimetic Membrane and Franz Cell Diffusion System

Strat-M® synthetic membrane (Sigma Aldrich, St. Louis, MO, USA) inside a glass Franz Cell Diffusion system (Permegear, Hellertown, PA, USA) was used to study the drug membrane permeation and retention of RocBr from RocBr solution (1% *w*/*v* RocBr solution prepared in PBS, pH 7.4, 200 µL) and lotion formulations. The membrane diameter available for diffusion was 5.0 cm. The RocBr formulation was prepared as described in the methods section. PBS (pH 7.4) mixed with 10% (*v*/*v*) ethanol was used as the receptor medium. The receptor compartment was filled with 5 mL of medium and maintained at 35 °C, the well-reported and generally accepted average human skin temperature, in a reciprocal shaking bath model 25 (Thermo Fisher Scientific, Fair Lawn, NJ, USA) at 30 oscillations/minute. A volume of 200 µL of RocBr solution and RocBr lotion were added onto the membrane and the effective diffusion area was 0.64 cm^2. At predetermined time intervals, 200 μL of the receptor medium was sampled and replaced with an equal volume of fresh medium. The flux at steady-state (J) was estimated as the slope of the linear regression analysis of the linear portion of the permeation curve. Lag time (Lt) was defined as the time intercept of the steady-state region of the permeation curve (i.e., x-intercept) [38]. The cumulative drug permeation and drug retention on the membrane were quantified with the HPLC method described in the Methods section.

4.16. In Vitro Permeation of RocBr by Using 3D Normal Human-Derived Epidermal Keratinocytes (EpiDerm^{TM}) and MatTek Permeation Device

Following Mat-Tek's protocol [39] and the MatTek Permeation Device (MatTek, Ashland, MA, USA), EpiDerm^{TM} samples were placed in tissue culture inserts and transferred onto a 6-well cell culture plate. Each well was pre-filled with 1 mL of Dulbecco's phosphate buffered saline without calcium chloride ($CaCl_2$) or magnesium chloride ($MgCl_2$) (Mat-Tek, Ashland, MA, USA). The plate was placed in a reciprocal shaking bath model 25 (Thermo Fisher Scientific, Fair Lawn, NJ, USA) at 30 oscillations per minute and maintained at 35 °C ± 0.05 °C, the well-reported and generally accepted average human skin temperature. A volume of 400 μL of RocBr lotion was added onto the EpiDerm^{TM} and the effective diffusion area was 0.256 cm^2. The same HPLC method described earlier was used.

4.17. Statistical Analysis

The data are presented as the mean ± standard deviation, derived from three independent experiments (n = 3). The statistical difference between the results of cell viability and drug retention were compared by one-way analysis of variance (ANOVA) with Tukey's post hoc test for comparisons (Prism 9.0, GraphPad Software, San Diego, CA, USA). In all cases, the p values of 0.05 or less were considered significant.

5. Conclusions

In conclusion, this systematic and comprehensive study reports several new findings for the first time. These include comprehensive physicochemical characterization, thermal analysis, imaging by electron microscopy with energy dispersive spectroscopy X-ray spectroscopy, imaging by hot-stage microscopy, molecular fingerprinting by spectroscopy and in vitro properties of RocBr. These in vitro properties include oil/water partition coefficient at two different temperatures, showing equal distribution of drug molecules in the octanol and water phases, consistent which drug amphilicity, Also observed were low toxicity in 2D human skin cell culture of the HaCaT human keratinocyte cell line over a wide drug concentration, low toxicity in 2D normal human epidermal keratinocytes (NHEK®) primary cells over a wide drug concentration, drug permeation and membrane retention using Strat-M® synthetic biomimetic membrane and drug permeation and membrane drug retention using EpiDerm ^{TM} human skin tissue.

A topical oil/water emulsion lotion formulation was developed and evaluated. The in vitro permeation behavior of RocBr from its lotion formulation was quantified with Strat-M® synthetic biomimetic membrane and EpiDerm^{TM} 3D human skin tissue. Significant membrane retention of RocBr drug was evident and more retention was obtained with the lotion formulation compared with the solution. Drug penetration of RocBr lotion was evaluated in two in vitro models, using STRAT-M® synthetic biomimetic membrane/Franz cell diffusion system and Epiderm® human tissue. Drug retention in the membrane was quantifiable and relatively high. Drug flux out of the membrane was relatively low, which is favorable for local skin delivery to treat non-melanoma skin cancer while minimizing systemic exposure. Clinical evaluation for treating non-melanoma skin cancer would be needed to assess clinical application.

Author Contributions: Conceptualization, V.H.R., C.C.-L., A.M.B. and H.M.M.; methodology, V.H.R., D.E.-B., B.S., B.B.E., E.R., N.O.A. and H.M.M.; formal analysis, V.H.R., D.E.-B., B.S., B.B.E., E.R., N.O.A., A.M.B. and H.M.M.; resources, C.C.-L., A.M.B. and H.M.M.; writing—original draft preparation, V.H.R., D.E.-B., B.S., B.B.E., E.R. and H.M.M.; writing—review and editing, V.H.R., D.E.-B., B.S., B.B.E., E.R., E.R., N.O.A., C.C.-L., A.M.B. and H.M.M.; project administration, C.C.-L., A.M.B. and H.M.M.; funding acquisition, C.C.-L., A.M.B. and H.M.M.; supervision, C.C.-L., A.M.B. and H.M.M. All authors have read and agreed to the published version of the manuscript.

Funding: This work was supported by federal grant award NIH NCI Project Program Grant (PPG) P01CA229112.

Institutional Review Board Statement: Not applicable.

Informed Consent Statement: Not applicable.

Data Availability Statement: The data presented in this study are available on request from the Corresponding Author.

Acknowledgments: All SEM images and data were collected in the W.M. Keck Center for Nano-Scale Imaging in the Department of Chemistry and Biochemistry at the University of Arizona, with funding from the W.M. Keck Foundation Grant. All FTIR spectra were collected in the W.M. Keck Center for Nano-Scale Imaging in the Department of Chemistry and Biochemistry at the University of Arizona. This instrument purchase was supported by Arizona Technology and Research Initiative Fund (A.R.S.§15-1648). The authors thank the Imaging Cores Materials Imaging and Characterization Facility supported by the University of Arizona Office of Research, Discovery and Innovation and the X-Ray Diffraction Facility of the Department of Chemistry and Biochemistry at The University of Arizona. The authors thank Jianqin Lu for access to the SpectraMax M3 multimode plate reader. The authors sincerely thank Brooke Beam-Masani and Andrei Astachkine for the core facility access and assistance.

Conflicts of Interest: The authors declare no potential conflict of interest with respect to the research, authorship and/or publication of this article.

References

1. Burton, K.A.; Ashack, K.A.; Khachemoune, A. Cutaneous squamous cell carcinoma: A review of high-risk and metastatic disease. *Am. J. Clin. Dermatol.* **2016**, *17*, 491–508. [CrossRef] [PubMed]
2. Wehner, M.R. Underestimation of Cutaneous Squamous Cell Carcinoma Incidence, Even in Cancer Registries. *JAMA Dermatol.* **2020**, *156*, 1290–1291. [CrossRef] [PubMed]
3. Tokez, S.; Hollestein, L.; Louwman, M.; Nijsten, T.; Wakkee, M. Incidence of Multiple vs First Cutaneous Squamous Cell Carcinoma on a Nationwide Scale and Estimation of Future Incidences of Cutaneous Squamous Cell Carcinoma. *JAMA Dermatol.* **2020**, *156*, 1300–1306. [CrossRef] [PubMed]
4. US Department of Health and Human Services. Skin cancer as a major public health problem. In *The Surgeon General's Call to Action to Prevent Skin Cancer*; Office of the Surgeon General (US): Washington, DC, USA, 2014.
5. Roh, E.; Lee, M.-H.; Zykova, T.A.; Zhu, F.; Nadas, J.; Kim, H.-G.; Bae, K.B.; Li, Y.; Cho, Y.Y.; Curiel-Lewandrowski, C.; et al. Targeting PRPK and TOPK for skin cancer prevention and therapy. *Oncogene* **2018**, *37*, 5633–5647. [CrossRef]
6. Gellrich, F.F.; Huning, S.; Beissert, S.; Eigentler, T.; Stockfleth, E.; Gutzmer, R.; Meier, F. Medical treatment of advanced cutaneous squamous-cell carcinoma. *J. Eur. Acad. Dermatol. Venereol.* **2019**, *33* (Suppl. 8), 38–43. [CrossRef]
7. Work, G.; Invited, R.; Kim, J.Y.S.; Kozlow, J.H.; Mittal, B.; Moyer, J.; Olenecki, T.; Rodgers, P. Guidelines of care for the management of cutaneous squamous cell carcinoma. *J. Am. Acad. Dermatol.* **2018**, *78*, 560–578. [CrossRef]
8. Capalbo, C.; Belardinilli, F.; Filetti, M.; Parisi, C.; Petroni, M.; Colicchia, V.; Tessitore, A.; Santoni, M.; Coppa, A.; Giannini, G.; et al. Effective treatment of a platinum-resistant cutaneous squamous cell carcinoma case by EGFR pathway inhibition. *Mol. Clin. Oncol.* **2018**, *9*, 30–34. [CrossRef]
9. Swick, A.D.; Prabakaran, P.J.; Miller, M.C.; Javaid, A.M.; Fisher, M.M.; Sampene, E.; Ong, I.M.; Hu, R.; Iida, M.; Nickel, K.P.; et al. Cotargeting mTORC and EGFR Signaling as a Therapeutic Strategy in HNSCC. *Mol. Cancer Ther.* **2017**, *16*, 1257–1268. [CrossRef]
10. Zan, U.; Topaktas, M.; Istifli, E.S. In vitro genotoxicity of rocuronium bromide in human peripheral lymphocytes. *Cytotechnology* **2011**, *63*, 239–245. [CrossRef]
11. Eedara, B.B.; Rangnekar, B.; Sinha, S.; Doyle, C.; Cavallaro, A.; Das, S.C. Development and characterization of high payload combination dry powders of anti-tubercular drugs for treating pulmonary tuberculosis. *Eur. J. Pharm. Sci.* **2018**, *118*, 216–226. [CrossRef]
12. Gomez, A.I.; Acosta, M.F.; Muralidharan, P.; Yuan, J.X.; Black, S.M.; Hayes, D., Jr.; Mansour, H.M. Advanced spray dried proliposomes of amphotericin B lung surfactant-mimic phospholipid microparticles/nanoparticles as dry powder inhalers for targeted pulmonary drug delivery. *Pulm. Pharmacol. Ther.* **2020**, *64*, 101975. [CrossRef] [PubMed]

13. Nyquist, R.A. (Ed.) Chapter 4-Alkenes and Other Compounds Containing C=C Double Bonds. In *Interpreting Infrared, Raman, and Nuclear Magnetic Resonance Spectra*; Academic Press: San Diego, CA, USA, 2001; pp. 55–91.
14. Larkin, P. *Infrared and Raman Spectroscopy: Principles and Spectral Interpretation*; Elsevier: Amsterdam, The Netherlands, 2017.
15. Lin-Vien, D. *The Handbook of Infrared and Raman Characteristic Frequencies of Organic Molecules*; Nachdr, Ed.; Academic Press: San Diego, CA, USA, 2006.
16. Wicks, T.C. The Pharmacology of Rocuronium Bromide (ORG 9426). *AANA J.* **1994**, *62*, 33–38. [PubMed]
17. Barbieri, J.S.; Wanat, K.; Seykora, J. Skin: Basic Structure and Function. In *Pathobiology of Human Disease*; McManus, L.M., Mitchell, R.N., Eds.; Academic Press: San Diego, CA, USA, 2014; pp. 1134–1144.
18. Afaq, F.; Adhami, V.M.; Ahmad, N.; Mukhtar, H. Inhibition of ultraviolet B-mediated activation of nuclear factor κB in normal human epidermal keratinocytes by green tea Constituent (-)-epigallocatechin-3-gallate. *Oncogene* **2003**, *22*, 1035–1044. [CrossRef]
19. Fukawa, T.; Kajiya, H.; Ozeki, S.; Ikebe, T.; Okabe, K. Reactive oxygen species stimulates epithelial mesenchymal transition in normal human epidermal keratinocytes via TGF-beta secretion. *Exp. Cell Res.* **2012**, *318*, 1926–1932. [CrossRef] [PubMed]
20. Meephansan, J.; Tsuda, H.; Komine, M.; Tominaga, S.-i.; Ohtsuki, M. Regulation of IL-33 Expression by IFN-γ and Tumor Necrosis Factor-α in Normal Human Epidermal Keratinocytes. *J. Investig. Dermatol.* **2012**, *132*, 2593–2600. [CrossRef]
21. Liu, L.; Xie, H.; Chen, X.; Shi, W.; Xiao, X.; Lei, D.; Li, J. Differential response of normal human epidermal keratinocytes and HaCaT cells to hydrogen peroxide-induced oxidative stress. *Clin. Exp. Dermatol.* **2012**, *37*, 772–780. [CrossRef]
22. Dazard, J.-E.; Gal, H.; Amariglio, N.; Rechavi, G.; Domany, E.; Givol, D. Genome-wide comparison of human keratinocyte and squamous cell carcinoma responses to UVB irradiation: Implications for skin and epithelial cancer. *Oncogene* **2003**, *22*, 2993–3006. [CrossRef]
23. Lehmann, B. HaCaT cell line as a model system for vitamin D3 metabolism in human skin. *J. Investig. Dermatol.* **1997**, *108*, 78–82. [CrossRef]
24. Schürer, N.; Köhne, A.; Schliep, V.; Barlag, K.; Goerz, G. Lipid composition and synthesis of HaCaT cells, an immortalized human keratinocyte line, in comparison with normal human adult keratinocytes. *Exp. Dermatol.* **1993**, *2*, 179–185. [CrossRef]
25. Colombo, I.; Sangiovanni, E.; Maggio, R.; Mattozzi, C.; Zava, S.; Corbett, Y.; Fumagalli, M.; Carlino, C.; Corsetto, P.A.; Scaccabarozzi, D.; et al. HaCaT Cells as a Reliable In Vitro Differentiation Model to Dissect the Inflammatory/Repair Response of Human Keratinocytes. *Mediators Inflamm.* **2017**, *2017*, 7435621. [CrossRef]
26. Zhang, N.; Liang, H.; Farese, R.V.; Li, J.; Musi, N.; Hussey, S.E. Pharmacological TLR4 Inhibition Protects against Acute and Chronic Fat-Induced Insulin Resistance in Rats. *PLoS ONE* **2015**, *10*, e0132575. [CrossRef] [PubMed]
27. Pavez Lorie, E.; Stricker, N.; Plitta-Michalak, B.; Chen, I.P.; Volkmer, B.; Greinert, R.; Jauch, A.; Boukamp, P.; Rapp, A. Characterisation of the novel spontaneously immortalized and invasively growing human skin keratinocyte line HaSKpw. *Sci. Rep.* **2020**, *10*, 15196. [CrossRef] [PubMed]
28. Uchida, T.; Kadhum, W.R.; Kanai, S.; Todo, H.; Oshizaka, T.; Sugibayashi, K. Prediction of skin permeation by chemical compounds using the artificial membrane, Strat-M™. *Eur. J. Pharm. Sci.* **2015**, *67*, 113–118. [CrossRef]
29. Haq, A.; Dorrani, M.; Goodyear, B.; Joshi, V.; Michniak-Kohn, B. Membrane properties for permeability testing: Skin versus synthetic membranes. *Int. J. Pharm.* **2018**, *539*, 58–64. [CrossRef] [PubMed]
30. Haq, A.; Goodyear, B.; Ameen, D.; Joshi, V.; Michniak-Kohn, B. Strat-M® synthetic membrane: Permeability comparison to human cadaver skin. *Int. J. Pharm.* **2018**, *547*, 432–437. [CrossRef]
31. Kaur, L.; Singh, K.; Paul, S.; Singh, S.; Singh, S.; Jain, S.K. A Mechanistic Study to Determine the Structural Similarities Between Artificial Membrane Strat-M™ and Biological Membranes and Its Application to Carry Out Skin Permeation Study of Amphotericin B Nanoformulations. *AAPS PharmSciTech* **2018**, *19*, 1606–1624. [CrossRef]
32. Nair, R.S.; Billa, N.; Leong, C.-O.; Morris, A.P. An evaluation of tocotrienol ethosomes for transdermal delivery using Strat-M® membrane and excised human skin. *Pharm. Dev. Technol.* **2021**, *26*, 243–251. [CrossRef]
33. Available online: https://mattek.com/products/epiderm/ (accessed on 6 December 2021).
34. Netzlaff, F.; Lehr, C.M.; Wertz, P.W.; Schaefer, U.F. The human epidermis models EpiSkin®, SkinEthic® and EpiDerm®: An evaluation of morphology and their suitability for testing phototoxicity, irritancy, corrosivity, and substance transport. *European J. Pharm. Biopharm.* **2005**, *60*, 167–178. [CrossRef]
35. Bode, A.M.; Dong, Z.; Roh, E. Skin Care Formulations and Skin Cancer Treatment. U.S. Patent US-2020179404-A1, 11 June 2020. Available online: https://patents.google.com/patent/US20200179404A1#patentCitations (accessed on 4 March 2023).
36. Błazewicz, A.; Fijałek, Z.; Warowna-Grześkiewicz, M.; Boruta, M. Simultaneous determination of rocuronium and its eight impurities in pharmaceutical preparation using high-performance liquid chromatography with amperometric detection. *J. Chromatogr. A* **2007**, *1149*, 66–72. [CrossRef]
37. *United States Pharmacopoeia 33 National Formulary 28*; The United States Pharmacopoeial Convention: Rockville, MD, USA, 2010.
38. Park, C.-W.; Mansour, H.M.; Oh, T.-O.; Kim, J.-Y.; Ha, J.-M.; Lee, B.-J.; Chi, S.-C.; Rhee, Y.-S.; Park, E.-S. Phase behavior of itraconazole–phenol mixtures and its pharmaceutical applications. *Int. J. Pharm.* **2012**, *436*, 652–658. [CrossRef]
39. Sciences, M.L. Download the EpiDerm Percutaneous Absorption Protocol. Available online: https://mattek.com/download-the-epiderm-percutaneous-absorption-protocol/ (accessed on 13 September 2021).

MDPI
St. Alban-Anlage 66
4052 Basel
Switzerland
www.mdpi.com

International Journal of Molecular Sciences Editorial Office
E-mail: ijms@mdpi.com
www.mdpi.com/journal/ijms

www.ingramcontent.com/pod-product-compliance
Lightning Source LLC
LaVergne TN
LVHW070417100526
838202LV00014B/1476
* 9 7 8 3 7 2 5 8 0 8 6 8 7 *